# Art Therapy Research

*Art Therapy Research* is a clear and intuitive guide for educators, students, and practitioners on the procedures for conducting art therapy research. Presented using a balanced view of paradigms that reflect the pluralism of art therapy research, this exciting new resource offers clarity while maintaining the complexity of research approaches and considering the various epistemologies and their associated methods. This text brings research to life through the inclusion of sample experientials in every chapter and student worksheets, as well as a full chapter on report writing that includes a completed sample report. This comprehensive guide is essential reading for educators looking to further the application of learning outcomes such as teamwork, communication, and critical thinking in their practice.

**Donna J. Betts, PhD, ATR-BC,** is the Clinical Research Advisor for Creative Forces®: NEA Military Healing Arts Network, an initiative of the National Endowment for the Arts in partnership with the US Departments of Defense and Veterans Affairs and state and local arts agencies with administrative support provided by Americans for the Arts. Dr. Betts is an adjunct Associate Professor at the George Washington University Graduate Art Therapy Program. From 2015 to 2017 she was President of the American Art Therapy Association and presently serves on the Research Committee. An award-winning scholar, Dr. Betts has presented internationally on art therapy practice, policy, and research.

**Sarah P. Deaver, PhD, ATR-BC, HLM,** is in private practice at The Psychotherapy Center in Norfolk, VA. She was appointed to the faculty of the Graduate Art Therapy and Counseling Program at Eastern Virginia Medical School in 1981, was its Research Director from 1996 to 2017, and was Professor from 2012 to 2018. Her clinical and research interests include assessment, visual journaling, and trauma informed art therapy. Dr. Deaver has been active in the American Art Therapy Association (AATA) in numerous capacities and was its President from 2013 to 2015. In 2014, the AATA recognized her as Distinguished Educator, and she was granted Honorary Life Membership in 2017.

# Art Therapy Research

## A Practical Guide

Donna J. Betts and
Sarah P. Deaver

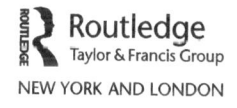

Routledge
Taylor & Francis Group
NEW YORK AND LONDON

First published 2019
by Routledge
52 Vanderbilt Avenue, New York, NY 10017

and by Routledge
2 Park Square, Milton Park, Abingdon, Oxon, OX14 4RN

*Routledge is an imprint of the Taylor & Francis Group, an informa business.*

© 2019 Taylor & Francis

The right of Donna J. Betts and Sarah P. Deaver to be identified as authors of this work has been asserted by them in accordance with sections 77 and 78 of the Copyright, Designs and Patents Act 1988.

All rights reserved. No part of this book may be reprinted or reproduced or utilised in any form or by any electronic, mechanical, or other means, now known or hereafter invented, including photocopying and recording, or in any information storage or retrieval system, without permission in writing from the publishers.

*Trademark notice*: Product or corporate names may be trademarks or registered trademarks, and are used only for identification and explanation without intent to infringe.

*Library of Congress Cataloging-in-Publication Data*
Names: Betts, Donna J., author. | Deaver, Sarah P., author.
Title: Art therapy research : a practical guide / Donna J. Betts & Sarah P. Deaver.
Description: New York, NY : Routledge, 2019. | "Introduction to art therapy research – Ethics and oversight in art therapy research – Quantitative research methods in art therapy – Qualitative research methods in art therapy (Theresa Van Lith) – Arts-based research in art therapy (Jordan Potash) – Mixed methods research in art therapy – Assessment research in art therapy – Designing and executing an art therapy research study." | Includes bibliographical references and index.
Identifiers: LCCN 2018042251 (print) | LCCN 2018043190 (ebook) | ISBN 9781315647081 (E-book) | ISBN 9781138126107 (hbk) | ISBN 9781138126114 (pbk) | ISBN 9781315647081 (ebk)
Subjects: LCSH: Art therapy–Research.
Classification: LCC RC489.A7 (ebook) | LCC RC489.A7 B487 2019 (print) | DDC 616.89/1656–dc23
LC record available at https://lccn.loc.gov/2018042251

ISBN: 9781138126107 (hbk)
ISBN: 9781138126114 (pbk)
ISBN: 9781315647081 (ebk)

Typeset in Sabon
by Newgen Publishing UK

In honor of our own teachers, and to all educators, students, and practitioners whose curiosity and creativity drive their passion to propel research, inform best practices, and ultimately benefit all people whose lives are touched by art therapy.

# Contents

*About the Authors*   viii
*Contributors*   x
*Acknowledgments*   xi
*How to Cite This Book and Its Contents*   xii

1. Introduction to Art Therapy Research   1
2. Ethics and Oversight in Art Therapy Research   18
3. Quantitative Research Methods in Art Therapy   41
4. Qualitative Research Methods in Art Therapy   83
   THERESA VAN LITH
5. Arts-Based Research in Art Therapy   119
   JORDAN S. POTASH
6. Mixed Methods Research in Art Therapy   147
7. Assessment Research in Art Therapy   167
8. Designing and Executing an Art Therapy Research Study   201

*Appendices*   229
*Glossary*   262
*Index*   281

# About the Authors

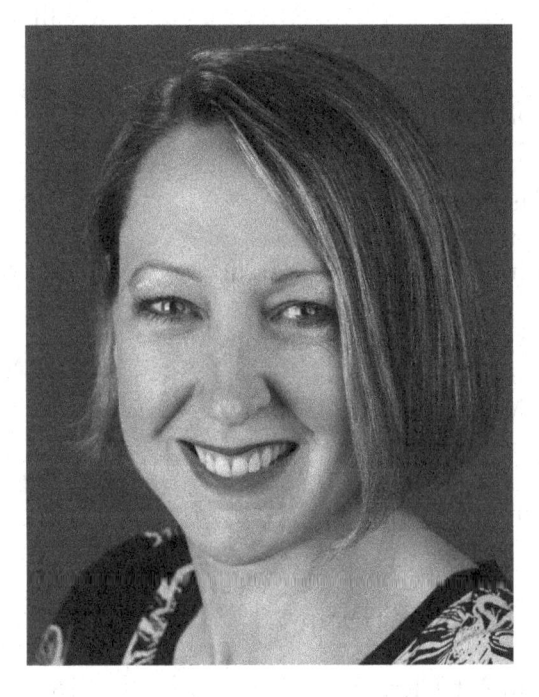

**Donna J. Betts, PhD, ATR-BC,** is the Clinical Research Advisor for Creative Forces®: National Endowment for the Arts Military (NEA) Healing Arts Network. Dr. Betts holds a PhD in Art Education and Art Therapy from Florida State University (FSU). She was on the faculty of the George Washington University Graduate Art Therapy Program from 2009 to 2018 and in 2016 was promoted to Associate Professor and Research Director. From 2015 to 2017 she was President of the American Art Therapy Association (AATA) and has served the organization in many capacities, including as a member of the Research Committee. An award-winning scholar, Dr. Betts has presented internationally on art therapy practice, policy, and research.

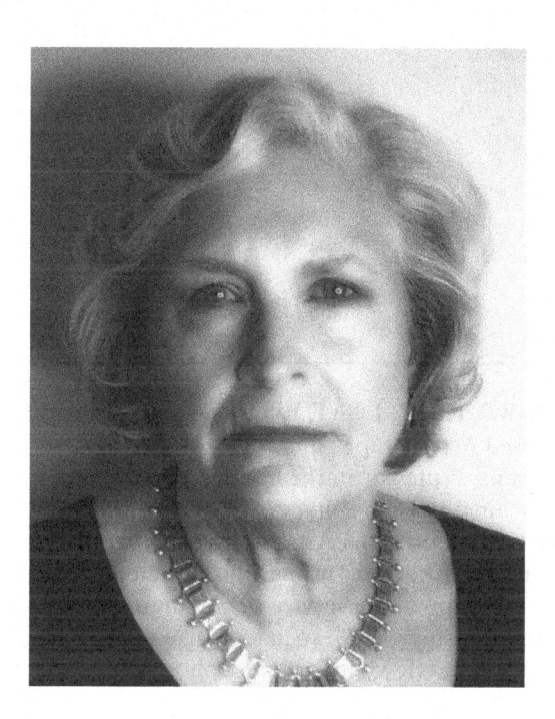

**Sarah P. Deaver, PhD, ATR-BC, HLM,** is in private practice at The Psychotherapy Center in Norfolk, VA. She was appointed to the faculty of the Graduate Art Therapy and Counseling Program at Eastern Virginia Medical School in 1981, was its Research Director from 1996 to 2017, and was Professor from 2012 to 2018. Her clinical and research interests include assessment, visual journaling, and trauma informed art therapy. Dr. Deaver has been active in the American Art Therapy Association (AATA) in numerous capacities and was its President from 2013 to 2015. In 2014, the AATA recognized her as Distinguished Educator, and she was awarded Honorary Life Membership in 2017.

# Contributors

**Jordan S. Potash, PhD, ATR-BC, REAT, LCAT, LPCAT,** is a Registered, Board Certified, and Licensed Art Therapist and Registered Expressive Arts Therapist. He is Assistant Professor in the Graduate Art Therapy Program at the George Washington University and Honorary Assistant Professor in the Masters of Expressive Arts Therapy Program at the University of Hong Kong. Jordan is primarily interested in the applications of art and art therapy in the service of community development, cross-cultural relationships, and social change. For more information about Jordan or to view his art portfolio, visit www.jordanpotash.com.

**Theresa Van Lith, PhD, ATR-BC, AThR,** is Assistant Professor and Clinical Coordinator in the Art Therapy Program at Florida State University. Her research interests have stemmed from working in the mental health system in her home country, Australia. She has since investigated art therapy professional development and service delivery models in the United States. Dr. Van Lith has published over 20 peer-reviewed articles, as well as presented nationally and internationally. Most recently her research interests have focused on collaborative initiatives with art therapists from Iran and Ukraine, children with Autism Spectrum Disorder, and children from Latino farmworker families.

# Acknowledgments

We wish to thank the friends, family members, and colleagues who provided support throughout each phase of the book's development. To our dear friend and colleague, Marcia Rosal, who reviewed the manuscript prior to publication – we are indebted. Gratitude is extended to Theresa Van Lith for her important contribution as the author of Chapter 4, "Qualitative Research Methods in Art Therapy." We also thank Jordan Potash, author of Chapter 5, "Arts-Based Research in Art Therapy," and appreciate his unique voice on this methodology. Readers will find these rich chapters to be invaluable in augmenting students' understanding of the applications of qualitative and arts-based research in graduate art therapy education. Dr. Potash's contributions to the experientially based components that complement the book as supplemental materials are also appreciated. We are grateful for the assistance of Robert Bornstein in reviewing and providing specific input on Chapter 7, "Assessment Research in Art Therapy." Finally, we wish to acknowledge the contributions of Donna Kaiser and Steven Johnson during the early stages of the book's development.

Art therapy research today builds upon the perseverance of pioneering art therapy researchers, many of whom we have had the honor of working with, and the good fortune to know. We are grateful for their efforts, which are a tremendous source of inspiration to us: Linda Gantt, Nancy Gerber, Val Huet, Lynn Kapitan, Girija Kaimal, Donna Kaiser, Marcia Rosal, and Neil Springham. It is the collective contributions of these eminent scholars that we endeavored to build upon in this book. To this end, future students and researchers will in turn expand the knowledge base, further advancing the profession, and more people will be helped by art therapists.

# How to Cite This Book and Its Contents

This work is a co-authored book and should be cited as follows:

Betts, D. J. & Deaver, S. P. (2019). *Art therapy research: A practical guide.* New York, NY: Routledge.

The two chapters written by those other than the book's lead authors should be cited as follows:

Potash, J. S. (2019). Arts-based research in art therapy. In D. J. Betts & S. P. Deaver, *Art therapy research: A practical guide* (pp. 119–146). New York, NY: Routledge.

Van Lith, T. (2019). Qualitative research methods in art therapy. In D. J. Betts & S. P. Deaver, *Art therapy research: A practical guide* (pp. 83–118). New York, NY: Routledge.

# Chapter 1

# Introduction to Art Therapy Research

The idea for writing this book came about based upon our experiences as art therapists and educators who have taught research at graduate art therapy programs in the United States. We had developed our own teaching materials over the years, and decided it was time to consolidate our ideas and pedagogical techniques, and to disseminate them. This book is the combined result of our experiences, materials, and knowledge, informed by our objective to provide a clear, definitive guide for educators, students, and practitioners on the procedures for conducting art therapy research, and presenting a balanced view of paradigms that reflect the pluralism of art therapy research.

As educators, we strive to prepare our students for work, citizenship, and life. This book was written with a commitment to this goal, as we believe that a strong art therapy research curriculum plays an important role in student preparation for the workforce, to enable them to become clinicians with an expanded worldview who are well-equipped as "research sensitive practitioners" (Huet, Springham, & Evans, 2014, p. 175). This approach is in keeping with the recent missive of the National Academies of Sciences, Engineering, and Medicine (2018), which set out to promote an integrative approach to higher education. It thereby furthers the application of learning outcomes such as teamwork, communication, and critical thinking – skills to prepare students to become adept in ways that translate to lifelong learning.

This chapter describes the importance of research, factors impacting the growth of the art therapy profession as related to research, and how research is shaped by government agencies and other entities. Research methods and implications for clinical practice are explored, including foundations of art therapy research and the types of inquiry that will be most valuable for moving the field forward. The continuum of paradigms and research designs and types of research are also delineated to set a context for the ensuing chapters, which are outlined in the final section, "Text Organization."

## The Importance of Research

Research is a major source of knowledge for guiding our work with clients and helps us learn the best ways to orient our approach for addressing particular conditions or concerns. The ultimate aim of art therapy research is to understand more comprehensively how art therapy is beneficial, which improves the services we provide (Deaver, 2002; Rosal, 2011). Practitioners possess knowledge accrued over years of working directly with people seeking art therapy services. Thus, research is enhanced through input from art therapists actively providing clinical work, and both research and practice contribute to theory development. Practice, research, and theory together underlie what we do, how we know it is helpful, and what it means in terms of a theoretical framework.

For many decades research in art therapy has been declared a priority by leading scholars. A brief historical review reflects the evolution of research in the field, and how the American Art Therapy Association (AATA) has concomitantly supported and advocated for research initiatives (Rosal, 2011). During AATA's formation in the 1960s, only four research articles were published. Later in the decade and into the 1970s, three emphases in research surfaced: assessment research – using individuals' art to differentiate diagnoses or conditions (Levy & Ulman, 1967; Silver & Lavin, 1977), study of the effectiveness of art therapy or understanding the art therapy process (Kagin & Lusebrink, 1978; Wadeson, 1978), and investigations of professional settings such as art therapy educational programs and workplaces (Anderson & Landgarten, 1974; Landgarten, 1978). Scholarly contributions have of course increased beyond the 1970s, and as eminent authors have written about the importance of research in art therapy (Carolan, 2001; Deaver, 2002; Gantt, 1986, 1998; Kaplan, 2001) so the scholarly base has continued to evolve.

More recently, studies are emerging that provide support for claims that art therapy is a valuable and cost-effective treatment. For example, in a pivotal study by Monti et al. (2006), art therapy for women with cancer was demonstrated to provide a significant decrease in distress and significant improvements in health-related quality of life compared to a wait-list control group. A small randomized controlled trial (RCT) with veterans with post-traumatic stress disorder (PTSD) determined that art therapy in conjunction with treatment as usual (Cognitive Processing Therapy) at a VA (Veterans Affairs) hospital improved patients' trauma processing by providing healthy distancing, enhanced trauma recall, and increased access to emotions, even though there were no statistical differences on standardized measures between experimental and control groups (Campbell, Decker, Kruk, & Deaver, 2016). Finally, a systematic review of several studies of patients with different clinical profiles by Uttley et al. (2015) found that, in ten of 15 RCTs ($N = 777$), art therapy was associated with positive outcomes in terms of mental health symptoms compared with controls. These three examples showcase recent advances, and also reflect that art therapy research is beginning to make the kind of impact that is needed to demonstrate efficacy of the profession to government bodies, legislators, healthcare agencies, and other decision-makers and stakeholders. Despite the advances, however, more needs to be done.

### *Factors Impacting the Growth of the Art Therapy Profession: How Research Can Help*

This book was written during a time when the American Art Therapy Association (AATA, 2016) was striving to "advocate for expansion of access to professional art therapists and lead the nation in the advancement of art therapy as a regulated mental health and human services profession." Many factors impact the AATA's ability to achieve its mission, and the following delineates factors related to research efforts to advance the profession.

Efforts to professionalize art therapy have included the establishment of an external accreditation process for graduate art therapy programs through the Commission on Accreditation of Allied Health Education (CAAHEP). The CAAHEP Standards and Guidelines for the Accreditation of Educational Programs in Art Therapy (S&Gs), adopted in 2016, include guidelines related to required course content for research, as is shown in Box 1.1.

Another factor influencing the need to professionalize art therapy includes the impact of funding agency mandates on research endeavors. Increasing pressure is being imposed upon mental health professions to demonstrate treatment efficacy, through evidence-based research, to US government bodies, insurance companies, and other regulatory entities (Betts, 2016). Art therapy educators and students should be aware of factors shaping art therapists' research pursuits and clinical practice. This is illustrated in the following section.

### *How Research Is Shaped by Government Agencies and Other Entities*

Researchers who seek recognition and endeavor to access funding must comply with a given agency's specifications. In doing so, they yield to the dominating factors that influence research pursuits, and the consequential

> **Box 1.1 Standards and Guidelines for Art Therapy Educational Program Accreditation in "Content Area m: Research"**
>
> This book is designed to support the adherence of graduate art therapy programs to the Standards and Guidelines for the Accreditation of Educational Programs in Art Therapy (S&Gs) of the Commission on Accreditation of Allied Health Education Programs (CAAHEP, 2016). In 2016, CAAHEP adopted S&Gs based upon the recommendation of the American Art Therapy Association (AATA) and the Accreditation Council for Art Therapy Education (ACATE). The S&Gs represent the minimum standards of quality used in accrediting graduate art therapy programs that prepare individuals to practice art therapy. The criteria for the content area "m" of "Research" are:
>
>> The curriculum must provide students with the opportunity to understand the purposes, methods, and ethical, legal, and cultural considerations of research and demonstrate the necessary skills to design and conduct a research study. Additional areas of coverage include the use of research to assess effectiveness of mental health and art therapy services by becoming an informed consumer of art therapy research. CAAHEP further delineates the required knowledge, skills, and behaviors that students must develop for competency in "Research."
>>
>> (p. 27)
>
> In terms of *Knowledge*: (1) Recognize foundational purposes of research with emphasis on applications to the field; (2) Define research methodologies (e.g., quantitative, qualitative, mixed methods) and research design formats used in the field; (3) Describe art-based research methodologies as related to art therapy; and (4) Understand concepts of validity and reliability and applications to selection and application of assessments and tests.
>
> In terms of *Skills*: (1) Apply methods used to conduct a review and critique of the literature on a topic of interest; (2) Perform basic steps required to design and conduct a research study; and (3) Demonstrate basic statistical concepts such as scales of measurement, measures of central tendency, variability, distribution of data, and relationships among data as applied in research studies.
>
> In terms of *Affective/Behavior*: (1) Recognize ethical and legal considerations used to design, conduct, interpret, and report research; and (2) Recognize cultural considerations used when conducting, interpreting, and reporting research.

ethical implications. For example, successful applicants for funds from the National Institute of Mental Health (NIMH) are encouraged to submit proposals that are in keeping with the NIMH's current research taxonomy, the Research Domain Criteria (RDoC) initiative (NIMH, n.d.), which prioritizes quantitative evidence-based research. The RDoC incorporates information ranging from social factors to genomics, toward a more accurate description of a client's presenting problems. Thus, the RDoC presents a very different approach as compared to the systems that have traditionally been used in symptom-oriented methods of diagnosis and treatment, such as the *Diagnostic and Statistical Manual of Mental Disorders* (*DSM*; American Psychiatric Association [APA], 2013).

The RDoC initiative was implemented by the NIMH based on its divergent perspective on the *DSM* (APA, 2013), as well as on the International Classification of Diseases, ICD-10 (World Health Organization, 1992). Although the *DSM* is the most widely used tool available in the US to inform diagnosis and treatment planning, it has been criticized for failing to reflect the complexity of many disorders. Its critics also caution that the *DSM*'s method of categorizing mental illnesses should not guide research, citing its lack of validity (Lane, 2013). Rather, it is suggested that researchers should be looking at what leads to richer and more fulfilling lives, which requires moving away from a symptom reduction approach. This is in line with Rose, Fleischman, and Wykes (2008), who examined priorities identified by mental health service users (clients or consumers) for research. As explained by Springham (2016), Rose et al. (2008) found that many service users perceived "professional research as biased and driven by career advancement, power and control" (p. 106). This underscores the clients' perceptions of research as disconnected from their lived experiences and failing to lead to improvements in treatment services.

Dr. Thomas Insel, former Director of the NIMH, promoted the RDoC as a project that promises to reshape the direction of psychiatric research with this new taxonomy that focuses on biology, genetics, and neuroscience. It enables scientists to define disorders by their *causes* rather than their symptoms. The RDoC integrates many levels of information (from genomics to social factors) for each patient to provide a precise characterization. The five RDoC construct domains consist of Negative Valence Systems, Positive Valence Systems, Cognitive Systems, Social Processes, and Arousal and Regulatory Systems. The eight units of analysis by which these constructs are measured are genes, molecules, cells, circuits, physiology, behaviors, self-reports, and paradigms.

It is increasingly evident that mental illness is best understood as disorders of brain structure and function that implicate specific domains of cognition, emotion, and behavior (NIMH, n.d.). Information from the RDoC project is being aggregated into a common, comprehensive database that will allow researchers to share and mine the results of

NIMH-funded research. As research findings emerge from the RDoC effort, the idea is to incorporate them into future *DSM* revisions and clinical practice guidelines. However, it will be several years before this ambitious effort will have a meaningful impact on the diagnosis and treatment of mental disorders.

The RDoC initiative has implications for art therapy practitioners and researchers. For instance, the NIMH (2016) encourages applications aimed at developing more thorough assessment of clinical outcomes, and particularly those that can enrich understanding of treatment efficacy and individual variation in response. In conjunction with this initiative, NIMH grant applications that include assessments of biological measures and markers, behavioral measures, and psychometric instruments are prioritized, especially those that address individual variables that presumably moderate treatment response. As such, the NIMH is pushing for the development of psychometrically sophisticated assessments that provide sensitive, *quantitative*, and *objective* measures of specific domains of function for use in RDoC-informed treatment research. The NIMH (n.d.) further recommends that researchers develop and validate "objective methods for stratifying subjects in order to optimally match individuals to interventions."

This discussion also echoes the experiences of art therapists in the UK. Springham (2016) discussed the need to "consider what is involved when a profession attempts to research its own practice" (p. 105) in the context of agency expectations. For example, the National Institute of Clinical Excellence (NICE), the UK entity that provides guidance as to the most reliable evidence for treatment efficacy, may be perceived as favoring particular patient population types and research methods – namely, quantitative.

## Research Methods and Implications for Clinical Practice: A Closer Look

The push for quantitative research methods by influential entities is of concern to social science and art therapy researchers who value the importance of qualitative and mixed methods approaches. The imperative for qualitative data and its relevance to clinical practice is gaining momentum, with clinician-researchers promoting the ways in which qualitative data lead to better understanding of a client's lived experience. For example, consider the contributions of notable clinician scholars such as Stephen Finn, creator of Therapeutic Assessment (Finn & Tonsager, 1997); Connie Fischer, who developed collaborative assessment (1994); and Robert Bornstein, known for the process-based approach to psychological assessment (2011). Each of these client-centered approaches to psychological assessment includes traditional psychological assessment with various standardized instruments, but was developed with an emphasis on individual narratives and anecdotal evidence and is known to enhance the therapeutic relationship and inform clinical practice. Based on the evidence gleaned from qualitative, humanistic approaches to research in the social sciences, investigators are encouraged to pursue this line of inquiry in mental health research. Funding agencies have their own priorities but, ultimately, they want to fund high quality studies that can include qualitative methods yielding data that complements and extends traditional quantitative approaches.

Qualitative research as we now know it had its beginnings in the early years of the psychology profession, based upon the methods employed by founders such as Freud, Piaget, Wundt, and others (Gough & Lyons, 2016). Citing "introspection, clinical interviews and close observation … including a focus on meaning and interpretation" (p. 235), Gough and Lyons underscored the fundamental importance of subjectivity in psychological science. Furthermore, the early psychologists encouraged us to consider qualitative research as a mindset – a "sensibility and a set of practices oriented towards eliciting psychological meaning" (p. 235). Notably, qualitative approaches and their ability to aid in the collection of socially relevant information are valuable in mental health professions that are steered by social justice values, such as art therapy. Denzin and Lincoln (2011) encouraged us to embrace a *critical social science*, based on the actuality that others cannot be truly known by outside groups.

Erard (2010) discussed using a qualitative approach to maximize the validity of clinical judgments. He urged practitioners to scrutinize their clinical judgments and to make the most of their scientific validity, cautioning:

> We are most likely to be seduced by overconfidence in our clinical intuitions when there is much redundant or homogeneous, low-quality information pointing to a certain conclusion. For example, we might administer two or three face-valid, self-report measures and conduct a structured interview, all covering more or less the same limited content domain associated with depression. If all of them seem to indicate that the patient is not depressed, we might assume that we have strong convergent evidence that the patient is not depressed. Or, we might get a Rorschach with a DEPI of 5 and three Morbid responses, a figure drawing with a sad looking expression, and some TAT stories about people who have suffered from significant losses, and believe that we have ample evidence that the patient is depressed.
>
> (p. 11)

However, Erard asserted, in using these methods the clinician has failed to comprehensively determine whether the client is actually depressed, what the client's experience has been, and how he has been impacted by the quality of his depression. To overcome this, one needs to consider the quality of the therapeutic relationship, the client's self-image, his or her willingness to self-disclose, defenses, and capacity for insight. Additionally, the clinician should be open to the possibility that the client may not be willing to discuss his or her depression. "Here we must bring much of our clinical experience to bear" (ibid.). Erard urged us to move beyond the results gleaned from assessments to consider the possibility that the client's dysphoria and depressive ideation are manifested in other contexts such as behavior and functioning, to contrast how this client is perceived with others who had confirmed depression, and to consider the input of another clinician who has worked with the client.

A UK-based review of 18 sources notably found that "high-quality quantitative articles provided inconclusive evidence for the effectiveness of art therapy in adults with psychosis" (Attard & Larkin, 2016, p. 1). Conversely, though based on a small number of articles, rigorous qualitative studies showed that art therapy was considered by clients and therapists to be a "beneficial, meaningful, and acceptable intervention" (p. 1). Attard and Larkin encouraged the pursuit of more robust research in order to "corroborate individuals' experiences and guide evidence-based practice" (p. 1).

In a subsequent *Lancet* review by Junne and Zipfel (2016), Attard and Larkin's (2016) findings were cited for underscoring the considerable efforts needed toward their recommendation of augmenting the art therapy evidence base. Junne and Zipfel (2016) emphasized the need "to bridge the gap between the ethical imperative of evidence-based mental health practice and the most relevant subjective needs and preferences of patients" (p. 1007), further underscoring the importance of both quantitative and qualitative research approaches. Toward that end, they put forth suggestions to support future efforts related to such areas as integration of research methods into the curriculum for art therapy training programs, study of how theory informs practice (and vice versa), and pursuit of research that permits "differential indications" for art therapy based on phases of treatment for various disorders, to name a few examples.

Junne and Zipfel's recommendations for furthering the evidence base are not foreign to experienced art therapy researchers, however. In 2002, Deaver cited the AATA's (1999) recommendations on the following three most researchable topic areas: "improving the quality of the services we deliver (practical research), the theoretical underpinnings of our field (theory-building research), and the professional lives of art therapists (institutional research)" (p. 24). Furthermore, Deaver offered suggestions intended to inspire directions for research undertakings within four categories: the therapeutic relationship, intervention, assessment, and art therapists themselves.

A Delphi study of expert American art therapy researchers yielded survey results that identified research priorities for the profession (Kaiser & Deaver, 2013). Multi-site randomized controlled trials (RCTs), studies that incorporate mixed methods, assessment research, and multicultural studies were deemed priorities. The same high endorsement was designated to quasi-experimental research, which can be more readily executed by clinicians, such as single-subject research designs.

So, there is a place for what art therapists have known for quite some time to be true – the importance of pursing research "within different epistemologies and methodologies," moving beyond the quantitative/qualitative dichotomy (Gough & Lyons, 2016, p. 242). Furthermore, if as clinicians we understand the need for rich data gathering from multiple sources to inform our research, if only one aspect of art therapy is studied (such as the effects of coloring), we must consider human subjects research ethics around participants' experience while coloring, or in their immersion in the creative process. Although studies that look at the effects of using art materials are useful, they only just scratch the surface of what we need to be really examining – the relational aspects of art therapy, the processes, the mechanisms of change. Thus, if we are not looking in depth at clients' experience, we need to consider the ethical implications of this oversight. Indeed, the imperative for qualitative information that helps a clinician to understand a client's lived experience, and the need to demonstrate how it can be linked to improving client outcome, is clearer than ever.

Not only is more research needed to demonstrate the efficacy of art therapy, but we also need to be able to show what it is about art therapy that makes it distinct as a profession. This is important in part because art therapy encompasses both the arts and mental health. We need to be able to state, with clarity, that art therapy is different from other mental health fields, and that it's also different from the way in which artists use the healing arts. This relates to advocacy efforts on the part of the AATA, which works to advance the profession by educating policy makers and the public as to how and why art therapy's scope of practice is distinct and effective.

One meaningful direction to this end is efforts to study mechanisms of change in art therapy. What is it that makes art therapy unique? Under what circumstances should a client seek the services of an art therapist instead of a counselor or a healing arts practitioner, for instance? Investigation of mechanisms of change is crucial to the furtherance of art therapy. To study this question, and other questions of relevance to art therapy, appropriate selection of a research approach needs to be determined.

## Guidelines for Choosing a Research Approach

Several factors inform development of a research approach suitable for a proposed investigation. These include the researcher's own philosophical worldview, consideration of strategies of inquiry, the suitability of the research problem for a particular paradigm, elements of design related to data collection procedures, techniques for interpretation and analysis of results, and the intended audience (Creswell, 2009). Research approaches vary along a continuum from quantitative to qualitative, and each approach is associated with a specific paradigm. A research paradigm is a worldview, characterized by a set of fundamental assumptions and beliefs, that guides researchers as they approach a topic of study. Paradigms have evolved as humankind has evolved and have been influenced over the years by advances in science, the arts, and society. Paradigms are anchored philosophically in the concepts of ontology, epistemology, axiology, and methodology (Ponterotto, 2005). *Ontology* is a branch of philosophy concerned with the nature of reality. For example, reality may be considered by some as consisting of universal truths that can be discovered through applying deductive logic as in the scientific method. Others may consider reality to be co-constructed from the truths of individual persons. *Epistemology* has to do with ways of knowing and what qualifies as acceptable knowledge. It also is concerned with the researcher-participant relationship.

*Axiology* is concerned with researcher values as they manifest in the research process. A researcher may believe that it is important to remain objective, value free, and unbiased throughout a study, remaining distant from research participants (Wahyuni, 2012). But can a researcher's values remain entirely outside of the research process? Some would say not, and instead acknowledge that the researcher's own lived experience is an important aspect in collaborative relationships with research participants, with the hope that the researcher's personal values will influence the process and results (Ponterotto, 2005). *Methodology* refers to the processes involved in the research.

In this text, we present chapters on quantitative, qualitative, arts-based, and mixed methods research. As shown in Table 1.1, the paradigm *postpositivism* relates to quantitative research, *constructivism* is associated with qualitative research, and *pragmatism* is aligned with mixed methods design. Each of these paradigms is elaborated upon in the respective chapters (3, 4, and 6). A note on arts-based research – some scholars have positioned it as a form of qualitative research, whereas others have claimed that it is a distinct paradigm or theoretical perspective. The challenges of convincing the research community that it is a viable investigative method were discussed by Eisner (2005), who referred to arts-based research as a "soft-form" of qualitative inquiry

Table 1.1 Paradigms and associated characteristics

|  | Quantitative | Qualitative | Mixed Methods |
| --- | --- | --- | --- |
| Paradigm | Postpositivism | Constructivism | Pragmatism |
| Ontology | There is an objective reality that can be only imperfectly known | Reality is subjective and contextual rather than universal | Single and multiple realities exist |
| Epistemology | Knowledge is based on observed phenomena | Knowledge is socially constructed through the multiple realities of individuals | There are multiple ways to know: both through observation and subjective experience |
| Axiology | Research is value-free, researcher independent of data and objective | Researcher's values cannot be separated from the process, subjective | Multiple stances on values: both biased and value free |
| Purpose | Explanation of interrelationships of variables | In-depth understanding of phenomena or experience | Logically combine inductive and deductive approaches for depth and breadth |
| Methods | Deductive: experimental, quasi-experimental, non-experimental | Inductive: ethnography, grounded theory, case studies, phenomenological, narrative | Combining both deductive and inductive: sequential, concurrent, transformative |
| Researcher-participant relationship | Objective, distant | Subjective, relational, collaborative | Combined objective and subjective approaches |
| How to determine rigor | Descriptive statistics Inferential statistics | Triangulation, member checking, external auditor, peer debriefing | Both statistics and qualitative techniques for trustworthiness and credibility |

(p. 5). In this book, Potash provides a cogent discussion on this aspect of arts-based research (see Chapter 5).

## Text Organization

We set out to create a practical guide for the teaching and learning of art therapy research methods, beginning with this chapter offering an introduction to art therapy research, which conveys important foundational and contextual information. The book is intended to be read sequentially, although after reading this chapter, we advise reading Chapter 8 before proceeding through the other parts of the book, as it includes important practical information on designing and executing a research study.

Given the necessity of research ethics and oversight to the effective practice of art therapy and as spanning all stages of the research process, this content is presented in Chapter 2. Each subsequent chapter provides a practical guide to research methods most conducive to the study of art therapy, brought to life with examples from the literature and research simulation experientials developed in collaboration with Jordan Potash. Chapter 3 presents quantitative research methods, and is followed by Chapter 4 on qualitative research methods, Chapter 5 on arts-based research, and Chapter 6 on mixed methods research. We are also pleased to provide a guide to assessment research in Chapter 7, where you'll find the most comprehensive content on art therapy assessment research published to date.

Chapter 8 is divided into three sections: Section I gets to the heart of student engagement in research and how to cultivate it, and serves as a bridge to detailing the stages of research proposal development. This includes practical content related to research questions and the subsequent stages of conducting the literature review, determining research design, sampling, ethical considerations, rigor and integrity, and data interpretation and analysis. In Section II, the steps involved in seeing a study through to completion are described and information about preparing the report for publication is briefly presented. These steps are illustrated with an in-depth example of how to conduct an art therapy investigation: Educators will find Section III of this chapter particularly useful in teaching students to write good research reports that can later be publishable.

The book is complemented by various supplemental materials both in the appendices as well as in the online course materials to support educators' use of this text, and to support students embarking upon their research journeys. They are designed as recommendations, and the resources can be tailored to suit the needs of individual graduate education programs. As you progress through the book, please bear in mind that, whereas the chapters on the methodologies are by necessity presented in a linear fashion, the development of research proposals is a circular, multi-layered process. You may approach the book accordingly!

This chapter emphasized the importance of research, factors impacting the growth of the art therapy profession as related to research, and how research is shaped by government agencies and other entities. Research methods and implications for clinical practice were explored, including foundations of art therapy research and the types of inquiry that will be most valuable for moving the field forward. Postpositivism, Constructivism, and Pragmatism worldviews were briefly explained as associated with quantitative, qualitative, and mixed methods research. Finally, an overview of the book's contents and organization was provided.

Bringing Research to Life!, a research simulation experiential developed by Betts and Potash (2018) for teaching research to graduate art therapy students, is used throughout this text to illustrate an effective means for making research methods and concepts relevant and interesting for students. The overview is described in Box 1.2.

---

### Box 1.2 Bringing Research to Life!

**Objective:** This experiential simulates components of a scientific investigation to enable the teaching and learning of research approaches for art therapy students. Through the use of the materials associated with this experiential (Appendix A), students can gain the experience of being mock research participants, and instructors can use the following collected "data" to refer back to over the duration of the course to illustrate various research methods and concepts:

| Research Method | Experiential "Data" | "Findings" |
|---|---|---|
| **Quantitative** Non-directional hypothesis: *An immersive art experience will have an effect on the mood state of graduate art therapy students.* Directional hypothesis: *An immersive art experience will improve the mood state of graduate art therapy students.* | Pre, post and follow-up measures (aggregated scores yield *t*-test results) (BMIS scale). Nominal scales (art characteristics). Ordinal scales (relational aesthetic questionnaire). | Degree of change that reflects effectiveness of activity on mood. Survey of art characteristics deemed meaningful. Ranking of what makes art perceived to be meaningful. |

**Mixed methods** *content is also taught in conjunction with this experiential, as it employs both quantitative and qualitative data, but is clarified as a distinct method. See Chapter 6 on mixed methods.*

| | | |
|---|---|---|
| **Qualitative** Research question: *What is the lived experience of graduate art therapy students' engagement in an immersive art experience?* | Content analysis of reflective writing on why the selected art is meaningful. | In-depth understanding of how exhibit attendees understand art that is meaningful. |

| Research Method | Experiential "Data" | "Findings" |
| --- | --- | --- |
| **Program Development/ Action Research** | Content analysis of relational aesthetics questionnaire and reflective writing. | How to design more meaningful exhibits in the future. |
| **Case Study/ Ethnography** | Thematic analysis of facilitator notes on one participant during their time in the exhibit. | In-depth description of process. |
| **Arts-Based/ Heuristic** <br> Research question: *What is the lived experience of graduate art therapy students' engagement in an immersive art experience?* | Thematic analysis of response art and content analysis of accompanying reflective writing. | In-depth understanding of one's own experiences, thoughts, and emotions. |

**Procedure:** Give the student participants about 40 minutes to complete the activities for the research simulation experiential (see Appendix A). This mock experiment simulates *pre-experimental* (not randomized, no control group), *one group pretest-posttest design* (see also Chapter 3):

| Informed consent | Pretest ($O_1$) <br> BMIS | Treatment (X)"intervention" (immersive art experience & research packet) | Posttest ($O_2$) <br> BMIS |
| --- | --- | --- | --- |

Source: Betts and Potash (2018).

## References

American Art Therapy Association (AATA). (1999). *Art therapy research initiative* [Brochure]. Mundelein, IL: Author.

American Art Therapy Association (AATA). (2016, August). *Mission statement*. Retrieved from http://arttherapy.org/aata-aboutus/

American Psychiatric Association (APA). (2013). *Diagnostic and statistical manual of mental disorders* (5th ed.). Washington, DC: Author.

Anderson, F. E. & Landgarten, H. (1974). Art in mental health: Survey on the utilization of art therapy. *Studies in Art Education, 15*(3), 44–48.

Attard, A. & Larkin, M. (2016). Art therapy for people with psychosis: A narrative review of the literature. *Lancet Psychiatry, 3*(11), 1067–1078. Retrieved from https://doi.org/10.1016/S2215-0366(16)30146-8

Betts, D. J. (2016, December). *Applications of attachment theory in American art therapy practice illustrated through the Bird's Nest Drawing and story.* Keynote paper presented at the British Association of Art Therapists Attachment & the Arts Conference: Trusting closeness: Advances in art therapy for attachment trauma, Regent's University, London.

Betts, D. J. & Potash, J. (2018). Research simulation experiential: Bringing research to life! (personal collection of D. Betts and J. Potash, the George Washington University, Washington, DC).

Bornstein, R. F. (2011). Toward a process-focused model of test score validity: Improving psychological assessment in science and practice. *Psychological Assessment, 23*(2), 532–544. Retrieved from https://doi.org/10.1037/a0022402

CAAHEP (Commission on Accreditation of Allied Health Education Programs). (2016). *Standards and guidelines for the accreditation of educational programs in art therapy.* Clearwater, FL: Author.

Campbell, M., Decker, K. P., Kruk, K., & Deaver, S. P. (2016). Art therapy and cognitive processing therapy for combat PTSD: A randomized, controlled trial. *Art Therapy: Journal of the American Art Therapy Association, 33*(4), 169–177. Retrieved from https://doi.org/10.1080/07421656.2016.1226643

Carolan, R. (2001). Models and paradigms of art therapy research. *Art Therapy: Journal of the American Art Therapy Association, 18*(4), 190–206. Retrieved from https://doi.org/10.1080/07421656.2001.10129537

Creswell, J. W. (2009). *Research design: Qualitative, quantitative, and mixed methods approaches* (3rd ed.). Los Angeles, CA: Sage.

Deaver, S. (2002). What constitutes art therapy research? *Art Therapy, Journal of the American Art Therapy Association, 19*(1), 23–27. Retrieved from https://doi.org/10.1080/07421656.2002.10129721

Denzin, N. K. & Lincoln, Y. S. (Eds.) (2011). *The SAGE handbook of qualitative research* (4th ed.). Thousand Oaks, CA: Sage.

Eisner, E. (2005, April). *Persistent tensions in arts based research.* Retrieved from http://med646.weebly.com/uploads/1/7/1/8/17184224/eisner.pdf

Erard, R. E. (2010, March). *How to cook without a book.* Presidential address presented at the annual meeting of the Society for Personality Assessment, San Jose, CA.

Finn, S. E. & Tonsager, M. E. (1997). Information-gathering and therapeutic models of assessment: Complementary paradigms. *Psychological Assessment, 9*(4), 374–385. Retrieved from https://doi.org/10.1037/1040-3590.9.4.374

Fischer, C. T. (1994). *Individualizing psychological assessment.* Mahwah, NJ: Lawrence Erlbaum.

Gantt, L. (1986). Systematic investigations of art works: Some research models drawn from neighboring fields. *American Journal of Art Therapy, 24*(4), 111–118.

Gantt, L. (1998). A discussion of art therapy as a science. *Art Therapy: Journal of the American Art Therapy Association, 15*(1), 3–12. Retrieved from https://doi.org/10.1080/07421656.1989.10759306

Gough, B. & Lyons, A. (2016). The future of qualitative research in psychology: Accentuating the positive. *Integrative Psychological and Behavioral Science, 50*, 234–243. Retrieved from https://doi.org/10.1007/s12124-015-9320-8

Huet, V., Springham, N., & Evans, C. (2014). The Art Therapy Practice Research Network: Hurdles, pitfalls and achievements. *Counselling and Psychotherapy Research, 14*(3), 174–180. Retrieved from https://doi.org/10.1080/14733145.2014.929416

Junne, F. & Zipfel, S. (2016). The art of healing: art therapy in the mental health realm. *Lancet Psychiatry, 3*(11),1006–1007. Retrieved from https://doi.org/10.1016/S2215-0366(16)30210-3

Kagin, S. L. & Lusebrink, V. B. (1978). The Expressive Therapies Continuum. *The Arts in Psychotherapy, 5*, 171–180. Retrieved from https://doi.org/10.1016/0090-9092(78)90031-5

Kaiser, D. & Deaver, S. (2013). Establishing a research agenda for art therapy: A Delphi study. *Art Therapy: Journal of the American Art Therapy Association, 30*(3), 114–121. Retrieved from https://doi.org/10.1080/07421656.2013.819281

Kaplan, F. F. (2001). Areas of inquiry for art therapy research. *Art Therapy: Journal of the American Art Therapy Association, 18*(3), 142–147. Retrieved from https://doi.org/10.1080/07421656.2001.10129734

Landgarten, H. (1978). The state of art therapy in greater Los Angeles, 1974: Two year follow-up study. *Art Psychotherapy, 5*, 227–233.

Lane, C. (2013). *The NIMH withdraws support for* DSM-5. Retrieved from: www.psychologytoday.com/blog/side-effects/201305/the-nimh-withdraws-support-dsm-5

Levy, B. & Ulman, E. (1967). Judging psychopathology from paintings. *Journal of Abnormal Psychology, 72*, 182–187. Retrieved from https://doi.org/10.1037/h0024440

Monti, D. A., Peterson, C., Shakin-Kunkel, E. J., Hauck, W. W., Pequignot, E., Rhodes, L., & Brainard, G. (2006). A randomized, controlled trial of mindfulness-based art therapy (MBAT) for women with cancer. *Psycho-Oncology, 15*, 363–373. Retrieved from https://doi.org/10.1002/pon.988

National Academies of Sciences, Engineering, and Medicine. (2010). *The integration of the humanities and arts with sciences, engineering, and medicine in higher education: Branches from the same tree.* Washington, DC: National Academies Press. Retrieved from https://doi.org/10.17226/24988

National Institute of Mental Health (NIMH). (n.d.). *Research Domain Criteria (RDoC).* Retrieved from www.nimh.nih.gov/research-priorities/rdoc/index.shtml

National Institute of Mental Health (NIMH). (2016, September). *NIMH strategic plan for research, strategic objective 3.2: Develop ways to tailor existing and new interventions to optimize outcomes.* Retrieved from www.nimh.nih.gov/about/strategic-planning-reports/strategic-research-priorities/srp-objective-3/priorities-for-strategy-32.shtml

Ponterotto, H. G. (2005). Qualitative research in counseling psychology: A primer on research paradigms and philosophy of science. *Journal of Counseling Psychology, 52*, 126–136.

Rosal, M. (2011, July). *Celebrating 50 years of art therapy research.* Paper presented at the 42nd Annual AATA conference, Washington, DC.

Rose, D., Fleischman, P., & Wykes, T. (2008). What are mental health service users' priorities for research in the UK? *Journal of Mental Health, 17*(5), 520–530. Retrieved from https://doi.org/10.1080/09638230701878724

Silver, R. & Lavin, C. (1977). The role of art in developing and evaluating cognitive skills. *Journal of Learning Disabilities, 10*(7), 27–35.

Springham, N. (2016). Description as social construction in UK art therapy research. *International Journal of Art Therapy, 21*(3), 104–115. Retrieved from https://doi.org/10.1080/17454832.2016.1220399

Uttley, L., Scope, A., Stevenson, M., Rawdin, A., Taylor Buck, E., Sutton, A., ... Wood, C. (2015). Systematic review and economic modelling of the clinical effectiveness and cost-effectiveness of art therapy among people with non-psychotic mental health disorders. *Health Technology Assessment, 19*(18), 1–120. Retrieved from https://doi.org/10.3310/hta19180

Wadeson, H. (1978). Some uses of art therapy data in research. *American Journal of Art Therapy, 18*, 11–18.

Wahyuni, D. (2012). The research design maze: Understanding paradigms, cases, methods and methodologies. *Journal of Applied Management Accounting Research, 10*(1), 69–80. Retrieved from http://hdl.handle.net/10536/DRO/DU:30057483

World Health Organization. (1992). *The ICD-10 Classification of Mental and Behavioural Disorders: Clinical Descriptions and Diagnostic Guidelines.* Geneva: Author.

Chapter 2

# Ethics and Oversight in Art Therapy Research

## Foundational Ethical Principles

Through a survey, a group of expert American art therapy researchers identified critical research priorities of the field (Kaiser & Deaver, 2013). Among the priorities are explorations of which art therapy processes and materials are most effective with various populations of clients, comparing the effectiveness of art therapy versus verbal therapies, the neuroscience underlying art therapy, and validity and reliability of art therapy assessments. Populations to prioritize through research studies included, for example, those with major psychiatric illnesses, individuals on the autism spectrum, and traumatized individuals such as veterans with PTSD. What are some of the ethical considerations for art therapists when designing and executing studies of these and other topics that would involve varying amounts of risk when working with vulnerable research participants? Foundational principles provide a structure and helpful guidelines for ethical research practice and decision making in the research process. This chapter introduces the ethical principles underlying art therapy research practice, as well as the aspects of art therapy professional codes that embody these principles. In addition, the functions of research review boards are discussed, and concerns unique to art therapy research, namely, the use of art in research and published research reports, are discussed in regard to the art materials used in studies, ownership of art produced in research studies, and secure storage of digital images and other study-related materials.

In our Western culture, rules regarding ethical research with human beings were first codified in the mid-twentieth century after the trials of Nazi physicians who performed medical atrocities upon individuals in concentration camps (Deaver, 2011; Perlman, 2004). The document, called the Nuremburg Code, that emerged in 1947 in response to the trials, was directed at physicians and included items such as the necessity for obtaining consent from research participants and the importance of minimizing risk to research participants (Perlman, 2004). The next iteration of a code for ethical research with human beings was the 1964 Declaration of Helsinki, which added many more guidelines for physician researchers. Nevertheless, in the US, notable unethical practices continued, including the notorious Tuskegee Syphilis Study in which the natural course of syphilis in 399 disadvantaged African American men was studied over 40 years – without providing the men medicine that would have cured their disease (Corbie-Smith, 1999). In response, the US government published the Belmont Report (US Department of Health, Education, & Welfare, 1979), which underlies current research ethics and regulation in the US. The Belmont Report describes three moral principles underlying research with human beings, and the application of the principles in research practice (Miracle, 2016). These three principles are *Respect for Persons*, *Beneficence*, and *Justice*. In addition to these, the American Psychological Association added *Integrity, Fidelity, and Responsibility* to their ethics document (American Psychological Association [APA], 2010). The American Art Therapy Association also includes in its Ethical Principles for Art Therapists (American Art Therapy Association [AATA], 2013) the core values of *Nonmaleficence, Fidelity*, and *Creativity*, all of which can be applied to art therapy research practice. Five principles that collectively embody those in the Belmont Report, the APA, and AATA are defined below, along with examples of their application in research. These principles are based on universal values held by the art therapy profession, and must be considered in all phases of research, from conceptualization through dissemination of results (Sieber, 2000).

## Respect for Persons

Respect for persons – called *autonomy* in the AATA Ethical Principles – refers to researchers' acknowledgement that individuals have the capacity to make decisions for themselves when it comes to participating in or declining to be in a research study, and that if persons lack the capacity to make such decisions, they are entitled to protection (US Department of Health, Education, & Welfare, 1979). In most cases, this principle is actualized in research studies through the process – not just documentation – of informed consent. It is imperative that potential research participants be fully informed of the purposes of the research study they are contemplating being in, what they will undergo during the study, and what possible risks are involved through participating, as well as their right to withdraw from a study at any time, with no negative consequences.

Thus, applied in practice, when there is the potential for risk through participation in a research study, art therapy researchers must prepare consent documents that explain study details in clear language that the potential research participant can read and understand, discuss these details in a face to face conversation with the potential participant that allows opportunities to have questions answered, and provide the participant with a copy of the consent form with researcher contact information for reference if at any time questions or concerns arise. If a potential participant does not have the capacity to make autonomous decisions, for example due to immaturity or mental disability, according to the principle of respect for persons, that individual deserves protection. In these cases, such as if an art therapy researcher wanted to engage persons with advanced dementia in an art therapy assessment study, or a child in an intervention study, a legally authorized representative, such as someone with power of attorney or a parent, would be recruited to participate in the consent process, sign the consent form, and make decisions for the participant if necessary throughout the course of the study. On the other hand, there may be no potential risk involved in participating in a study consisting of, for example, an electronic survey to which a participant can respond anonymously. Even in this case, however, the potential participant must nonetheless be provided with information about the goals and methods of the survey as well as contact information for the researchers, and be given the opportunity to decline participation, with no negative consequences for doing so.

The principle of respect for persons is also applied in practice through sensitive approaches to research with those from cultures different from the culture of the researchers. Culturally determined notions of privacy, confidentiality, collectivism, and family must be taken into account (Kapitan, 2015; Kitchener & Anderson, 2011; Marzano, 2007). For example, Gubrium, Hill, and Flicker (2014) described a study involving First Nations adolescents in Canada, where the plan for researchers from the dominant culture to obtain signatures on paper consent forms was considered a vestige of colonialism. To address this, the researchers underwent training regarding how to obtain verbal consent in a culturally alert manner, and how to vary standard consenting procedures to include obtaining ongoing verbal consent throughout various stages of the study, thus providing the teens multiple opportunities to consent or decline to participate, depending on the expectations of each phase of the study. Kapitan (2015) strongly advocated for art therapists' reflexivity and ethnorelativistic attitudes and behaviors when engaged in cross-cultural encounters such as those described by Gubrium et al. Zappa (2017), citing Ansara and Hegarty (2013), clarified that "research cannot be divorced from the context within which it was created" (p. 130). Thus, an ethical stance in cultures different from the researcher's includes the awareness of cultural norms and acclimating to them when designing and executing research studies. Furthermore, particular care must be taken with research participants who have been oppressed historically, so that a researcher-participant hierarchy does not contribute to continued oppression and to ensure that their voices can be heard (Zappa, 2017).

## Beneficence and Nonmaleficence

The principle of beneficence suggests that researchers have an obligation to assure the safety and well-being of research participants, and the principle of nonmaleficence means "do no harm." Taken together, these principles must be weighed when developing a research design that will minimize risks for participants while at the same time maximize benefits. Beneficence and nonmaleficence are additionally actualized through oversight by university research review committees, called research ethics committees (Farrant, Pavlicevic, & Tsiris, 2014), human subjects committees, or "institutional review boards" (IRBs) (Deaver, 2011; Miracle, 2016). Because beneficence is an *obligation* when considering whether to approve a researcher's proposed study involving human participants (US Department of Health, Education, & Welfare, 1979), IRBs assess the "risk/benefit ratio" regarding whether the benefits to the participants and potentially others in the future outweigh the inherent risks of research procedures. It is not difficult to imagine this assessment being made regarding experimental surgical procedures or untested drugs; however, in art therapy research, which typically involves participants who are *psychologically* vulnerable, assessing that ratio may be more challenging. IRBs also consider the risks to participants' privacy, and possible social and economic risks for participants (Sieber, 2000). Sometimes, the risks of a study may be unknown and unforeseeable, which must be made clear to potential participants during the informed consent process.

Furthermore, art therapy researchers must acknowledge the power of art – both looking at it and making it – to elicit strong reactions from research participants. Soft pedaling the risk of participants' possibly strong and disturbing reactions to art making in an art therapy research proposal, in order to obtain approval from an IRB, is noncompliant with the principles of creativity, beneficence and nonmaleficence, and fidelity (Deaver, 2011; Knapp, 1992). Thus, the methodology of any proposed art therapy research study that has the potential for emotional disruption in participants must include a plan for addressing disturbing responses to art making: During the informed consent process, potential participants must be alerted to this risk and assured that the researcher is prepared to address any discomfort they may experience, provide them with a referral list to mental health professionals in the area, or allow them to withdraw from the study if they choose.

The research design itself can embody these principles. Using randomization is effective in ensuring that all participants have an equal chance of being in either the experimental or control group. For example, in a randomized controlled pilot study, Campbell, Decker, Kruk, and Deaver (2016) compared the effect of art therapy as an adjunct to cognitive processing therapy (CPT) versus CPT alone in veterans with combat-related posttraumatic stress disorder (PTSD). Because art therapy's effectiveness in ameliorating PTSD symptoms is not yet established through rigorous research studies, the researchers increased the benefit and reduced the risk to participants by having all of them participate in CPT, which does have strong research support for its effectiveness (Watts et al., 2014). Other examples of research designs supporting beneficence and nonmaleficence include studies that use a "wait list" control group (Beebe, Gelfand, & Bender, 2010; Monti et al., 2006). In these studies, the experimental group that is engaged in art therapy completes the study including pretest and posttest measures, and the control group, although not engaging in the art therapy intervention, takes the pre and post measures at the same time as the experimental group. At the conclusion of the study, depending on the experimental group's outcome, the intervention is then offered to those on the wait list.

## Justice

In research, justice pertains to fairness regarding who bears the burden of research and who benefits from the gains made through research, which is described as "distributive justice" (Kitchener & Anderson, 2011; Smith, 2000). Historically, in medical research, poor patients in hospital wards served as research subjects in studies that ultimately benefited wealthier, private patients (Smith, 2000; US Department of Health, Education, & Welfare, 1979). To support the principle of justice, investigators working from positivist and postpositive perspectives must acknowledge the inherently hierarchical relationship between the researcher and the research participant and diligently pursue recruitment procedures for all potential participants that are fair rather than exploitative or under representative of specific groups of people (Smith, 2000). Furthermore, it is unjust to select research participants simply due to their vulnerable positions as, for example, confined patients or easily manipulated prisoners, rather than for reasons specifically related to the topic under study (US Department of Health, Education, & Welfare, 1979). Finally, according to the Belmont Report:

> Whenever research supported by public funds leads to the development of therapeutic devices and procedures, justice demands both that these not provide advantages only to those who can afford them and that such research should not unduly involve persons from groups unlikely to be among the beneficiaries of subsequent applications of the research.
>
> (para. 21)

## Vulnerable Populations

The US Code of Federal Regulations Title 45 Part 46 (45CFR46) (US Department of Health and Human Services, 2009) pertaining to research with human participants identifies pregnant women, children, and prisoners as "vulnerable populations" that require special attention and protections in research. These and other vulnerable persons, such as those suffering from mental illness, people lacking sufficient basic resources, stigmatized individuals, historically oppressed groups of people, and individuals with autism or learning disabilities, are some of the very individuals that art therapists serve, and who therefore are often the focus of research efforts. In light of this, Kapitan (2010) emphasized that "how art therapist researchers view, describe, and interpret artworks, and how they apply the knowledge gained, must be ethically sensitive to the people and phenomena that contributed to the study" (p. 33). Furthermore, Deaver (2011) asserted that "art therapists, who work regularly with clients and their artwork, may be especially knowledgeable and prepared for working with [clients and their] artwork in a research context" (p. 175), emphasizing the ethical necessity of ensuring that practitioners who are uniquely skilled with art materials, processes, and products – i.e., *art therapists* – are included as part of research teams investigating therapeutic implications of artmaking. Such inclusion lies within art therapists' unique scope of practice.

## Fidelity

Fidelity relates both to researchers' trustworthiness with research participants and to their scientific integrity. Trustworthiness is demonstrated through researchers' honesty with potential research participants regarding what a study involves, and the accurate reporting of research results. Researchers' scientific integrity entails in-depth and current knowledge of laws and rules about human subjects' protections, use of sound and appropriate research designs and methods, upholding participants' privacy and confidentiality, sensitivity to all aspects of participants' experiences in research studies, and not deviating from study procedures that have been approved by the IRB (Kitchener & Anderson, 2011; Smith, 2000). Regarding scientific integrity, Farrant et al. (2014) addressed the issue of scientific justification of art therapy research studies. They asserted that ethical rigor in research mandates strongly designed studies and logical, appropriate methods that are justified by their potential contribution to the field, to individuals served by art therapists, and to society at large. Furthermore, they averred that, "if there is no reasonable justification for a study to take place, it could be argued that it is not ethical to involve participants and invest time and expenses in the implementation of that study" (p. 34). In other words, at the conceptualization stage, an art therapy researcher must answer the "So what?" questions about the value of the proposed study: Will it likely add new knowledge to the field? Is it justified in terms of human and financial costs? Is it designed with integrity and does it honor the autonomy of research participants?

The principle of fidelity also addresses the widely debated practice of deception in research, which involves deliberately misleading research participants regarding purposes and methods involved in studies. A well-known example of this is Milgram's 1963 study of obedience, in which research participants naïve to the study design were deceived into following orders to administer what they thought were high voltage electric shocks to a "victim" (a confederate of the researcher who was role playing) (Nestor & Schutt, 2015). Based on the idea that obedience to authority is a basic tenet of civilization, Milgram's study explored the willingness of participants to blindly obey orders to shock the victim, despite the victim's apparent great pain and discomfort. Some of the participants' anxieties and conflicts regarding the experimental procedures were assuaged through post experiment debriefing, and discussion with the "victim." Within the field of experimental psychology, controversy continues over Milgram's study, including doubts regarding his claims about the results (ibid.). Clearly, by today's standards, Milgram's experimental methods did not honor the principles of fidelity and nonmaleficence. Although the AATA, Art Therapy Credentials Board, British Association of Art Therapists, and Canadian Art Therapy Association ethics and practice standards documents do not refer specifically to deception in research, each of these documents states specifically that art therapist researchers must fully disclose to potential research participants all details of studies for which they have been recruited. Eyde (2000), arguing that there are certain constructs and situations that cannot plausibly be researched if participants are fully aware of all study details, also asserted the need for researchers to very carefully consider the possible ramifications of deception in research, such as unanticipated psychological harm, because researchers and participants may differ in their evaluation of what is harmful. Eyde advocated for post-study debriefing sessions with participants as a strategy to alleviate some of the stressors associated with using deception in research.

## Creativity

The AATA's (2013) Ethical Principles for Art Therapists includes the value of creativity, including artmaking, to deepen self-understanding and knowledge of others and the world. Furthermore, these principles state that, "art therapists support creative processes for decision making and problem solving, as well as meaning making and healing." In considering the addition of creativity to the 2013 update of the AATA Ethical Principles, Hinz (2017) conceptualized creativity as the basic human right to freedom of expression and a "force for positive change" (p. 143). She noted that, "across the life span, participation in creative activities is associated with increased psychological, emotional, social, and physiological well-being" (p. 144). The principle of creativity is upheld in art therapy research through the respect paid to research participants' art processes and products and the care taken in handling these (Hinz, 2013; Kapitan, 2010; Moon, 2015), the use of non-toxic art materials in research studies, secure storage of participant art, and the value that art produced in research studies belongs to research participants unless otherwise specified in the study consent form (AATA, 2013; Robb, Potash, Deaver, & Furman, 2015). These concerns are explored more fully later in this chapter.

## Ethical Codes and Decision Making about Research

Guidelines and rules for ethical research practices in art therapy are listed in the American Art Therapy Association Ethical Principles for Art Therapists (2013), the British Association of Art Therapists (BAAT) Code of Ethics and Principles of Professional Practice (2014), the Canadian Art Therapy Association (CATA) Standards of Practice (n.d.), and the Art Therapy Credentials Board (ATCB) Code of Ethics, Conduct, and Disciplinary Procedures (2016). Box 2.1 illustrates that specific items in the AATA Ethical Principles embody the foundational ethical principles above. For example, principle 9.1 is directly related to researcher fidelity and scientific integrity, 9.2 to beneficence and nonmaleficence, 9.4 to respect for persons, and 9.6 and 9.7 to creativity and respect for persons. Ethical codes and guidelines, which comprise "principle ethics," provide answers to the question, "What should I do?" In other words, professionals are *obligated* to follow their code of ethical conduct. Guillemin and Gillam (2004) questioned the relevance of ethical codes to actual research practice, however, because often when an ethical dilemma arises, such as when designing a research study involving vulnerable participants, or when considering recruiting one's peers as research participants (as in heuristic models of research), ethical guidelines and codes may not provide the specificity necessary for making choices with confidence. In these cases, art therapists may follow any of a number of decision-making models to address the dilemma.

## Box 2.1 Comparison of AATA Ethical Principles to Foundational Principles

| AATA Ethical Principle | Foundational Principle |
| --- | --- |
| **Responsibility to research participants** | |
| 9.1 Researchers are guided by laws, regulations, and professional standards governing the conduct of research. When institutional review and approval is required for the conduct of research with human subjects, art therapists provide accurate information about their proposed research, obtain approval from the relevant institutional review board (or equivalent) prior to initiating research activities, and adhere to the institutionally approved protocol at every stage of the research. | Fidelity |
| 9.2 To the extent that research participants may be compromised by participation in research, art therapist researchers seek the ethical advice of qualified professionals not directly involved in their investigations and observe safeguards to protect the rights of research participants. | Nonmaleficence |
| 9.3 Researchers requesting participants' involvement in research inform them of all aspects of the research that might reasonably be expected to influence willingness to participate. Researchers take all reasonable steps necessary to ensure that full and informed consent has been obtained from all participants. Particular attention is paid to the informed consent process with research participants who are also receiving clinical services, have limited understanding and/or communication, or are minors. | Respect for persons Beneficence Justice |
| 9.4 Researchers respect participants' freedom to decline participation in, or to withdraw from, a research study at any time with no negative consequences to their treatment. | Respect for persons |
| 9.5 Information obtained about research participants during the course of an investigation is confidential unless there is authorization previously obtained in writing. When there is a risk that others, including family members, may obtain access to such information, this risk, together with the plan for protecting confidentiality, is explained as part of the procedure for obtaining informed consent. | Fidelity |
| 9.6 Artwork created by research participants as a part of a research study belongs to the research participants, unless otherwise specified through the research study informed consent document. | Fidelity Creativity Respect for persons |

| AATA Ethical Principle | Foundational Principle |
|---|---|
| 9.7 Art therapy researchers fulfill federal, state, and institutional laws and regulations that pertain to the duration and location of retaining raw data. Original artwork and/or digital photographs of participant artwork are de-identified and securely stored. Audio- or video-recordings are stored according to compliant procedures in a password-protected electronic folder. Any artwork and/or photographs of artwork may be saved indefinitely for potential use in future research, presentations, publications, and related educational forums, as specified in the informed consent document. | Fidelity Creativity Respect for persons |
| **Responsibility to clients** 1.8 Art therapists strive to provide a safe, functional environment in which to offer art therapy services. This includes proper ventilation, adequate lighting, access to water, knowledge of hazards or toxicity of art materials and the effort needed to safeguard the health of clients, storage space for artwork and secured areas for any hazardous materials, allowance for privacy and confidentiality, and compliance with any other health and safety requirements according to state and federal agencies that regulate comparable businesses. | Creativity Beneficence Nonmaleficence |
| **Professional competence and integrity** 6.2 Art therapists refrain from using art materials, creative processes, equipment, technology, or therapy practices that are beyond their scope of practice, experience, training, and education. | Fidelity Nonmaleficence |

## Decision-Making Models

Many decision-making models based upon the moral principles discussed above have been described in the scholarly literature (Cottone, 2001; Cottone & Claus, 2000; Garcia, Cartwright, Winston, & Borzuchowska, 2003). They provide clinicians with steps to take when confronted with ethical dilemmas, typically in the practice domain rather than specific to research. Steps may include intense study of professional ethics codes, consultation with professionals who have depth knowledge of ethics codes, and consideration of legal and professional consequences of various options. However, these models do not always provide clear answers, and often when designing and executing a research study, the researcher must weigh one ethical principle against another. For example, would the potential value to humankind of a research study's outcome outweigh the lack of respect for persons intrinsic in the use of deception? Were Milgram (1963) to present his research protocol to an IRB today, this ethical dilemma inherent in the study design would likely be considered in depth by the IRB reviewers considering whether or not to grant approval to such a study.

The American Counseling Association's Center for Counseling Practice, Policy, and Research has published a decision-making model based on the principles of autonomy, justice, beneficence, nonmaleficence, and fidelity (Forester-Miller & Davis, 2016) that is clear, succinct, and useful to art therapist practitioners and researchers. Its steps are summarized in Box 2.2.

---

**Box 2.2 Summary of Forester-Miller and Davis' Ethical Decision-Making Model, Adapted to Art Therapy**

**1. Identify the problem.**

Collect information and separate fact from assumptions or anxieties. Identify if the problem area is in the realm of ethics, the law, clinical practice, or professional standards. Is the problem primarily related to the practitioner, client, other entity such as an agency or employer?

**2. Apply the relevant ethical guidelines: AATA, ATCB, or other source.**

Read codes to discover whether or not the problem is addressed. Consider aspects of the problem related to cultural competency, or use of technology, including social media. If the problem is clearly addressed in applicable ethics documents, following relevant ethical standards as written should resolve the issue. If the problem is unclear or not fully addressed in ethics documents, the problem is identified as more complex, requiring further action.

**3. Determine the type of dilemma and its extent.**

Consider the problem in light of the foundational principles of respect for persons, beneficence and nonmaleficence, justice, fidelity, and creativity. Decide which principle takes priority, or if more than one is relevant and important. Review current professional literature regarding similar situations. Consult with experienced art therapists, as well as with national or state professional associations, to ensure objectivity in addressing the issue.

### 4. Outline possible courses of action.

Brainstorm with at least one professional art therapist to develop several potential courses of action.

### 5. Consider consequences of each possible course of action, and select one.

Consider each option along with its consequences for all the persons involved in the situation. Eliminate those that would potentially lead to further problems, and then choose one or a combination of actions, keeping priorities or the outcome in mind.

### 6. Evaluate the chosen course of action.

Use three tests (Stadler, 1986) to evaluate the wisdom of the course of action.
   Justice: Would you treat others the same if they were in this dilemma?
   Publicity: Would you want this situation to be publicized in the media?
   Universality: Would you recommend this course of action to other art therapists in similar ethical dilemmas?
If these tests can all be answered "yes," then it is possible to proceed to the final step. If not, one must go back to the beginning to reevaluate all the steps in ethical decision making.

### 7. Implement the course of action.

Implementing the plan is difficult and requires strength and perseverance. After the course of action has been taken, follow up to evaluate the consequences.

Forester-Miller and Davis' decision-making model is an example of a linear approach, based on the ethics principles discussed above, that is compatible with quantitative research studies, which are typically hypothesis driven and based on the traditional scientific method, including deductively discovering a singular truth or explanation about the matter under study. Qualitative research is less linear, often with emergent and situational designs and procedures, with the aim of *understanding* a phenomenon rather than explaining it. In qualitative approaches, the relationship between researcher and participant or "co-researcher" may involve the researcher delving deeply into research participants' personal experiences; this may present a host of ethical questions regarding roles, boundaries, and the potential for researcher exploitation of participants. Qualitative research often evolves and changes direction or focus while studies are underway, making it impossible to predict and describe in a consent form all of the procedures or experiences in which study participants would engage. To navigate these and other ethical conundrums in both qualitative and quantitative research, the art therapist may reflect upon his or her inner moral code for guidance in the decision-making process. Guillemin and Gillam (2004) referred to this process of thinking on one's feet in the midst of a real-time ethical conundrum as "ethics in practice," and suggested that the researcher's reflexive stance is a crucial aspect of her or his fidelity to the research process and participants. According to the Qualitative Research Guidelines Report (n.d.), reflexivity in research is defined as "an attitude of attending systematically to the context of knowledge construction, especially to the effect of the researcher, at every step of the research process." Guillemin and Gillam stated:

> Reflexivity in research is not a single or universal entity but a process – an active, ongoing process that saturates every stage of the research ... Our research interests and the research questions we pose, as well as the questions we discard, reveal something about who we are. Our choice of research design, the research methodology, and the theoretical framework that informs our research are governed by our values and reciprocally, help to shape these values. Who we include and who we exclude as participants in our research are revealing. Moreover, our interpretations and analyses, and how we choose to present our findings, together with whom we make our findings available to, are all constitutive of reflexive research. Reflexivity in research is thus a process of critical reflection both on the kind of knowledge produced from research and how that knowledge is generated.
>
> (p. 274)

Incorporating a reflexive attitude throughout the process of any research study involves the use of both principle ethics and virtue ethics.

## Virtue Ethics

To date, only two ethical decision-making models have been published in the art therapy scholarly literature (Hauck & Ling, 2016; Hinz, 2011). Although Hauck and Ling's "DO ART" model is applicable to art therapy practice and includes steps to take when faced with an ethical dilemma, it does not include art therapy-specific steps; for example, the model does not specifically address ethical aspects of media choices or resolving issues around the disposition of client artwork that has been left behind after termination or after a research study is completed. Because of the lack of specificity regarding art therapy decision making, when using this and other ethical decision-making models, art therapists may apply virtue ethics while resolving ethical dilemmas.

As opposed to principle ethics, virtue ethics pertains to personality traits and ideals that characterize ethical, virtuous, individuals. Whereas professionals have an obligation to comply with their ethical codes, virtue ethics are aspirational. Meara, Schmidt, and Day (1996) identified five characteristics of virtuous professionals and four virtues to which they aspire. The five characteristics are motivation for doing good, ability to discern ethical aspects of professional situations, recognition of the effect of emotion upon judgment, great self-awareness (achieved through reflexivity throughout the research process), and deep understanding and awareness of the values and mores of the community. The four virtues identified by Meara et al. include "practical wisdom" (p. 38), integrity, respectfulness, and benevolence or compassion. These aspirational virtues are embodied in all of the ethical principles underlying research that are discussed above. When employing virtue ethics, art therapists ask themselves, "What moral and honorable personal traits within myself can I rely upon when addressing ethical dilemmas?" Hinz (2011) took this approach, couched in positive psychology, in advocating for a less linear, rule-bound approach in favor of a more excellence-driven way for art therapists to navigate ethical dilemmas. Along these lines, Kapitan (2010) asserted that:

> The art therapy lens predisposes the art therapist to be ethically sensitive toward the artworks created in therapy and research. Where many social scientists see only inert "data" that takes the form of an image, art therapists often extend their compassionate regard for the ethical treatment of people they serve in therapy to the images created.
>
> (p. 33)

The following discussion of the dimensions of using art in art therapy research includes references to both principle ethics and virtue ethics.

## Ethical Use of Art in Art Therapy Research

Regarding the use of art forms in research, there is a great deal of literature from the fields of social science, visual anthropology, and visual sociology, in which researchers' photographs are a main source of study data. The literature describes ethical dilemmas inherent in the use of photographs of identifiable people in published research reports, including concerns about informed consent and copyright laws (Balmer, Griffiths, & Dunn, 2015; Boxall & Ralph, 2009; Pauwels, 2008; Wiles, Coffey, Robinson, & Heath, 2012). The central issue seems to be the problem of maintaining confidentiality of those photographed through digital alterations versus authentic photographic records of cultural phenomena or events. On the other hand, there is relatively little scholarly literature about the ethics surrounding the use of participants' art generated in art therapy research studies, yet some aspects of the social science image-based research literature regarding photographs are applicable to art therapy. For example, the principles underlying research ethics in all of these fields are the same, and the need for clarity in the participant consent form regarding ownership of imagery and use in publications, presentations, and public display is common to both visual sociology and art therapy (Clark, Prosser, & Wiles, 2010). However, in art therapy research, study design and ethical decision making typically center on the factors that distinguish art therapy research from other types of psychological research: the effects of participants' engagement in art making during art therapy interventions, and the art produced in the course of research studies. In compliance with ethical principles regarding beneficence and respect for persons, at the conceptualization stage of a study, decisions regarding types of art media used in research, ownership of art produced by research participants, maintaining participants' confidentiality, and secure storage of study-related data must be considered. Art therapy researchers' attitudes toward the art therapy process and products may shape their approach to these concerns (Hinz, 2013; Moon, 2015; Temple & McVittie, 2005).

Robb et al. (2015) discussed many of these matters at a conference presentation by members of the AATA Ethics and Research committees. They asserted that, in addition to the AATA (2013) ethics principles directly addressing art therapy research, principle 1.8 regarding providing a safe art therapy space, including proper ventilation, and tending to the health of clients through knowledge of toxicity of various art media, addresses the obligation for researchers to do no harm to participants. Furthermore, principle 6.2 states that ethical art therapists don't practice with materials with which they are unfamiliar or inexperienced. Some institutions and research review boards require art therapists to describe, in the methodology section of research proposals submitted for review, specific materials, brands, and styles of art materials to be used in research studies that have been approved as non-toxic by the Art and Creative Materials Institute. IRB approval of such materials ensures the safety of research participants when they are engaged in art therapy research involving art making (ibid.).

Regarding ownership of art created during research studies, AATA principle 4.0 states that, "art therapists regard client artwork as a form of protected information and the property of the client" (AATA, 2013, p. 4) unless the practice site considers the art or representations of the art to be part of the clinical or medical record. The notion that art produced in art therapy belongs to the artist/client is widely held throughout the profession. However, this principle refers to art generated in clinical or other settings where art therapists practice, not necessarily to art generated in research studies. To support the respect for persons inherent in AATA principle 4.0 for research participants, principle 9.6 states that, "artwork created by research participants as a part of a research study belongs to the research participants, unless otherwise specified through the research study consent form" (p. 9). Thus, art therapy researchers must clarify in the informed consent process and specify exactly what will happen to the art produced in the study: Will it be photographed and the original art given to the participant? If photographed, what will happen to the digital images of the participant's art? Will they be analyzed in some way? Identifiable? Kept in perpetuity by the researcher? Researchers can seek clarity regarding these questions by referring to principle 9.7, which states that,

> original artwork and/or digital photographs of participant artwork are de-identified and securely stored ... Any artwork and/or photographs of artwork may be saved indefinitely for potential use in future research, presentations, publications, and related educational forums, as specified in the informed consent document.
>
> (pp. 9–10)

What does secure storage of research-related data involve? Typically, IRBs require that all study-related data, such as signed consent forms, completed standardized instruments, transcribed interviews, original or digital copies of participant-generated artwork, and the like, be saved for at least three years in password-protected storage (Office for Human Research Protections, n.d.). This can be defined as a locked file cabinet to which only the principal investigator has the key, a password-protected computer, or encrypted files to which only the principal investigator has the password – or a combination of these systems.

The life of the image as a matter of ethical concern has been discussed by art therapists and researchers that use visual imagery (Boxall & Ralph,

2009; Hinz, 2013; Moon, 2015; Temple & McVittie, 2015). According to Hinz (2013), the human life cycle applied to images created in art therapy is an ethical way to conceptualize their treatment, and this metaphor may also be applicable to imagery created by research participants. She likened art created in phases of treatment to the birth, infancy, adolescence, adulthood, old age, and death of humans: The image is brought into the world/produced in a research context; lives from infancy through old age/is worked with throughout an experiment or intervention; and passes away/is photographed and then returned to the research participant. Moon (2015) also considered art images as living entities that deserve respectful treatment by researchers.

Temple and McVittie (2005) conducted a qualitative study of six art therapists' understanding of their role regarding artwork produced in clinical sessions that was not taken by the client at the end of treatment, and discussed their results as applied to research. The art therapists, all in the UK, were interviewed, data were analyzed using a modified grounded theory approach, and four themes emerged from the data analysis. The participants were unclear about professional guidelines regarding storage or disposal of artworks at the end of treatment; but were aware of their differing roles regarding protecting the artworks created in sessions versus storage or disposal of artworks that remained after termination. The participants experienced a sense of loss if they disposed of the artworks, even if they had photographed them. Finally, the artworks that remained beyond the end of treatment seemed to take on a life of their own, including creating for the therapists tension associated with the artworks' past existence versus what the future held for them. These results were discussed in the context of research; at the time the study was conducted there were no ethical guidelines in the UK regarding resolving the fate of images beyond three years after they were produced. Thus, Temple and McVittie were rightly concerned about issues such as storage and disposal of imagery and the rights of research participants when it came to imagery they produced or photographs of them. They were mindful of the applicability of the study results to researchers, and recognized that these concerns would become more vexing for visual researchers as long as the issues remained unresolved. Fortunately for art therapist researchers, clear guidelines are in place at this time in the US and the UK, both in the AATA Ethical Principles (2013) and in the laws and regulations regarding research with human subjects (Farrant et al., 2014; Furman, 2013).

## Research Review Board Oversight

In the United States, laws governing the practice of research with human beings are codified under Title 45 Code of Federal Regulations

Part 46 (45 CFR 46) (US Department of Health and Human Services). Collectively, these laws are called "the Common Rule." Institutions that receive federal funding for research must comply with the Common Rule, including establishing research review committees called institutional review boards to approve and monitor all human subjects research emanating from these institutions. Regardless of whether they receive federal funding, however, many universities and medical centers in the US have research review committees in place, the main purpose of which is to protect the public from unsound research practices (Deaver, 2011). Such committees have more recently been established in multiple countries around the world, and information about international human subjects research can be found here: www.hhs.gov/ohrp/international/index.html. In the UK, these committees are called research ethics committees (RECs), and a good amount of controversy exists among arts therapy and visual researchers in the UK regarding the rules, standards for compliance, participant anonymity, and possible lack of fit between biomedically oriented IRBs/RECs and the arts (Clark et al., 2010; Farrant et al., 2014; Prosser & Burke, 2008). Prosser and Burke (2008) emphasized the importance of research participants' voices being heard through their photos and drawings in published research reports, and criticized the US for its "restrictive research codes of practice" that can deny research participants' choice regarding whether to be named in research reports and "their work celebrated" (p. 417).

Controversial or not, IRBs and RECs and similar committees in other countries are the entities that decide whether a research proposal gets approved. In the US, IRBs consist of more than four members, from inside and outside the academic or medical institution housing the committee, who are charged with reviewing proposed research for compliance with the Common Rule, approving or denying protocols, and monitoring approved studies through completion (Deaver, 2011). Deaver explained that there are three levels of IRB approval: (a) exempt from review, (b) expedited review, which entails review by only one or a small group of IRB members, and (c) full board review. IRB members determine the level of review based on the risk/benefit ratio explained earlier in this chapter. Because art therapy research typically involves human participants, but with no more than minimal risk, such protocols are often categorized as expedited. But no matter how benign an art therapist may consider his or her research proposal to be, it is not up to the art therapist to determine whether or not the project requires IRB oversight. Thus, to ensure compliance with the AATA Ethical Principles (AATA, 2013), as well as to ensure the ethical and legal protections of an IRB, it is wise for art therapy researchers to consult with their university IRB or to make a connection with a university or medical center IRB, become oriented to current rules and procedures, and to submit proposals for approval (Deaver, 2011).

Typically, training in research practices and laws governing research with human subjects is required for researchers' proposals to be reviewed by an IRB; in the US, training from the Collaborative Institutional Training Program is typically the required course, which can be accessed at https://about.citipropram.org/en/homepage/.

## Summary

Ethical principles underlying art therapy research include respect for persons, beneficence and nonmaleficence, justice, fidelity, and creativity. These principles are actualized in research practice through, for example, informed consent, scientific integrity, and sensitive treatment of artworks produced by research participants. Art therapy researchers are obligated to abide by these principles. In the face of ethical dilemmas in research, professional codes of ethics do not always have solutions. In these cases, art therapists can follow ethical decision-making models that involve steps to take toward finding solutions.

Ethical codes embody "principle ethics," whereas "virtue ethics" call upon the art therapist's character and inner moral code for finding solutions to ethical dilemmas in research. Art therapists are encouraged to implement a reflexive stance throughout all research endeavors. The art produced by research participants, and the ethical and sensitive treatment of it, is a primary focus of art therapy research. Review, approval, and oversight of art therapy research by a research review committee ensure the integrity of the study and protect research participants from harm.

## References

American Art Therapy Association (AATA). (2013). *Ethical principles for art therapists*. Retrieved from www.arttherapy.org/upload/ethicalprinciples.pdf

American Psychological Association (APA). (2010). *Ethical principles of psychologists and code of conduct*. Retrieved from www.apa.org/ethics/code/

Ansara, Y. & Hegarty, P. (2013). Misgendering in English language contexts: Applying non-cisgenderist methods to feminist research. *International Journal of Multiple Research Approaches, 7*, 160–177. Retrieved from https://doi.org/10.5172/mra.2013.7.2.160

Art Therapy Credentials Board. (2016). *Code of ethics, conduct, and disciplinary procedures*. Retrieved from www.atcb.org/Ethics/ATCBCode

Balmer, C., Griffiths, F., & Dunn, J. (2015). A review of the issues and challenges involved in using participant-produced photographs in nursing research. *Journal of Advanced Nursing, 71*(7), 1726–1737. Retrieved from https://doi.org/10.1111/jan.12627

Beebe, A, Gelfand, E., & Bender, B. (2010). A randomized trial to test the effectiveness of art therapy for children with asthma. *Journal of Allergy and*

*Clinical Immunology, 126*, 263–266. Retrieved from https://doi.org/10.1016/j.jaci.2010.03.019

Boxall, K. & Ralph, S. (2009). Research ethics and the use of visual images in research with people with intellectual disability. *Journal of Intellectual & Developmental Disabilities, 34*(1), 45–54. Retrieved from https://doi.org/10.1080/13668250802688306

British Association of Art Therapists. (2014). *Code of ethics and principles of professional practice*. Retrieved from www.baat.org/Assets/Docs/General/BAAT%20CODE%20OF%20ETHICS%202014.pdf

Campbell, M., Decker, K., Kruk, K., & Deaver, S. (2016). Art therapy and Cognitive Processing Therapy for combat PTSD: A randomized, controlled trial. *Art Therapy: Journal of the American Art Therapy Association, 33*(4), 1–9. Retrieved from https://doi.org/10.1080/07421656.2016.1226643

Canadian Art Therapy Association. (n.d.). *Standards of practice*. Retrieved from https://cata15.wildapricot.org/about-cata/code-of-ethics

Clark, A., Prosser, J., & Wiles, R. (2010). Ethical issues in image-based research. *Arts & Health, 2*(1), 81–93. Retrieved from https://doi.org/10.1080/17533010903495298

Corbie-Smith, G. (1999). The continuing legacy of the Tuskegee Syphilis Study: Considerations for clinical investigation. *American Journal of the Medical Sciences, 317*(1), 5–8. Retrieved from www.columbia.akadns.net/itc/history/rothman/COL479E4252.pdf

Cottone, R. (2001). A social constructivism model of ethical decision making. *Journal of Counseling & Development, 79*, 39–45. Retrieved from https://doi.org/10.1002/j.1556-6676.2001.tb01941.x

Cottone, R. & Claus, R. (2000). Ethical decision-making models: A review of the literature. *Journal of Counseling & Development, 78*, 275–283. Retrieved from https://doi.org/10.1002/j.1556-6676.2000.tb01908.x

Deaver, S. (2011). Research ethics: Institutional review board oversight of art therapy research. *Art Therapy: Journal of the American Art Therapy Association, 28*(4), 171–176. Retrieved from https://doi.org/10.1080/07421656.2011.622685

Eyde, L. (2000). Other responsibilities to participants. In B. Sales & S. Folkman (Eds.), *Ethics in research with human participants* (pp. 61–73.). Washington, DC: American Psychological Association.

Farrant, C., Pavlicevic, M., & Tsiris, G. (2014). *A guide to research ethics for arts therapists and arts and health practitioners*. London: Jessica Kingsley.

Forester-Miller, H. & Davis, T. (2016). *Practitioner's guide to ethical decision making*. Retrieved from www.counseling.org/docs/default-source/ethics/practitioner-39-s-guide-to-ethical-decision-making.pdf?sfvrsn=2

Furman, L. (2013). *Ethics in art therapy: Challenging topics for a complex modality*. Philadelphia, PA: Jessica Kingsley.

Garcia, J., Cartwright, B., Winston, S., & Borzuchowska, B. (2003). A transcultural integrative model for ethical decision making. *Journal of Counseling & Development, 81*, 268–277. Retrieved from https://doi.org/10.1002/j.1556-6678.2003.tb00253.x

Gubrium, A., Hill, H., & Flicker, S. (2014). A situated practice of ethics for participatory visual and digital methods in public health research and practice: A focus on digital storytelling. *American Journal of Public Health, 104*(9), 1606–1614. Retrieved from https://doi.org/10.2105/AJPH.2013.301310

Guillemin, M. & Gillam, L. (2004). Ethics, reflexivity, and "ethically important moments" in research. *Qualitative Inquiry, 10*(2), 261–280. Retrieved from https://doi.org/10.1177/1077800403262360

Hauck, J. & Ling, T. (2016). The DO ART model: An ethical decision-making model applicable to art therapy. *Art Therapy: Journal of the American Art Therapy Association, 33*(4), 1–6. Retrieved from https://doi.org/10.1080/07421656.2016.1231544

Hinz, L. (2011). Embracing excellence: A positive approach to ethical decision making. *Art Therapy: Journal of the American Art Therapy Association, 28*(4), 185–188. Retrieved from https://doi.org/10.1080/07421656.2011.622693

Hinz, L. (2013). The life cycle of images: Revisiting the ethical treatment of the art therapy image. *Art Therapy: Journal of the American Art Therapy Association, 30*(1), 46–49. Retrieved from https://doi.org/10.1080/07421656.2013.757757

Hinz, L. (2017). The ethics of art therapy: Promoting creativity as a force for positive change. *Art Therapy: Journal of the American Art Therapy Association, 34*(3), 142–145. Retrieved from https://doi.org/10.1080/07421656.2017.1343073

Kaiser, D. & Deaver, S. (2013). Establishing a research agenda for art therapy: A Delphi study. *Art Therapy: Journal of the American Art Therapy Association, 30*(3), 114–121. Retrieved from https://doi.org/10.1080/07421656.2013.819281

Kapitan, L. (2010). *Introduction to art therapy research*. New York, NY: Routledge.

Kapitan, L. (2015). Social action in practice: Shifting the ethnocentric lens in cross-cultural art therapy encounters. *Art Therapy: Journal of the American Art Therapy Association, 32*(3), 104–111. Retrieved from https://doi.org/10.1080/07421656.2015.1060403

Kitchener, K. & Anderson, S. (2011). *Foundations of ethical practice, research, and teaching in psychology and counseling* (2nd ed.). New York, NY: Routledge.

Knapp, N. (1992). Ethics in research with human subjects. In H. Wadeson (Ed.), *A guide to conducting art therapy research* (pp. 39–51). Mundelein, IL: American Art Therapy Association.

Marzano, M. (2007). Informed consent, deception, and research freedom in qualitative research: A cross-cultural comparison. *Qualitative Inquiry, 13*(3), 417–436. Retrieved from https://doi.org/10.1177/1077800406297665

Meara, N., Schmidt, L., & Day, J. (1996). Principles and virtues: A foundation for ethical decisions, policies, and character. *Counseling Psychologist, 24*(1), 4–77. Retrieved from https://doi.org/10.1177/0011000096241002

Milgram, S. (1963). Behavioral study of obedience. *Journal of Abnormal and Social Psychology, 67*, 371–378. Retrieved from https://doi.org/10.1037/h0040525

Miracle, V. (2016). The Belmont Report: The triple crown of research ethics. *Dimensions of Critical Care Nursing, 35*(4), 223–228.

Monti, D., Peterson, C., Kunkel, E., Hauck, W., Pequignot, E., Rhodes, L., & Brainard, G. (2006). A randomized, controlled trial of mindfulness-based art therapy (MBAT) for women with cancer. *Psycho-Oncology, 15,* 363–373. Retrieved from https://doi.org/10.1002/pon.988

Moon, B. (2015). *Ethical issues in art therapy* (3rd ed.). Springfield, IL: Charles C Thomas.

Nestor, P. & Schutt, R. (2015). *Research methods in psychology: Investigating human behavior* (2nd ed.). Los Angeles, CA: Sage.

Office for Human Research Protections. (n.d.). *Investigator responsibilities FAQs.* Retrieved from www.hhs.gov/ohrp/regulations-and-policy/guidance/faq/investigator-responsibilities/index.html US govt dept of hhs

Pauwels, L. (2008). Taking and using: Ethical issues of photographs for research purposes. *Visual Communication Quarterly, 15,* 243–257. Retrieved from https://doi.org/10.1080/15551390802415071

Perlman, D. (2004). Ethics in clinical research: A history of human subjects protections and practical implementation of ethical standards. *SoCRA Source, 40,* 37–42. Retrieved from http://materiais.dbio.uevora.pt/MA/Modulo2/Artigos/SoCRA-Perlman.pdf

Prosser, J. & Burke, C. (2008). Image-based research: Childlike perspectives. In J. G. Knowles & A. Cole (Eds.), *Handbook of arts in qualitative research: Perspectives, methodologies, examples, and issues* (pp. 407–419). Los Angeles, CA: Sage.

Qualitative Research Guidelines Report (n.d.). *Reflexivity.* Retrieved from www.qualres.org/HomeRefl-3703.html

Robb, M., Potash, J., Deaver, S., & Furman, L. (2015). *What are ethical practices in research?* Panel presented at the American Art Therapy Association annual conference, Minneapolis, MN.

Sieber, J. (2000). Planning research: Basic ethical decision making. In B. Sales & S. Folkman (Eds.), *Ethics in research with human participants* (pp. 13–26). Washington, DC: American Psychological Association.

Smith, M. B. (2000). Moral foundations in research with human participants. In B. Sales & S. Folkman (Eds.), *Ethics in research with human participants* (pp. 3–10). Washington, DC: American Psychological Association.

Stadler, H. A. (1986). Making hard choices: Clarifying controversial ethical issues. *Counseling and Human Development, 19,* 1–10.

Temple, M. & McVittie, C. (2005). Ethical and practical issues in using visual methodologies: The legacy of research-originating visual products. *Qualitative Research in Psychology, 2,* 227–239. Retrieved from https://doi.org/10.1191/1478088705qp040oa

US Department of Health and Human Services (2009). *Code of Federal Regulations Title 45 Part 46 (45 CFR 46).* Retrieved from www.hhs.gov/ohrp/regulations-and-policy/regulations/45-cfr-46/

US Department of Health, Education, & Welfare (1979). *The Belmont Report: Ethical principles for the protection of human subjects of research.* Retrieved from www.hhs.gov/ohrp/regulations-and-policy/belmont-report/

Watts, B. V., Shiner, B., Zubkoff, L., Carpenter-Song, E., Ronconi, J. M., & Coldwell, C. M. (2014). Implementation of evidence-based psychotherapies for posttraumatic stress disorder in VA specialty clinics. *Psychiatric Services, 65,* 648–653. Retrieved from https://doi.org/10.1176/appi.ps.201300176

Wiles, R., Coffey, A., Robinson, J., & Heath, S. (2012). Anonymisation and visual images: Issues of respect, "voice" and protection. *International Journal of Social Research Methodology, 15*(1), 41–53. Retrieved from https://doi.org/10.1080/13645579.2011.564423

Zappa, A. (2017). Beyond erasure: The ethics of art therapy research with trans and gender-independent people. *Art Therapy: Journal of the American Art Therapy Association, 34*(3), 129–134. Retrieved from https://doi.org/10.1080/07421656.2017.1343074

# Chapter 3

# Quantitative Research Methods in Art Therapy

Art therapy research can be conducted using approaches that vary along a continuum from quantitative to qualitative. Because the process involved in research is akin to the creative process, in pursuing either research or art making, the art therapist has a question or becomes aware of a problem and is internally motivated to find an answer to the question or to investigate the problem. The same basic steps are taken in either the creative process of art making or research: Become aware of what has been learned before about the problem, develop an approach to finding a solution, collect useful and appropriate tools for the pursuit, embark on the pursuit, and arrive at a conclusion (Carolan, 2001; Deaver, 2002; Franklin, 2012; Kaplan, 1998). This chapter introduces quantitative methodologies, often considered the most traditional or "scientific" research approach. In quantitative research, to structure the inquiry process, the researcher typically employs the scientific method of hypothesis testing through deductive reasoning. This logical, positivist approach purports that, to understand the world around us, we must engage in systematic inquiry by employing the scientific method.

The scientific method is based on the premise that phenomena under investigation occur with regularity or predictability and are not entirely comprised of random events. Due to this regularity or predictability, an assumption of the scientific method is that there is a common truth to be found through systematic investigation. This way of thinking about phenomena – that regularity and predictability characterize our world and the people in it, and that it is possible to discover universal truths – characterizes positivism. The positivist worldview has dominated scientific thinking since the late 1800s (Ponterotto, 2005), and continues to dominate research in many fields, particularly those characterized as "hard science" such as biochemistry, neurology, and physics. However, when it comes to human beings and their infinite variety of feelings, senses, and experiences, it appears that universal truths may not be fully discoverable, and that truth may only be approximated through using the scientific method; this notion that human observation of social phenomena is fallible characterizes the paradigm of postpositivism. Postpositivism as applied to research embraces the scientific method while simultaneously acknowledging that researchers are inherently biased based upon their own life experiences and that therefore total objectivity in research is not possible.

The scientific method of inquiry is characterized by three overarching principles: objectivity, generalization, and replication (Erford, 2008). *Objectivity* pertains to the principle that researchers must minimize the influence of their assumptions, feelings, and emotions by distancing themselves from the mechanics and processes involved in their own research studies. In this way, researchers assure that personal opinions and research expectations do not influence the results of a study. Objectivity is also gained through use of data that are quantified through numbers, which clarifies research results in specific ways. *Generalizability* refers to the usefulness of research findings to greater numbers of people than those individuals who actually participated in a particular study. This requires carefully constructed research designs and methodology, and application of appropriate statistical methods to analyze data generated through the study. Use of such a rigorous methodology will allow for replication of studies by other researchers, which is the third principle underlying quantitative research. *Replication* refers to consistency in research findings across numerous studies that examine the same phenomenon, using the same methodology and research procedures as the original study. Replication adds to the body of art therapy research and supports the development of theory. Thus, quantitative research approaches allow art therapists to generate new knowledge through collecting large amounts of data, reducing the data to numbers, and using statistics to express the results of the study; the methodology used is rigorous, permitting generalization and replication.

Art therapy theory has not been rigorously tested and thus there are opportunities for researching several assumptions that underlie the profession. The concept of isomorphism (Cohen & Cox, 1995), the concepts delineated in the Expressive Therapies Continuum (Hinz, 2009; Lusebrink, 1990), and the theory that focused art making is inherently reflective and meaning making (Dahlmann, 2007; Deaver & McAuliffe, 2009; Deaver & Shiflett, 2011; Marshall, 2007) all underpin art therapy practice, yet despite "the processes and mechanisms in art therapy" and "principles of art therapy" being identified by expert art therapy researchers (Kaiser & Deaver, 2013, p. 116) as among the most important topics to research in our field, none of these theoretical concepts has been systematically and rigorously researched.

## Quantitative Research Concepts and Definitions

A number of specific concepts associated with quantitative research are defined below. These terms are essential to understand, not only to conduct scientific research successfully, but also to clearly grasp the meaning and value of published research reports. With an eye to applying the results of published research studies to better help those we serve, being a wise consumer of art therapy research helps to ensure an ethical approach to art therapy practice.

### *Variable*

Key to the conceptualization and conduct of scientific research, a variable is a characteristic, attribute, or behavior that may vary or change in at least two ways, depending upon conditions. Variables can be measured. There are many types of variables in research, the most important of which are independent and dependent variables. Independent variables are assumed to be the main cause of effects in an experiment. The variables affected by the independent variable are the dependent variables. The investigator attempts to control other variables that may impact the dependent variable. Take the example of a researcher who is primarily interested in the impact of three-dimensional artmaking on adolescents' engagement in art therapy: The independent variable is "three-dimensional artmaking," and the researcher examines its impact on the dependent variable, "engagement in art therapy." The dependent variable "depends" on the independent variable(s).

However, in addition to the dependent and independent variables that are the focus of study, when designing an experiment, researchers also consider extraneous, confounding, and intervening variables. In our example, the teens' engagement in the art therapy session is understood to be affected by other factors such as how long they slept the night before the session, the art materials offered, or whether the art therapist is a man or a woman; these are additional (extraneous) independent variables that, unless controlled, would make it impossible to determine a cause and effect relationship between "three-dimensional art" and "engagement in art therapy." Confounding and intervening variables are variables that are not part of an experiment – that is, they are not controlled or manipulated by the researcher – but which nonetheless may affect the dependent variable. They obscure the effects of other variables and make it impossible to determine if outcomes are caused by one or more independent variables. In our case, confounding variables would include everyday situations in adolescents' lives such as school schedules and family conflicts. An intervening variable explains a link between variables, a link that exists entirely separately from the study.

For example, research points to a relationship between greater income and living longer, but just having more money does not explain a longer life; more money results in greater access to healthcare, which then results in longer life. Access to healthcare is the variable that intervenes between money and long life (Indiana University Bloomington, n.d.).

## Hypothesis Testing

Hypothesis testing is unique to quantitative research. The system of generating a research hypothesis that predicts a study outcome as well as a null hypothesis that predicts that the research hypothesis will not be supported is currently a matter of discussion by scholars and researchers in neuroscience, medicine, and psychology, with the recommendation that null hypothesis significance testing be phased out (Szucs & Ioannidis, 2017). Thus, our discussion is limited to research hypothesis development and testing. A research hypothesis is an "educated guess" or prediction of the results of a study, particularly regarding the way in which the variables of interest interrelate. It is generated from the researcher's knowledge of theory and of what research in the topic area has been done before. The hypothesis is formulated before the study begins, and thus the study is focused on and designed around supporting the hypothesis, that is, demonstrating it to be true. A hypothesis is written as a statement. Sometimes, researchers distinguish between *directional* and *nondirectional* hypotheses, depending upon how much they know about the topic under study; the more theoretical underpinning and previous research on the topic there is, the easier it is to develop a directional hypothesis (Fraenkel, Wallen, & Hyun, 2012). Using the example of adolescents' engagement in art therapy, and narrowing the variables down to type of art materials offered by the art therapist, a nondirectional hypothesis might be stated this way:

> *It is hypothesized that adolescents making two-dimensional art in art therapy and adolescents making three-dimensional art in art therapy will differ in how they engage in the sessions.*

On the other hand, this would be a way to state a directional hypothesis for the same study:

> *It is hypothesized that adolescents making three-dimensional art in art therapy will be more engaged in the sessions than adolescents making two-dimensional art in art therapy.*

In this example, since independent and dependent variables must be measurable, the dependent variable "engagement" must be defined in a way in which it can be represented by numbers. This process is called *operationalization*. "Engagement" might be operationalized as the number of minutes each adolescent is actively making art in each session, or as scored responses to a questionnaire completed by each teen after each session, or by scored responses to a questionnaire completed by the art therapist in each session based on observations of engagement, or by a combination of these. To design a study testing either of the above hypothesis, the following additional terms (or independent variables) must be clearly defined: adolescent, three-dimensional art, two-dimensional art, and session. As hypotheses are repeatedly tested through replication with various populations of people, a body of research is built, and what began as theory is gradually supported as true. For example, researchers from several fields, including art therapy, have examined the effect upon stress of creating mandalas or of coloring in predesigned mandalas (Curry & Kasser, 2005; Drake, Searight, & Olson-Pupek, 2014; Henderson, Rosen, & Mascaro, 2007; Schrade, Tronsky, & Kaiser, 2011; van der Vennet & Serice, 2012), and the collective evidence seems to support the usefulness of coloring in predesigned mandalas for stress reduction. Furthermore, a small number of carefully designed and executed studies collectively point to art therapy's efficacy in reducing negative psychological symptoms and increasing quality of life in individuals with serious medical illness (Beebe, Gelfand, & Bender, 2010; Monti et al., 2006; Öster et al., 2006; Svensk et al., 2009). These and other similar studies require replication to establish art therapy as an evidence-based field.

## *Sampling*

Sampling pertains to specific procedures for recruiting individuals to participate in a research study. The goal of sampling is to obtain a group of research participants – or "subjects" – who represent the larger population of people to whom the results of the study are to be generalized. To guarantee generalizability of study results, researchers would want to study an entire population (such as all the children in the US who have autism), but as this is impossible, they will seek a sample. A "sample" is a subset of the group of people of interest to the researcher, and how well the sample represents the larger population has a bearing upon how study results may be interpreted. When designing studies, researchers specify demographic characteristics of the subjects they are seeking, such as age range, trauma history, and diagnosis; these are referred to as inclusion criteria. Likewise, they specify demographic characteristics that would disqualify a person from participating in their studies; these are called exclusion criteria. Examples of exclusion criteria might include current engagement in verbal therapy, or higher or lower scores on a standardized test than are specified in the research design. Sampling – or methods for participant selection based on inclusion and exclusion criteria – can take several forms. Probability sampling employs random selection of research participants whereas nonprobability sampling does not. The purpose of probability sampling is to have chance dictate the selection of research participants, to the greatest degree possible, which improves generalizability of study results. Of the approaches listed below, random, stratified random, and cluster random sampling are probability sampling approaches; purposive and convenience sampling are nonprobability approaches.

*Random Sampling*

Random sampling (or selection) is the process whereby researchers draw the sample of people for their studies from a larger population. Random sampling allows researchers to obtain a sample representative of the population to be participants. Therefore, results of the study can be generalized to the population (random sampling is not to be confused with random assignment [randomization], which involves how researchers assign individuals in the sample to different groups or treatments in a study, as is further detailed later in this chapter; see "Experimental Research"). When employing random sampling, each person in the larger population is given an equal probability of being selected for participation in a study, and no person's selection has any influence upon any other person's selection. Examples of random sampling techniques include selecting every tenth name from a list of all names in the population or using a random numbers table. Both of these techniques, however, have the disadvantage of the requirement to identify and assign a number to all persons in a population – impossible to accomplish in situations when the population of interest is widespread geographically or otherwise unavailable to the researcher. Other forms of sampling listed below are more typically used – stratified random, cluster random, purposive, and convenience.

STRATIFIED RANDOM SAMPLING

This approach to sampling results in subgroups of a larger population being represented in the study sample proportionate to their representation in the larger population. The population is divided into subgroups, or *strata*, and random sampling is employed for each stratum. Strata represent different ways of classifying the larger group, for example grade level, gender, income level, and ethnic identity. If an art therapy researcher in an ethnically diverse community were interested in examining the effect of culturally informed artistic traditions on children's responses to a particular art therapy approach or directive, the researcher would need to include subgroups of child participants of different ethnic identities in the same proportions as they exist in the larger community. This approach would strengthen the research design and potential for generalization of study results to each of the subgroups (or strata) within the sample.

## CLUSTER RANDOM SAMPLING

Faced with situations in which researchers cannot access entire populations of potential research participants for randomization purposes, they might employ cluster random sampling in which they access groups (or "clusters") of individuals rather than the entire population of interest. For example, there are 24 state-operated juvenile detention facilities in Virginia, most of which employ an art therapist to use a specific curriculum to deliver therapeutic art education that facilitates social and emotional learning through psychoeducation that focuses on character development, interpersonal skills development, transitions, and prevention (Roberts & McChesney, 2012). If an art therapist researcher were interested in studying the therapeutic and educational outcomes of this statewide program, rather than study every art therapy classroom in Virginia, the researcher might randomly select three of the facilities, and study the outcomes of those three art therapy programs. In this approach, it is not the individuals who are studied, it is the groups (or clusters) of individuals in the art therapy programs. A problem inherent with cluster random sampling is that there is no assurance that the clusters selected represent the entire population; thus, generalizability is not guaranteed. The more clusters that are randomly sampled, the greater confidence that the clusters represent the entire population.

## PURPOSIVE SAMPLING

Researchers using purposive sampling, also called "maximum variation sampling" (Patton, 2003), attempt to recruit volunteers who represent as much diversity as possible. This sampling approach is more characteristic of qualitative research but may also be used in quantitative studies. Obviously with this approach, generalization to groups outside of the study participants is not possible as there is no effort to recruit subjects who proportionately represent the larger population.

## CONVENIENCE SAMPLING

This sampling strategy involves seeking available volunteers who fit the inclusion and exclusion criteria for the study. Without the rigor of the previous methods, convenience sampling often limits the generalizability of results to the sample studied because representation of the larger population is not assured. Because convenience sampling is so often used in published research reports, careful consideration of the limits of generalizability is warranted when applying the results of such research to practice.

### *Instrumentation*

Instrumentation refers to standardized measures (*instruments*) such as scales, tests, or structured observations that are used in research studies for data collection, and the ways in which these measures are implemented in the research design. In quantitative research, these instruments must yield data in the form of numbers. Information about standardized instruments is widely available online and in university libraries; the Buros Center for Testing is a useful resource containing thousands of reviews and critiques of standardized tests (http://buros.org/test-reviews-information). Other sources include test publishers' catalogues and peer-reviewed journals devoted to psychological assessment. Carefully selecting measurement tools is essential to good research design. Ways in which they can be used in art therapy research include as prescreens for inclusion or exclusion of potential study participants, and as ways to measure change from before an intervention begins until after it ends. In addition, in correlational research, standardized instruments can be used as measures of the amount of a specific psychological construct (such as depression level or attachment category) in individual research participants to discover if relationships exist between that particular variable of interest and specific drawing characteristics. For further information about assessment development and how to determine rigor and quality when selecting standardized instruments for use in research, see Chapter 7 in this book.

## Quantitative Methods

There are two categories of quantitative methodology: experimental and non-experimental. Experimental research is designed to discover cause and effect relationships through the researcher's control of all extraneous and potentially confounding variables and by manipulation of the independent variable(s). Conversely, in non-experimental designs, there is no manipulation of variables, and, although relationships between or among variables can be established, cause and effect cannot.

### *Experimental Research*

Depending upon whether probability sampling is utilized in participant selection, experimental research may be categorized as *true* experimental or *quasi*-experimental. In true experimental research, participants are randomly assigned (randomized) to experimental and control groups. Random assignment (randomization) is the process researchers undertake to assign individuals in the sample to different groups or treatments in a study. Random assignment ensures that the only difference between the various treatment groups is the variables under study. Random assignment helps create treatment groups that are similar to each other, with the only difference between them being the treatment. Therefore, causality can be inferred. The increased rigor inherent in this method, particularly when the sample is large, permits generalization of study results to individuals beyond those who participated in the study, and cause and effect can be established (i. e., the intervention caused the results).

However, often researchers find it impossible to use random assignment; for example, an art therapy researcher's plan to disrupt established classrooms in a school through randomizing students into experimental and control groups would likely not get far with school officials who want to maintain order and consistency in the classroom. In these cases, a quasi-experimental design may be used; in such designs, because randomization is not possible, existing groups are assigned to experimental and control conditions. In the example of school art therapy research, students in one classroom would participate in art therapy and same-aged students in a similar classroom would engage in the control activity. However, it may or may not be true that the students in the existing classrooms are essentially equal; thus, absence of randomization in quasi-experimental designs negatively affects the ability to generalize results, attribute them to the experimental intervention, and establish cause and effect between the independent and dependent variables.

Control is a basic concept underlying experimental research. It refers to the researcher manipulating the study design to ensure maximum control over variables. The most obvious and clear example of experimental control is a study examining the effect of the independent variable (such as an art therapy intervention) on the dependent variable (for example, depression) in two groups of research participants: the experimental group (art therapy) and a control group. The control group would be designed to approximate the experience of the experimental participants, but without art therapy. For example, control participants might engage only in verbal therapy, or be assigned art tasks to complete without attending any group at all, or be placed in a "wait group condition." In a wait group condition, the control group participants would do nothing other than their normal daily activities except take pretest and posttest measures at the same times as the experimental group does, and then have an opportunity to take part in the art therapy group after all data are collected. If this hypothetical study was designed to evaluate the effect of art therapy upon depression levels in participants, the researcher might administer a depression inventory to research participants before (pretest) and after (posttest) the art therapy and control groups. The purpose of the pretest is to gather baseline data regarding group members' depression levels. The outcome in this hypothetical research study could be evaluated by statistically analyzing the differences in pretest and posttest depression scores of both groups. If in this study the participants receiving the art therapy intervention made significant gains over those in the control group as seen in lower depression levels, we might be tempted to attribute those gains to the art therapy intervention. However, it is impossible to do so without considering threats to both the internal and external validity of our study design.

Internal validity in experimental research design assures researchers that the results of the study and inferences drawn from them may be attributed to the experimental treatment or interventions, whereas external validity pertains to the extent to which study results can be generalized to populations greater than the sample participants. Ideally, both types of validity are built into the research design to the extent possible.

## Internal Validity

Internal validity is increased when extraneous and confounding variables are controlled. A number of threats to internal validity, and ways to address them to strengthen the research design, are described below.

### Selection

Selection bias results when differences between experimental and control groups exist before the study begins. For example, participants in one group may be less depressed, have greater exposure to art, or be more mature than participants in the other group. In art therapy research, bias may be manifested in the extent of research participants' previous art education or involvement in personal art making. Thus, individual attributes that may be different between experimental and control participants, rather than the art therapy treatment, may account for the outcome of the study. To control for selection bias, the researcher must randomize participants to experimental and control groups. An additional approach is to examine the pretest scores (or, specifically in art therapy research, the art involvement of all participants), match participants with similar scores or level of art involvement, and distribute those participants to the two groups equally. However, this approach only approximates randomization and is not a substitute for it.

### History

In addition to experiencing the experimental intervention between the pretest and posttest, other unanticipated external events may occur during that time span that may affect participants. Examples of unplanned events that might affect participant responses are natural disasters such as earthquakes or hurricanes, popular media events such as a movie or television special related to the study topic, or a community-wide health problem such as a flu epidemic. Randomization is a solution to this threat, as it would ensure that both experimental and control group participants have experienced the external event and that one group would not be differentially affected by it.

*Instrumentation*

Changes in the standardized tests used in a study or in the method of observation of participants may impact study results to the extent that the researcher is unable to attribute pre to post changes to the experimental intervention. If a standardized measure is unreliable, doesn't measure the variable of interest, or is administered incorrectly, we cannot be confident that study results can be attributed to the experimental intervention. Moreover, if an observer is used, his or her approach to systematic observations may vary over the duration of a study. To address these problems, researchers must correctly administer rigorously developed reliable and valid tests as both pretests and posttests, follow an observation protocol exactly, and ensure that the tests or observations measure the variable of interest, e.g., self-esteem versus self-concept. Assessments that are under development to establish rigor should not be used as the sole pretest and posttest measures in experimental research (Flanagan & Motta, 2007; Groth-Marnat, 1999), and this includes all art therapy assessments. For example, Beebe et al. (2010) conducted a randomized controlled study to evaluate the effectiveness of seven weeks of art therapy in helping children manage and cope with their chronic asthma. Before and after the art therapy intervention, in addition to using the Formal Elements Art Therapy Scale (FEATS; Gantt & Tabone, 1998) applied to the Person Picking an Apple from a Tree art therapy assessment, the researchers also used reliable and valid quality of life, depression, and anxiety scales to measure the children's responses to the art therapy intervention. The results reflected that, although the FEATS scores improved on several of the scales, it is the reliability and validity of the standardized tests, and the differences pre to post, that made the difference. These tests allowed the authors to conclude that art therapy effectively reduced the participants' anxiety and improved their self-concept and quality of life.

*Experimenter Bias*

This threat exists if the researcher's biases or opinions about study hypotheses affect the outcome. Such biases fly in the face of the objectivity critical to experimental research but can be addressed by having the intervention carried out by someone other than the researcher, someone who is "blind" to the expected or hoped for outcome. Another example of experimenter bias is the use of only one art therapist to provide the intervention to all participants in an art therapy study. Having several different art therapists facilitate the intervention controls for experimenter bias.

*Maturation*

Maturation refers to natural changes that occur in research participants, both long and short term, as a result of time passing. For example, changes in participants' energy and interest levels will likely fluctuate during an intervention and affect their responses to pretests and posttests; study outcomes may be the result of these changes rather than in response to the intervention. Randomization addresses this threat.

*Attrition*

As described in the previous chapter on ethics, participants may withdraw from a study at any time. There may be a difference between the participants who drop out of a study and those who complete the study, and this difference may affect the results to the extent that they are due to attrition rather than to the intervention itself. Attrition, or "mortality," is a very difficult threat to control and it may result in unexpected bias. By examining pretest scores of all participants, it may be possible to determine if those who leave a study are in some important ways different from those who finish. Simply replacing lost participants with new ones is not typically a successful strategy, as the researcher will never be able to determine what effect the lost participants may have had on the results.

*Statistical Regression*

This threat to internal validity pertains to "regression to the mean." It is a statistically supported fact that individuals with extreme scores (very high or very low) on standardized pretests tend to score closer to the mean (average) on subsequent testing. As art therapy researchers, we are often most interested in examining the effect of our work on the very individuals who might have these extreme scores. For example, if our research participants complete an anxiety inventory as a pretest that suggests that they are struggling with very high anxiety, and again after our art therapy intervention aimed at reducing anxiety, and their scores are lower, we are tempted to attribute their reduced anxiety to the art therapy intervention. However, because of regression to the mean, we cannot be sure that the lower posttest scores are not simply a result of this statistical phenomenon. The logical approach to addressing this threat to internal validity is to randomize participants to control and experimental groups. Both groups would likely experience regression to the mean in their posttest scores; however, if the art therapy group's posttest scores are lower than those of the control group, we are on firmer ground in inferring that it was our intervention that caused the reduction in anxiety.

## External Validity

Three overarching threats can potentially compromise generalizability of study findings: reactivity, order effects, and interaction effects (Erford, 2008). The setting of an experiment and the method of sampling have important bearing on the generalizability of results, so setting and recruitment of participants must be carefully considered when planning a study (Fraenkel et al., 2012). Obviously, random assignment to experimental and control groups improves external validity; nevertheless, generalization is always compromised by the impossibility of recruiting every member of a population under study. Thus, designing replicable studies is crucial for supporting art therapy research; replicating studies with different populations of participants and different art therapists administering interventions increases generalizability and supports the growth of knowledge in the field.

### Reactivity

Reactivity refers to the possibility that the results of a study are due to the participants' reactions to being in the study rather than to the intervention itself. For example, in biomedical research, participants in drug studies may be unaware of whether they are in the placebo group; they may report improvements despite not receiving any experimental drug at all. Or, participants may imagine that they know what the researcher's desired outcome is (or pick up on cues from the researcher) and behave in ways that they think will either achieve or sabotage that outcome. In addition, adult participants' anxiety about their perceived lack of art ability may significantly affect their involvement in the art therapy intervention (Kimport & Hartzell, 2015; Powers, 1999; Werner-Reap, 1995). To help control for this, participants can be asked about their perceived art ability in a post-intervention demographic questionnaire.

### Order Effects

Order effects refers to the likelihood that the order in which the intervention is presented to research participants has an effect on study results. For example, if a researcher devotes the first session of an art therapy intervention to reducing experimental participants' anxiety about their perceived lack of art skills, or to exploring ways to expand their capacity for artistic expression, and then proceeds with the rest of the intervention, the results will have limited generalizability because other populations beyond those in the study will not have experienced the preparatory session on anxiety reduction and learning about creative expression. Order effect also applies to the order in which pretest and posttest outcome measures are administered. An art therapy assessment administered first in a series of pretests could stimulate the research participant in ways that influence responses to the subsequent paper and pencil tests, and vice versa. The solution is to administer the pretest and posttest measures in a different order for every other participant; this washes out the order effect.

### Interaction Effects

Interaction effects result from selection biases: Characteristics of individual participants may predispose them to respond to an intervention in specific ways that the larger group to which we desire to generalize may not. For example, non-clients who volunteer for art therapy research may differ considerably from the population of non-volunteer clients or patients to whom we want to apply research results: In addition to not being clients, they may be curious about art therapy or eager to receive a financial incentive for consenting to be in the study. Furthermore, characteristics of the art therapy researcher administering the intervention, such as gender, enthusiasm, familiarity with specific art processes, or confidence level, may have an effect upon the results that would limit generalizability. To address this possibility, more than one art therapist should be involved in administering the intervention.

## Research Designs

Campbell and Stanley (1966) devised a visual method that uses symbols to diagram research designs, including reading from left to right to represent the passage of time from the beginning of a study until its end. Using this method, O represents an observation or measurement (such as a standardized test), and X represents exposure of research participants to an intervention or event (such as an art therapy group). When a pretest and posttest are used, or observations are made before and after an intervention, small numbers next to the Os indicate the order in which the tests are administered or the observations made. When there are two or more groups in a design, the Os and Xs of each group are lined up in columns and indicate that the intervention or event and the observations or measurements occur simultaneously in the groups. Finally, an R in these diagrams represents randomization, and thus distinguishes between true experimental and quasi-experimental designs. The figures below use this method to illustrate research designs.

## Pre-Experimental Designs

Some designs are considered pre-experimental because they don't include a control group, or if there is a control group, there is no randomization of participants. These designs are rife with validity problems, such as selection and experimenter bias and lack of generalizability, but in many fields, including art therapy, they often serve as preliminary explorations upon which to build larger studies with more sophisticated designs that have fewer threats to internal and external validity. Figure 3.1 illustrates three pre-experimental research designs.

| One Shot Case Study | X O |
| One-Group Pretest-Posttest Design | $O_1$ X $O_2$ |
| Static Group Comparison | X $O_1$ |
|  | $O_2$ |

*Figure 3.1* Three pre-experimental designs

### The One-Shot Case Study

This approach is often undertaken by art therapy practitioners or by researchers examining theoretical approaches or specific art therapy techniques. Typically, the case study will describe in detail the therapist's or researcher's work with an individual or group and, through a posttest or observation, the researcher makes inferences about the effect of the art therapy treatment. Despite pressures to support the field through traditional experimental research, Edwards (1999) advocated for well-written case studies that convey the depth and complexity of the therapeutic work, humanize research, prompt reexamination of art therapy theory, and include both the client's and art therapist's experience. However, in terms of experimental research, a case study entails no control over variables and outcome is determined by impressionistic means rather than by statistical analysis. For example, Nishida and Strobino (2005) conducted a case study exploring the effect of eight one-hour art therapy sessions upon the well-being and expressive capacity of a 57-year-old woman undergoing hemodialysis three times a week for several hours each time. The art therapy sessions were highly structured and focused on media exploration including paint and collage. After the last session, the patient was interviewed regarding her art therapy experience; she stated that the media exploration had given her a sense of mastery and control. The researchers noted that art therapy facilitated the patient's expression of various concerns, and that, despite the burden of her illnesses, she had an improved sense of well-being. Nishida and Strobino acknowledged the inability to generalize the findings of this study. It is possible that other factors such as experimenter bias or the subjectivity of the interview and observations may have been responsible for the results (Diamond, 1992). However, because of the favorable outcomes, further research of the effect of art therapy with hemodialysis patients is warranted.

*One Group Pretest-Posttest Design*

In this design, a standardized test of the variable of interest is given to research participants, the participants are exposed to an intervention, and then the standardized test is administered for a second time. The advantage of this design over the one-shot design is that there is a uniform measure of change in the same group of participants from before the intervention until after it (Isaac & Michael, 1995). However, although tempting when such a study yields statistically significant results supporting art therapy treatment, because of the many uncontrolled variables and threats to validity, it is impossible to attribute the change to the intervention.

The Bringing Research to Life! research simulation experiential (Betts & Potash, 2018) described in this book (see Chapter 1, Box 1.2, and Appendix A) involves student participation in a mock study that simulates a pre-experimental (not randomized, no control group), one group pretest-posttest design. The premise of the study is to investigate how students' engagement with an art exhibition may affect their well-being. First, students complete a pretest ($O_1$), the Brief Mood Introspection Scale (BMIS; Mayer & Gaschke, 1988). The treatment (X) phase involves the students' active participation in an immersive art experience, which includes a series of activities described in Appendix A. For the posttest ($O_2$) phase, the students complete the BMIS. During in-class experientials for the quantitative research unit, students are given the opportunity to analyze the de-identified data generated from their pre- and post-BMIS scores.

Kimport and Hartzell (2015) used the one group pretest-posttest design to test the effect of creating a pinch pot on levels of anxiety in 28 women and 28 men in a private psychiatric hospital. The researchers administered the State Trait Anxiety Inventory (Spielberger, 1989), which measures amounts of anxiety in respondents, before and after participants engaged for ten minutes in crafting a pinch pot with either acrylic clay or air-dry ceramic clay. The statistical results indicated that, after creating the pinch pot, participants' anxiety was significantly reduced, with the men in the experiment experiencing a greater reduction in anxiety than did the women. The limitations of this study are numerous, including using a small convenience sample of volunteer participants, rather than randomization of volunteers into experimental and control groups. Indeed, because of these limitations, it is possible that factors other than the clay work contributed to the reduction in anxiety. However, the significant reduction in anxiety that occurred in this study is worth researching using a more rigorous design, as described in the next section.

### Static Group Comparison

This design includes a control group in addition to the experimental group. The experimental group is exposed to a particular treatment and the control group is not, but both groups complete the same measure or test after the experimental group has received the treatment. For example, after eight weeks of facilitating an inpatient group, an art therapist might be interested in finding out whether the art therapy (experimental) group members' self-esteem has improved. The art therapist administers a self-esteem inventory to group members and to an equal number of inpatients who did not attend the group (who comprise the control group). When comparing the inventory scores from before and after the intervention, experimental group members' self-esteem is indeed higher compared to the control group, yet we are unable to infer that the improvement is due to the art therapy group, for two reasons. First, without randomization, it is not possible to assume that the two groups were essentially equal at the onset of the experiment; perhaps the individuals in the art therapy group had higher self-esteem to begin with. Second, there are countless other factors that may have impacted both groups and their scores on the self-esteem measure, such as the threats to internal and external validity described above.

## True Experimental Designs

True experimental designs are characterized by randomization of participants to experimental conditions. Most often, this means including a control group that does not experience the experimental (art therapy) condition, whose results are compared to those of the experimental participants. These designs offer ways to control for variables that are lacking in the pre-experimental approaches; in other words, there is greater internal and external validity in experimental designs than in the pre-experimental designs, and this greater validity permits inferences about cause and effect relationships between independent and dependent variables. Figure 3.2 illustrates three true experimental designs.

### Pretest-Posttest Control Group Design

In this design, participants are randomized to two groups, and both groups complete pretest and posttest measures of the dependent variable of interest, in the same sequence and at the same times. However, only the

| Pretest-Posttest Control Group Design | R  $O_1$  X  $O_2$ |
|---|---|
|  | R  $O_3$      $O_4$ |
| Control Group Posttest-Only Design | R          X  $O_1$ |
|  | R               $O_2$ |
| Solomon 4-Group Design | R  $O_1$  X  $O_2$ |
|  | R  $O_3$      $O_4$ |
|  | R          X  $O_5$ |
|  | R               $O_6$ |

*Figure 3.2* Three true experimental designs

experimental group receives the intervention. By insuring, through randomization, that the participants in both groups are essentially equal at the onset of a study, and exposing only experimental group participants to an art therapy intervention (i.e., the independent variable), we are in a good position to infer that the study outcomes may be attributed to the intervention. Art therapist Caroline Peterson developed the first known mindfulness-based art therapy (MBAT) program that includes various structured art therapy interventions, combined with mindfulness-based stress reduction, administered over eight weeks in a small group format. Working with colleagues, she conducted a randomized controlled trial that involved 111 women with various cancer diagnoses randomized to either an experimental group (MBAT) or a wait list condition (Monti et al., 2006). Ninety-three participants completed the entire study, which included administration pre and post of the Symptoms Checklist Revised (SCL-90-R) to measure psychological stress and stress-related physical complaints, and the Medical Outcomes Study Short-Form Health Survey (SF-36) to measure health-related quality of life (QOL). Through the use of sophisticated statistical analyses, the results indicated that, on every scale of the SCL-90-R, experimental subjects demonstrated statistically significant improvement compared to the control subjects, and on five of the eight scales of the SF-36, experimental subjects improved significantly compared to controls. Despite Monti et al.'s acknowledgment of the limitation of having a control group that was not involved in an activity that would compare to the MBAT condition, the rigor with which this study was conducted makes it an excellent example of a randomized control group pretest-posttest design with results that support the efficacy of the art therapy treatment developed for women with cancer.

## Control Group Posttest Only Design

This is a variation of the above design, in which only the posttest is administered. Often this design is used when it is impossible to obtain a pretest, for example if one wanted to research the effect of a human-made or natural disaster upon children's sense of safety in school (Leedy & Ormrod, 2005). Because of randomization, when implementing this design, the researcher can assume that the participants in both groups are essentially equal. The advantage of the posttest only design is the elimination of the pretest, which may have an influence due to order effect on participants' responses to the posttest. Despite this advantage, there are some inherent disadvantages: The intervention itself may impact the groups differently, negatively affecting the assumed equality of the two groups (Fraenkel et al., 2012).

Although there are no known art therapy studies using this design, a music therapy study conducted by Silverman (2009) compared the effect upon psychiatrically impaired hospitalized adults of a single session of psychoeducational music therapy (experimental group) versus a single session of verbal psychoeducation (control group). Having randomized the 105 participants to the two groups, the researcher assumed that the participants were essentially equal, and he conducted statistical tests that confirmed this to be true. The focus of both conditions was upon symptom management, life satisfaction, and responses to the particular psychoeducational interventions; these constructs were measured after the group sessions, using a wide variety of standardized and researcher-developed instruments. Using scripts in both conditions ensured that similar content was delivered to all participants, but, in addition to the scripted content, patients in the music therapy group were exposed to a song and lyrics that were discussed in terms of their relevance to the psychoeducational focus.

Analyses of the many posttests revealed few statistically significant differences between the two groups, although several measures revealed that the mean scores for the music therapy group were slightly higher than those of the verbal psychoeducational group, suggesting somewhat greater understanding of the educational goals of the groups, as well as enjoyment of the method of delivery (music therapy versus verbal only). Patients in the music therapy group tended to be more engaged in the intervention than those in the control group. Silverman (ibid.) was able to conclude that, "psychoeducational music therapy can be as effective as a proven psychosocial intervention such as psychoeducation on various measures" (p. 122).

*Solomon 4-Group Design*

By combining the two experimental designs above, the elegant Solomon 4-group design improves both internal and external validity by controlling for the effect of pretests (Erford, 2008; Fraenkel et al., 2012; Leedy & Ormrod, 2005). In this design, there are two groups (experimental and control) that are pretested and posttested, and two additional groups (experimental and control) that are tested only after the intervention.

If groups 3 and 4 differ in ways similar to how groups 1 and 2 do, the researcher can be confident that the study results are generalizable to situations in which there is no pretesting (Leedy & Ormrod, 2005). The researcher can also be confident that confounding variables and extraneous factors have not influenced the results. The disadvantage of this design relates to the increased number of participants who must be recruited to fill four groups, and the effort required of the researchers.

There are no known art therapy studies using a randomized Solomon 4-group design. However, Pretorius and Pfeifer (2010) utilized this design – *without randomization* – to study the effects of group art therapy upon sexually abused girls' depression, anxiety, and self-esteem. Although Pretorius and Pfeifer's study included control of variables by the researchers, the lack of randomization characterizes the study as *quasi-experimental*. Quasi-experimental designs are described below.

### Quasi-Experimental Designs

Quasi-experimental designs mimic experimental designs, but there is no randomization. However, often these designs are the only feasible possibility due to constraints on randomization in the natural setting of the participants, and thus many published quantitative research studies are quasi-experimental. Although researchers make every effort to address validity concerns, generalizability of results is limited.

Pretorius and Pfeifer (2010) used the Solomon 4-group design discussed above, but without randomization. The participants in their study were 25 South African sexually abused girls aged 8 to 11 years who were living in group homes with non-offending caretakers. For practical and logistical reasons, the researchers opted to assign their participants to groups according to which home they lived in; in other words, each group consisted of girls who lived together in a particular home. A trauma check list for children that measures depression, anxiety, and sexual trauma, and a Human Figure Drawing (HFD) to assess self-esteem were used as pretests and posttests according to the Solomon 4-group design. The two experimental groups (groups 1 and 3) engaged in eight sessions of art therapy using a variety of processes and materials, each addressing a specific theme such as establishing trust, expression of feelings associated with the children's history of abuse, and development of boundaries and strategies to avoid revictimization. With no art therapy intervention, pretests and posttests were collected from group 2 and posttests only were collected from group 4. All control group participants were provided the art therapy intervention after the study concluded. Differences between the groups were analyzed between pretest and posttest scores, in every possible combination to eliminate the effect of pretesting and determine whether the results could be attributed to the intervention. Differences between pretest scores indicated that groups 1 and 2 were not equal at the onset, a problem likely resulting from lack of randomization. However, other results indicated that, "following the intervention, the experimental groups demonstrated improvement in depression, anxiety and sexual trauma as compared to the control groups" (p. 70). The researchers also speculated that lack of differences in the self-esteem scores might be attributable to the inability of the HFD to identify changes in self-esteem.

*Nonrandomized Control Group Pretest-Posttest Design*

In this design, the researcher seeks two groups of research participants who are assumed to be equal, based upon recruitment criteria and the setting; for example, students in two fifth-grade classrooms in the same school, or adults in outpatient support groups. The design is similar to the one used by Monti et al. (2006) in that pretests and posttests are used to measure and compare change between groups' reactions to two different conditions, but participants are not randomized to the two groups. Hartz and Thick (2005) implemented a non-randomized control group pretest-posttest design to study differences between two groups of adolescent girls residing in a detention center. Unable to randomize the participants to experimental and control groups due to the inherent structure of the facility, the researchers nonetheless assumed that the two groups were as alike as possible because, upon admission, each detainee was carefully and intentionally assigned to a residential unit with the goal of maintaining overall diversity within the facility. Twelve girls participated in 10 weeks of "art psychotherapy" and 15 had 10 weeks of "art as therapy."

The researchers measured change by comparing scores on a standardized self-esteem questionnaire administered before and after the ten sessions, and through a self-designed posttreatment questionnaire about the girls' responses to the intervention. All participants significantly improved in "global self-worth" on the standardized measure, but they differed on subscales according to their group. The art psychotherapy group improved significantly in close friendship and conduct, and the art as therapy group improved significantly in social acceptance. According to Hartz and Thick (ibid.), these results are useful for treatment planning in that the two art therapy approaches studied appear to address different aspects of self-esteem. These researchers acknowledged several limitations to their study, including small sample size, the relatively short-term intervention, and the girls' concurrent participation in other therapies in the milieu. Although they carefully considered the purposeful placement of detainees to maintain diversity in the facility, lack of randomization and other limitations meant they were unable to isolate the art therapy treatment as the cause of the statistically significant results. However, on the posttreatment questionnaire, participants identified art therapy as extremely helpful in facilitating expression of feelings, developing coping skills, and increasing feelings of mastery and connection to others.

## Time-Series Designs

In the pretest-posttest research designs described so far, observations or tests are administered to groups of participants immediately before and immediately after the intervention. However, in time-series designs, observations are made and tests administered multiple times before and after the intervention. Similar to the one group pretest-posttest design seen in Figure 3.1, this design is an improvement since, with greater amounts of data collected, the likelihood increases that participant improvements on the posttests are caused by the intervention (Fraenkel et al., 2012). Miller (1993) examined the effect of a structured, art history-enriched art therapy intervention upon anxiety, time on task, and quality of art product in a small group of psychiatrically hospitalized adults. Miller's alternating treatment design, in which the same group undergoes two or more variations of a treatment, and the basic time-series design are seen in Figure 3.3.

In Miller's (1993) study, 13 research participants completed an anxiety inventory before and after making paintings in a minimally structured art therapy session. Then, a week later, the same group of people completed the same inventory before and after painting in a highly structured art history-based art therapy session. In both sessions, the amount of time participants spent on their paintings was calculated, and the paintings completed in each session were evaluated using a researcher-created form on which raters identified the structure and organization of the works. Statistical analysis revealed that the art history-enriched group facilitated significantly greater reduction in anxiety than did the minimally structured group. In addition, participants spent statistically significantly more time engaged in painting in the art history-enriched group. Although the art produced in the art history-enriched group was deemed more organized than that produced in the other group, the difference was not statistically significant. Miller recognized the limitations of her study: only 13 participants, short interval between art therapy sessions, and possible practice effect of the anxiety inventory; however, her study nonetheless points to the direct applicability of a time-series design study to clinical practice.

| Basic Time-Series Design | $O_1$ $O_2$ $O_3$ $O_4$ X $O_5$ $O_6$ $O_7$ $O_8$ |
|---|---|
| Alternating Treatment Time-Series Design | $O_1$ $X_1$ $O_2$ $O_3$ $X_2$ $O_4$ |

*Figure 3.3* Time-series and alternating treatment designs

## Single-Subject Designs

The research designs discussed thus far involve groups of participants. However, often there are occasions when an art therapist is interested in testing out a treatment strategy or art process with a particular client to determine its effect upon that client's functioning. Perhaps the client is so unique in presentation, diagnosis, or characteristics that recruiting similar participants for a group experiment would be impossible. Single-subject experiments are different from the previous designs in that typically only a single individual is involved. Using this approach, the researcher can test a client's response to an art therapy strategy using a specific design involving repeated and systematic measurement of one or more variables over time (Fraenkel et al., 2012). There are distinct benefits resulting from using single-subject designs in that this approach is easily implemented by practitioners in their work setting (Aldridge, 1994; Isaac & Michael, 1995; Kapitan, 2018). However, this research design differs from a narrative or descriptive case study in the rigor utilized; participant change is measured over time using a variety of different methods, and clinical replication is an essential part of the method (Diamond, 1992). Despite lack of generalizability due to weak external validity, the results of such studies are directly applicable to practice, and through replication, external validity is improved (Isaac & Michael, 1995). In other words, it is possible to apply single-subject designs simultaneously to small numbers of clients who are undergoing the same treatment, which improves our ability to draw cause and effect inferences, and thus provides an evidence base for our profession (Aldridge, 1994; Gallo, Comer, & Barlow, 2013).

In single-subject designs, participants serve as their own controls. This is possible through establishing a stable baseline of subject behaviors or symptoms, exposing the subject to several different conditions, and systematically measuring the response to each exposure. The idea is to use baseline measurement of the particular behavior that will be the focus of treatment, in order to predict what would happen should treatment not occur. In every single-subject design, the behavior of interest is measured before and after treatment (Diamond, 1992; Isaac & Michael, 1995; Purswell & Ray, 2014). The measurements may be analyzed statistically to demonstrate improvement or lack thereof, but instead are usually presented in the form of a graph, so that responses to treatment conditions are easily seen by simply viewing the graph.

The basic single-subject design is called the A-B design, with A representing the baseline phase of the experiment, and B representing the treatment phase. In the treatment phase, the baseline behavior is interrupted and affected in some way by the intervention, but, with such a simple design, positive or negative changes in behavior cannot be attributed to the intervention (Isaac & Michael, 1995). Pleasant-Metcalf and Rosal (1997) described a single-subject research study of a 12-year-old girl whose grades had fallen in reaction to her parents' divorce. In implementing an A-B design, the researchers used two earlier report cards and the child's scores on a self-concept scale as baseline measures, and the treatment phase consisted of ten individual art therapy sessions that focused on self-concept and problem solving. After the intervention, the researchers compared the child's next report card to the earlier ones and noted improvement in six of seven subjects; this difference was statistically significant ($p = 0.008$). Furthermore, scores on the self-concept scale indicated improvement in all subscales and substantial improvement in the total raw score. Despite the encouraging results of Pleasant-Metcalf and Rosal's study, due to weak internal validity inherent in the design it is not possible to attribute the changes to the intervention (Isaac & Michael, 1995; Kapitan, 2010).

Using a design that increases internal validity in single-subject research, Kuo and Plavnick (2015) studied the effect of engagement in an art activity on the classroom behavior of a three-year-old speech-impaired boy with autism. The child had difficulty with classroom tasks in three areas – motor activity, vocalizing, and not attending to task – and observation of the child in the classroom provided an opportunity to measure the frequencies of these behaviors of interest. This comprised the first phase of the A-B-A-B design. Then the researchers initiated the art activity (the first B phase), which consisted of facilitated manipulation of animal pictures and beads before the child joined the classroom. These two phases were then repeated, providing two baseline measurements and two administrations of the art activity, which allowed a comparison of the frequencies of baseline behaviors to the frequencies of behaviors after the facilitated art sessions. Because off-task behaviors decreased after the first facilitated art session, it was predicted that they would also decrease after the second facilitated art activity. This did in fact occur and demonstrated that there was a causal relationship between the art activity and the reduced off-task behaviors.

## *Factorial Designs*

To this point in this chapter, the research designs described study the effect of only a single independent variable (such as participation in group art therapy) upon dependent variables (such as level of depression or management of asthma symptoms). Factorial designs allow researchers to study the effect of *and interaction between* two or more independent variables, with or without randomization (Fraenkel et al., 2012), although clearly randomization enhances external validity. According to St John (2016), "a study using a single-variable design is easier to create and conduct, but the factorial design produces more information" (p. 108). Thus, these more complex designs yield deeper knowledge of the relationships between variables. Here, variables are referred to as "factors," hence the term "factorial design." In these designs, each factor has two levels (since variables can vary in at least two ways).

Within the context of a large body of music therapy literature pointing to the positive benefits of music therapy in combination with various other factors, Boothby and Robbins (2011) were interested in determining whether listening to music could be isolated as the "active ingredient" (p. 205) in mood improvement in patients, or whether other factors described in the literature, such as a music therapist's presence, concurrent relaxation induction, or imagery, were concomitant factors in patient mood improvement. They designed a factorial study in which they examined the effect of three factors upon research participants' mood. These factors were music (music versus no music), art (production versus sorting), and time (pre to post). Such a design is termed a "2 x 2 x 2 factorial design." Figure 3.4 illustrates the factorial design implemented by Boothby and Robbins.

Sixty adults were randomly assigned to four conditions: (a) listening to ten minutes of Bach's *Magnificat* + freely creating a drawing; (b) listening to ten minutes of Bach's *Magnificat* + sorting prints of famous art; (c) freely creating a drawing without music playing; and (d) sorting prints of famous art with no music playing. Negative mood was induced through participants listing ten negative life events, after which they completed mood and stress questionnaires (pretests). They then participated individually in their assigned task and completed the questionnaires again (posttests), followed by making a list of ten positive life events (to restore pretest mood). Using this design, Boothby and Robbins were able to control for the effect of a therapist's presence since there was no therapist involvement, and to compare changes in mood between music listening and no music, as well as to determine whether any combination of the art conditions and music listening had a different effect on mood than any one condition did alone. Statistical analysis involved comparing the pre to post scores on both mood instruments to music/no music and art production/art sorting conditions. Results indicated that, "listening to a

| Group A | R  O  $X_1 + X_2$  O |
| Group B | R  O  $X_1 + X_3$  O |
| Group C | R  O  $X_2$  O |
| Group D | R  O  $X_3$  O |

*Figure 3.4* Boothby and Robbins' (2011) factorial design

Notes: $X_1$ = music listening; $X_2$ = art production; $X_3$ = art sorting.

10-min segment of Bach's *Magnificat* significantly reduced negative mood levels ... compared to a no music condition. This effect was not affected by whether participants were sorting art prints or actively drawing" (p. 207). Thus, there was no effect of either art condition on mood level. Because Boothby and Robbins' study did not compare music therapy to art therapy, the findings of this study challenge art therapy researchers to devise studies to isolate the effect upon mood of artmaking while alone versus artmaking in the presence of an art therapist.

## Non-Experimental Designs

In non-experimental research, variables are not manipulated or controlled by the researcher and therefore no cause and effect conclusions can be drawn. However, relationships between variables can be established. This is reflected in the three types of non-experimental designs: descriptive survey research, correlational research, and causal comparative or ex post facto research.

### Descriptive Survey Research

The goal of survey research is to gain knowledge about a large population of people by asking questions of a smaller group that represents that population, and then using statistics or other mathematical means to summarize the responses (Leedy & Ormrod, 2005). Survey questions are constructed so that the results describe characteristics of the population of interest. The two basic types of surveys are longitudinal and cross-sectional (Fraenkel et al., 2012). Longitudinal surveys query the same population at several different points in time, to study changes over time. There are three basic types of longitudinal surveys: trend, cohort, and panel (Erford, 2008; Fraenkel et al., 2012). The numerous AATA membership surveys (see, for example, Elkins & Deaver, 2015) constitute a trend study, in which a population whose members may change is surveyed repeatedly to discover changes that have occurred over time. In a cohort study, the same persons are queried at different times over a specified time frame. For example, an art therapy educator could survey students three times over a semester to learn their responses to course content and teaching methods. A panel study involves studying the same group of individuals (the "panel") over time. Many studies of the life histories of gifted children exist and are examples of panel studies (see, for example, Gottfried, Gottfried, and Guerin's [2006] study).

Cross-sectional studies result in a snapshot of a population or populations at one point in time. A researcher may survey individuals of different ages at approximately the same point in time, in order to understand developmental issues; an art therapist might explore child, adolescent, and adult clients' responses to particular art therapy processes, to discover which are most valued by the different groups of survey respondents. More typically, a population is surveyed in order to describe its characteristics at a specific time. Patterson, Debate, Anju, Waller, and Crawford (2011) surveyed art therapists employed by the National Health Service (NHS) in England regarding theoretical approaches to treatment of patients with schizophrenia, job responsibilities, and the integration of art therapy services within the national healthcare system. Patterson et al.'s study exemplifies best practices in conducting a survey. The researchers carefully designed their study to obtain the answers to specific research questions. The development of questions was informed by existing scholarly literature, written job descriptions, and semi-structured interviews with a number of art therapists; after piloting a draft version, the final version was mailed to a random sample of the employed art therapists. The results captured the state of the profession for art therapists in the NHS at the time of the survey: Most respondents felt valued in their jobs, worked part time, delivered individual and group art therapy, used a psychoanalytic theoretical approach, and perceived that their clients with schizophrenia benefited from this approach. However, Patterson et al. noted that, based on the survey, individuals with schizophrenia are critically underserved due to the extreme shortage of art therapists in the NHS.

*Correlational Research*

Sometimes called "associational" research (Fraenkel et al., 2012, p. 331), correlational research investigates the relationship between two or more variables to determine whether there is a predictable relationship between them (Leedy & Ormrod, 2005). It is predictable that, for most students, minimal sleep the night before an examination results in a poor grade; it's also predictable that, in many men, hair loss is correlated with advancing age. These everyday examples show that, as one variable decreases or increases (hours of sleep, age), the other variable increases or decreases (exam grade, amount of hair) in a predictable manner. However, in research studies, no matter how strong these correlations are as determined by statistical analysis, no causality can be inferred.

Australian researchers Caddy, Crawford, and Page (2012) provide a useful example of an art therapy-related correlational study. They addressed the lack of published research support for creative therapeutic activity to improve mental health. Using de-identified data from the medical records of 403 adults who were inpatients in an acute psychiatric setting, they explored the relationship between participation in an inpatient group consisting of "art- and craft-based creative therapies" (p. 327) and mental health outcomes. The creative activities group was facilitated by a psychiatric nurse with postgraduate training in art therapy, who was being supervised by a professional art therapist. The medical records contained admission and discharge scores on standardized measures of depression and anxiety, quality of life, experience of illness (all self-rating measures), and overall patient functioning (clinician-rated). Analysis of the change from admission to discharge revealed that participants in the creative activity group demonstrated strong, statistically significant improvement in all four outcome measures.

Caddy et al. (ibid.) described the limitations inherent in their study that prevent interpreting the results as a causal relationship. Although the results clearly suggest that the positive treatment outcomes experienced by the participants are related to attendance in the creativity group, it is not possible to identify participation in the group as the cause of the positive outcomes. The anonymous patients whose data were used were simultaneously receiving nursing and psychiatric care, had differing treatment plans, and differing medications; these or other factors may have been responsible for the positive changes. Caddy et al. suggested that a randomized controlled trial would address many of the limitations of their study, as an experimental design would allow isolation of the variables that caused the positive changes in the group participants.

*Causal Comparative or Ex Post Facto*

Ex post facto (Latin for "after the fact") research – also known as causal comparative research – entails observing an existing group characteristic or behavior and conducting an investigation to determine its cause. Like correlational research, causal comparative research is associational in nature; there is no researcher manipulation of variables, and therefore causality cannot be inferred from study results. The methodology entails gathering data from two or more groups that differ only in terms of the phenomenon of interest. An example would be an investigation comparing twelfth-grade smokers to twelfth-grade nonsmokers at the same school along a number of variables such as parental smoking habits, religion, involvement in extracurricular activities and sports, and number of school absences due to illness. The goal of such a study would be to discover if there are relationships between specific familial and societal characteristics and adolescent smoking.

In an example from psychology, Schreiber and Schreiber (2002) studied the parents of children aged 6 to 15 to understand parental personality factors associated with violent children. Using a standardized list of questions, they interviewed 25 parents of violent children and 25 parents of same-aged nonviolent, well-behaved children. The violent children had been diagnosed with Oppositional Defiant Disorder or Conduct Disorder and had performed acts such as setting fires and killing animals. All children whose parents participated in the study attended special education classes in the same school district. Interviewers categorized parents' responses to interview questions according to six behaviors derived from the literature about violent children and adolescents: abusive, impulsive, immature, insecure, emotionally cold, and inconsistent behavior. Data analysis revealed that the parents of violent children demonstrated statistically significantly more of these six behaviors than did the parents of the control group. This was a well-designed study in its use of two groups of parents that differed only on the basis of the phenomenon of interest (violent versus nonviolent children).

There are no known art therapy ex post facto studies. However, Brown (1993) recognized a pattern in the content of drawings done by 47 adult acute care hospital patients; each had drawn a picture of a person fishing. Brown retrospectively examined the hospital charts of these patients and discovered that each had been diagnosed with major depression or was in a depressive phase of bipolar disorder. Immediately prior to hospitalization, each had experienced suicidal ideation or the death of a close relative. Furthermore, discharge was imminent for each patient who drew a fishing image. Based on an extensive literature review, and the pre-discharge timing of the drawings, Brown theorized about the meaning of the fishing drawings and concluded that the "fish symbol represents fulfillment, emotional nurturance – a means of sustaining life" (p. 170), and associated this meaning with successful treatment and hope regarding discharge. Although an interesting study, it failed to include a comparison group of depressed individuals near their discharge date who did not draw a fishing image. Including such a group would have constituted an ex post facto study as the two groups of individuals would differ only on the variable of interest: whether they drew a fishing image. However, Brown's study suggests that ex post facto studies are an interesting possibility for art therapy researchers.

## Quantitative Data Analysis: Introduction to Statistics

Students attending approved or accredited art therapy master's degree programs in the US are required to "demonstrate basic statistical concepts such as scales of measurement, measures of central tendency, variability, distribution of data, and relationships among data as applied in research studies" (CAAHEP, 2016). A basic knowledge of certain principles underlying statistics is useful not only for engaging in assessment and research, but also for understanding and evaluating tests used in clinical work and published research reports of quantitative and mixed methods studies regarding their applicability to practice. Moreover, because art therapy practitioners are typically not experts in statistics, we support consultation with a statistician or psychometrician through every stage of designing and executing studies that include quantitative data.

There are three purposes of statistics in research studies. First, statistics enables researchers to organize large amounts of data from multiple sources. Second, statistics helps researchers describe existing data. These describing and summarizing processes are called *descriptive statistics*. Third, through *inferential statistics*, data are compared and relationships between variables are discovered; through these techniques, researchers are also able to interpret results, including whether or not they occurred simply by chance or as a result of the particular design and execution of the study. Depending on the topic under study, researchers may incorporate both descriptive and inferential statistics in the research design. This section provides a brief overview of the basics of statistics use in research. Refer to Box 3.1 at the end of this chapter for an illustrative example of quantitative data analysis as related to the Bringing Research to Life! research simulation experiential (Betts & Potash, 2018).

### Numbers and Measurement

Measurement is a crucial concept that has to do with the organization and use of numbers because, in quantitative research, data are distilled to numbers and statistics are used to understand the data. Although the process of assigning numbers to data may be straightforward in some professions, it is more complicated in fields like psychology, social science, and art therapy, in which the topics of interest focus upon the complexities and abstract qualities of human nature and human behavior. How is it possible to quantify personality characteristics, artworks, the therapeutic relationship, or mental illness? Understanding the nature of variables provides some answers, because the types of variables used in a study determine the types of measurement scales used in data analysis. Discrete variables can be considered either/or variables; for example, in art therapy, media might be fluid or resistive (Hinz, 2009; Kagin & Lusebrink, 1978), or a research participant's status might be inpatient or outpatient. On the other hand, continuous variables change along a continuum, thus providing greater precision of measurement. For example, Likert scales that include a range of answers such as "never," "sometimes," and "always" provide research participants with the chance to choose one of several answers, each of which is assigned a number for data analysis purposes. One art therapy example of a continuous variable is the amount of space on a sheet of paper filled by a Human Figure Drawing, as determined by applying a modified FEATS (Gantt & Tabone, 1998) rating instrument (Deaver, 2009). By using grids on transparent plastic placed over the drawing, the amount of space occupied by the drawing can be easily ascertained as 25, 50, 75, or 100 percent.

The type of variable, discrete or continuous, determines the method of measurement and data analysis. There are four types of scaling methods for measuring variables used in quantitative research: nominal, ordinal, interval, and ratio. These four scales provide increasingly greater information about variables; that is, the nominal scale provides the least amount whereas the ratio scale provides the most (see Chapter 7 for a full description of these scales as applied to assessment research). Thus, when designing studies, researchers must consider which type of measurement will yield the most information to answer research questions (Fraenkel et al., 2012). A nominal scale simply identifies or names variables. Such a scale consists of classifying variables into mutually exclusive (discrete), non-ordered categories, each of which is assigned a numerical value. For example, a researcher interested in the variable of clay might group data into three categories: acrylic clay, terra cotta, and porcelain, and assign the number 1 to acrylic clay, 2 to terra cotta, and 3 to porcelain. These numbers are used for data analysis only; there is no implication that porcelain (3) is any "more" or "better" than terra cotta (2) or acrylic clay (1). The categories are simply different from each other (ibid.).

Ordinal scales rank order data, although the numerical differences between the rankings are not uniform. Kagin (Kagin & Lusebrink, 1978) coined the phrase "media dimension variables" to describe the effect of various art media upon the art therapy process (Hinz, 2009). These variables are categorized as ranging from fluid to resistive. An example is paint, which would range from most fluid (finger paint or water color on wet paper) to most resistive (paint sticks or sponge bottle paints); a researcher would assign numbers to each variable for use in data analysis, but, although the differences between the rankings are in order of increasing structure or control, those differences are not arithmetically uniform. In other words, if finger paint is assigned the value of 1, wet on wet watercolor is assigned 2, and sponge bottle paints are assigned 4, it does not mean that sponge bottle paints are four times more resistive than finger paint.

Interval scales are similar to ordinal scales but with one important difference: The spaces between the items on the scale are uniform. In addition, the zero point on the scale does not imply a complete absence of the variable or attribute being measured. The lack of the absolute zero point on the scale means that it is impossible to make absolute comparisons among values. These concepts are most easily understood through the examples of psychological tests of self-esteem, achievement, or other variables such as depression and anxiety. In using such tests, a score of 10 on a self-esteem scale does not mean that that research participant has ten times the amount of self-esteem than does a participant who scores a 1. Furthermore, the participant who scores 1 on such a test does not entirely lack self-esteem.

Ratio scales have all the attributes of the other three scales, with the addition that a ratio scale has an absolute zero, which indicates a total absence of the variable or attribute being measured. Physical measurements are examples of ratio scales; a person 5 feet tall is twice the height of a person who is 2.5 feet tall. Examples of ratio scales that might be used in art therapy research include amount of time participants spend on task and frequency counts of observed behaviors. Kuo and Plavnick's (2015) study, discussed above, utilized a ratio scale through counting the frequency of observed behaviors of a preschool student with attention and behavior problems, and then comparing those frequencies over the four phases of their single-subject study. Another example of use of a ratio scale in an art therapy study would be time on task. Miller (1993) counted the number of minutes participants in two groups spent on their paintings, and data analysis indicated that the structured art history-informed art therapy group spent statistically significantly more time engaged in painting than did the minimally structured art therapy group without art history stimulus.

## Descriptive Statistics

Descriptive statistics summarize data from a large sample into numerical or graphic form. Examples of such data include research participant characteristics like age and diagnosis, scores on pretests and posttests, responses to survey items, and the like. Data are most often summarized using frequency tables and graphs that show the number of responses in each category studied. For example, Elkins and Deaver's (2015) report on AATA's membership survey displays results in frequency tables and graphs, and compares current survey results to the results of three previous membership surveys, providing readers with information about trends in the field over a six-year period. Basic descriptive statistics include distribution of scores on standardized tests or responses to surveys, and the like; measures of central tendency; and measures of variability.

### Measures of Central Tendency

Measures of central tendency provide information about the middle of a distribution of data, which often represents the typical value attained by the entire population under study. There are three such measures: mean, median, and mode. The mean is the average value, the median is the middle value, and the mode is the value that occurs most frequently in a set of scores or responses. For example, Holmqvist, Roxberg, Larsson, and Lundqvist-Persson (2017) interviewed 38 art therapists regarding their conceptualizations of patients' inner change that occurred during art therapy treatment. They described the research participants using measures of central tendency: the mean number of years the participants had practiced art therapy was 17, with the median value being 16. Because these values were so close, we can infer that the group of art therapists was homogeneous in terms of work experience.

## Measures of Variability

Measures of variability describe how widely values are distributed or *dispersed* across a population or sample. The *range* and the *standard deviation* are measures of dispersion. The range is the distance between the lowest and highest values in a distribution; determining the range requires a minimum of ordinal-level data. If the range is large, there is great variability of scores. The standard deviation (SD) is a value that describes how close to or far away from the mean scores are dispersed. A low SD indicates that most of the values are close to the mean and a high SD indicates that values are widely dispersed. At minimum, interval data are required to calculate the SD. Patterson et al. (2011), discussed earlier in this chapter, included SDs in their table summarizing agreement among interviewees about survey items. Based on the SDs calculated for items, they determined that interviewees' views were consistent on most items but the large SDs on two items indicated a lack of agreement. These results illuminated important aspects of the organization and the process of group art therapy service delivery in England.

## Distribution of Data

The concept of the normal curve is crucial to understanding descriptive statistics. The normal curve depicts the distribution of values if the mean, median, and mode are all equal. It is a natural phenomenon that if such conditions exist (that is, if the mean, median, and mode are equal), the distribution of values will conform to the "68–95–99.7 rule" by which 68 percent of the values are within two SDs of the mean, 95 percent are within four SDs, and 99.7 percent (or estimated as 100 percent) are within six SDs. That is, the values would be evenly distributed around the mean, as seen in Figure 3.5.

Andsell and Pavlicevic (2001) stated, "Real life, however, isn't quite like that, but the normal curve is a standard distribution of frequency against

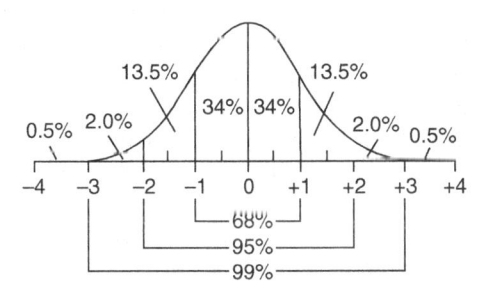

*Figure 3.5* Normal curve with standard deviations

which we can compare the distributions of our own data" (p. 173). In other words, it is likely that many participants in art therapy research studies are unique in terms of diagnoses, behaviors, and problem areas, whose data may lie outside of the normal distribution. The concept of the normal curve is helpful in understanding data related to participant characteristics, scores on standardized measures, and other relevant data.

## Inferential Statistics

Hypothesis testing, a foundational aspect of quantitative research, involves assessing the likelihood – or *probability* – that a study's result occurred either by chance or due to its carefully designed plan and execution. This is most readily accomplished when the participants in a study have been selected through random sampling (described earlier), when the total number of participants in the study (the "N") is large, and when the participants have been randomized to groups. Of course, a goal of quantitative research is to design studies with great care, to control variables and increase the likelihood that the study results do not result from chance, or put another way, increase the likelihood that the sample of study participants closely represents the broader population of interest. Statistical tests are then used to analyze relationships between numbers derived from a study's data, and answer research questions with a probability statement of the extent to which the results occurred by chance.

### Probability

The probability of whether study results are due to the design and execution of the study or merely due to chance is determined by statistical analysis and expressed as a "*p-value*." The $p$ value is a number expressed as a percentage that represents the level of statistical significance in terms of the likelihood that the study results are or are not due to chance. The larger the *p*-value, the greater the likelihood that results are due to chance. Significance levels are established by statisticians and are typically accepted benchmarks used by scholarly journals and academic institutions. In art therapy research, significance is established at the 0.05 level and expressed thus: $p \leq 0.05$; such a *p*-value means that at the 95 percent level (95 times out of 100), the study results are due to the research design and execution rather than to chance. A *p*-value of greater than 0.05, for example 0.10, is less desirable, and not considered to be statistically significant. On the other hand, a *p*-value of less than 0.05, such as 0.01 (99 times out of 100), is better, and represents a robust result highly likely to not be attributable to chance.

## Common Statistical Tests

There are two basic categories of statistical test: those that determine relationships among variables, and those that determine differences between groups. Choosing a statistical test that is appropriate depends on these factors and on the type of data (nominal, ordinal, interval, ratio) to be analyzed. A further classification of statistical procedures is *parametric or nonparametric*. Parametric tests assume a normal distribution in the population from which the research sample was drawn, whereas nonparametric tests do not rely on such assumptions. Nonparametric tests are sometimes called distribution-free tests. Here, we introduce examples of statistical tests that are commonly used to test for relationships between or among variables and to test for differences between groups. Table 3.1 shows applications of three commonly used statistical tests according to the type of data to be analyzed.

*Chi-square* is used to compare frequencies of data that are organized in categories, to discover the differences between expected frequencies and actual frequencies. The *Pearson product-moment correlation coefficient* ("Pearson's *r*") measures the strength and direction of the linear relationship between two variables. In her initial study of the Bird's Nest Drawing (BND), Kaiser (1996) developed a first version of the Attachment Rating Scale (ARS) to identify secure or insecure attachment through theorized graphic equivalents of secure or insecure attachment organization. She asked research participants to take a reliable and valid standardized test (the Attachment to Mother scale [ATM]) and to draw a picture of a bird's nest. For data analysis, participants were grouped into high and low groups (the two categories necessary for using a chi-square), depending on scores they obtained on the ATM. Kaiser first used chi-square analysis to discover the relationship between the test scores and the theorized graphic equivalents on the ARS; the results demonstrated that no relationships reached significance. Applying the Pearson product-moment correlation coefficient, it was discovered that only two of the indicators approached significance. Based on an earlier pilot study, additional theorized graphic equivalents were added to the ARS and, again,

*Table 3.1* Some basic statistical tests

| Type of Data | Testing for Relationships | Testing for Differences |
|---|---|---|
| Nominal | Chi-square | N/A |
| Ordinal | Spearman's rho | Analysis of Variance (ANOVA) |
|  |  | Kruskal–Wallis one-way Analysis of Variance (ANOVA) |
| Interval | Pearson's *r* | *t*-test for independent means; Analysis of Variance (ANOVA) |
| Ratio |  |  |

chi-square was used to determine differences between the BNDs drawn by participants in the high group and those in the low group. For those in the high group, the inclusion of either parent or baby birds was significant at the 0.01 level, and the inclusion of baby birds was significant at the 0.05 level. These results suggested an association between secure attachment and including birds in the BND. For greater detail regarding how Kaiser's research was conducted, see Chapter 8 in this book.

*Spearman's rho* is the nonparametric equivalent of Pearson's *r*, but it is used with ordinal data rather than with ratio or interval data. Like Pearson's *r*, Spearman's rho is utilized to measure the strength of relationships between two variables. In a study of self drawings and family drawings done by very young children from two widely differing cultures, Rübeling, Schwarzer, Keller, and Lenk (2011) explored the possible impact of culture upon the drawings. They developed a list of 13 "graphical elements" (p. 69) in the children's family and self drawings, and two raters blind to the nature of the study scored the drawings. Spearman's rho was used to calculate the inter-rater reliability of the two raters' scores on graphical diversity and closed forms, both of which were determined to be significant at the 0.001 level, allowing for reliable rating of the rest of the drawings.

The *t-test for independent means* is used to determine the significance of the difference between two sample means. In a mixed methods multiple case study, Streeter (Streeter & Deaver, 2018) studied the effect of six weekly sessions of individual art therapy on 13 women who were diagnosed with infertility and struggled with symptoms of depression. A *t*-test was used to measure the difference in scores on a reliable and valid depression inventory that was administered before and after the six weeks. The test results indicated a highly significant difference, with improved post-intervention scores ($p = 0.000006$), strongly suggesting the effectiveness of individual art therapy to address symptoms of depression in women diagnosed with infertility.

The *Analysis of Variance (ANOVA)* is also used to test the differences in group means but is typically used when three or more groups are being compared. With ANOVA, variation within groups and between groups is analyzed for significance. The *Kruskal–Wallis One-Way Analysis of Variance* is also a test for use when comparing more than two independent groups but is nonparametric; using this test, individual scores from all groups are rank ordered and then compared to the summed scores for each of the individual groups. For example, Pretorius and Pfeifer (2010), discussed earlier in this chapter, used a Solomon 4-group design to examine the effect of group art therapy upon abused girls' anxiety, depression, self-esteem, and trauma symptoms; their design had two experimental groups and two control groups. They implemented *t*-tests, ANOVA, and the Kruskal-Wallis test to compare the scores on outcome measures among the four groups; these analyses were chosen according to the level of data analyzed, ordinal, interval, or ratio. Their results indicated that the girls who participated in group art therapy improved in depression, anxiety, and trauma symptoms, compared to the girls in the two control groups.

## Summary

This chapter began by likening the research process to the creative process in terms of recognizing a problem or question that needs answering and pursuing that answer systematically. The chapter introduced quantitative research as associated with the postpositivist research paradigm, and as characterized by use of the scientific method of hypothesis testing through deductive reasoning. Quantitative research is based upon three principles: *objectivity* in the research process by researchers' distance from the workings of their own studies; *generalizability* of results to populations beyond the persons who participated in studies; and *replication* of studies to increase the body of research and support theory development. Terms associated with quantitative research were defined, and examples were provided.

Next, the types of quantitative research methods were introduced: true experimental, quasi-experimental, and non-experimental. True experimental and quasi-experimental studies strive to establish cause and effect relationships between variables through researcher manipulation of variables, whereas in non-experimental methods there is no researcher manipulation of variables so cause and effect cannot be established, although relationships among variables can be. Pre-experimental, true experimental, and quasi-experimental research designs were described and examples of each type of design were provided using examples from art therapy and other fields. In addition, non-experimental approaches including survey, correlational, and ex post facto designs were described together with examples. The chapter concluded with an introduction to descriptive and inferential statistics; a basic understanding of these terms assists art therapists in designing research studies and also permits them to be critical consumers of published research and its application to practice.

---

**Box 3.1 Bringing Research to Life! Quantitative Data Analysis Example**

**Objective:** Please refer to Box 1.1 (Chapter 1) and Appendix A for the purpose, set-up, and materials to guide the application of this experiential. The following provides information on the *quantitative* data analysis portion of the Bringing Research to Life! research simulation experiential (after the mock experiment and data collection has been completed):

| Research Method | Experiential "Data" | "Findings" |
|---|---|---|
| **Quantitative**<br>Non-directional hypothesis: *An immersive art experience will have an effect on the mood state of graduate art therapy students.*<br>Directional hypothesis: *An immersive art experience will improve the mood state of graduate art therapy students.* | Pre, post and follow-up measures (aggregated scores yield *t*-test results) (BMIS mood scale).<br>Nominal scales (art characteristics).<br>Ordinal scales (relational aesthetic questionnaire). | Degree of change that reflects effectiveness of activity on mood.<br>Survey of art characteristics deemed meaningful.<br>Ranking of what makes art perceived to be meaningful. |

Source: Betts and Potash (2018).

# References

Aldridge, D. (1994). Single-case research designs for the creative art therapist. *The Arts in Psychotherapy, 21*(5), 333–342. Retrieved from https://doi.org/10.1016/0197-4556(94)90061-2

Andsell, G. & Pavlicevic, M. (2001). *Beginning research in the arts therapies: A practical guide*. London: Jessica Kingsley.

Beebe, A., Gelfand, E., & Bender, B. (2010). A randomized trial to test the effectiveness of art therapy for children with asthma. *Journal of Allergy and Clinical Immunology, 126,* 263–266. Retrieved from https://doi.org/10.1016/j.jaci.2010.03.019

Betts, D. J. & Potash, J. (2018). Research simulation experiential: Bringing research to life! (personal collection of D. Betts and J. Potash, the George Washington University, Washington, DC).

Broothby, D. & Robbins, S. (2011). The effects of music listening and art production on negative mood: A randomized, controlled trial. *The Arts in Psychotherapy, 38,* 204–208. Retrieved from https://doi.org/10.1016/j.aip.2011.06.002

Brown, R. J. (1993). The fishing image: A preliminary study. *The Arts in Psychotherapy, 20,* 167–171. Retrieved from https://doi.org/10.1016/0197-4556(93)90006-N

CAAHEP (Commission on Accreditation of Allied Health Education Programs). (2016). *Standards and guidelines for the accreditation of educational programs in art therapy*. Clearwater, FL: Author.

Caddy, L., Crawford, F., & Page, A. (2012). "Painting a path to wellness": Correlations between participating in a creative activity group and improved measured mental health outcome. *Journal of Psychiatric and Mental Health Nursing, 19,* 327–333. Retrieved from https://doi.org/10.1111/j.1365-2850.2011.01785.x

Campbell, D. & Stanley, J. (1966). *Experimental and quasi-experimental designs for research*. Chicago, IL: Rand McNally.

Carolan, R. (2001). Models and paradigms of art therapy research. *Art Therapy: Journal of the American Art Therapy Association, 18*(4),190–206. Retrieved from https://doi.org/10.1080/07421656.2001.10129537

Cohen, B. & Cox, C. (1995). The integrative method: Making sense of art. In *Telling without talking: Art as a window into the world of multiple personality* (pp. 1–19). New York, NY: W.W. Norton.

Curry, N. & Kasser, T. (2005). Can coloring mandalas reduce anxiety? *Art Therapy: Journal of the American Art Therapy Association, 22*(2),81–85. Retrieved from https://doi.org/10.1080/07421656.2005.10129441

Dahlman, Y. (2007). Towards a theory that links experience in the arts with acquisition of knowledge. *International Journal of Art and Design Education, 26*(3), 274–284. Retrieved from https://doi.org/10.1111/j.1476-8070.2007.00538.x

Deaver, S. (2002). What constitutes art therapy research? *Art Therapy: Journal of the American Art Therapy Association, 19*(1), 23–27. Retrieved from https://doi.org/10.1080/07421656.2002.10129721

Deaver, S. (2009). A normative study of children's drawings: Preliminary research findings. *Art Therapy: Journal of the American Art Therapy Association, 26*(1), 4–11. Retrieved from https://doi.org/10.1080/07421656.2009.10129309

Deaver, S. & McAuliffe, G. (2009). Reflective visual journaling during art therapy and counselling internships: A qualitative study. *Reflective Practice, 10*(5), 615–632. Retrieved from https://doi.org/10.1080/14623940903290687

Deaver, S. & Shiflett, C. (2011). Art-based supervision techniques. *The Clinical Supervisor, 30*, 257–276. Retrieved from https://doi.org/10.1080/07325223.2011.619456

Diamond, P. (1992). The single case study. In H. Wadeson (Ed.), *A guide to conducting art therapy research* (pp. 107–119). Mundelein, IL: American Art Therapy Association.

Drake, C., Searight, H. R., & Olson-Pupek, K. (2014). The influence of art-making on negative mood states in university students. *American Journal of Applied Psychology, 2*(3), 69–72. Retrieved from https://doi.org/10.12691/ajap-2-3-3

Edwards, D. (1999). The role of case study in art therapy research. *Inscape, 4*(1), 2–9. Retrieved from https://doi.org/10.1080/17454839908413068

Elkins, D. & Deaver, S. (2015). American Art Therapy Association, Inc.: 2013 membership survey report. *Art Therapy: Journal of the American Art Therapy Association, 32*(2), 60–69. Retrieved from https://doi.org/10.1080/07421656.2015.1028313

Erford, B.T. (2008). *Research and evaluation in counseling*. Boston, MA: Houghton Mifflin.

Flanagan, R. & Motta, R. (2007). Figure drawings: A popular method. *Psychology in the Schools, 44*(3), 257–270. Retrieved from https://doi.org/10.1002/pits.20221

Fraenkel, J., Wallen, N., & Hyun, H. (2012). *How to design and evaluate research in education* (8th ed.). New York, NY: McGraw-Hill.

Franklin, M. (2012). Know thyself: Awakening self-referential awareness through art-based research. *Journal of Applied Arts & Health, 3*(1), 87–96. Retrieved from https://doi.org/10.1386/jaah.3.1.87_1

Gallo, K., Comer, J., & Barlow, D. (2013). Single-case experimental designs and small pilot trial designs. In J. Comer & P. Kendal (Eds.), *The Oxford handbook of research strategies for clinical psychology* (pp. 24–39). New York, NY: Oxford University Press.

Gantt, L. & Tabone, C. (1998). *Formal Elements Art Therapy Scale: The rating manual*. Morgantown, WV: Gargoyle Press.

Gottfried, A.W., Gottfried, A. E., & Guerin, D. (2006). The Fullerton Longitudinal Study: A long-term investigation of intellectual and motivational giftedness. *Journal for the Education of the Gifted, 29*(4), 430–450. Retrieved from https://doi.org/10.4219/jeg-2006-244

Groth-Marnat, G. (1999). Projective drawings. In *Handbook of psychological assessment* (pp. 499–533). New York, NY: Wiley.

Hartz, L. & Thick, L. (2005). Art therapy strategies to raise self-esteem in female juvenile offenders: A comparison of art psychotherapy and art as therapy approaches. *Art Therapy: Journal of the American Art Therapy Association, 22*(2), 70–80. Retrieved from https://doi.org/10.1080/07421656.2005.10129440

Henderson, P., Rosen, D., & Mascaro, N. (2007). Empirical study on the healing nature of mandalas. *Psychology of Aesthetics, Creativity, and the Arts, 1*(3), 148–154. Retrieved from https://doi.org/10.1037/1931-3896.1.3.148

Hinz, L. (2009). *Expressive Therapies Continuum: A framework for using art in therapy*. New York, NY: Routledge.

Holmqvist, G., Roxberg, A., Larsson, I., & Lundqvist-Persson, C. (2017). What art therapists consider to be patients' inner change and how it may appear in art therapy. *The Arts in Psychotherapy, 56*, 45–52. Retrieved from https://doi.org/10.1016/j.aip.2017.07.005

Indiana University Bloomington. (n.d.) *Types of variables*. Retrieved from www.indiana.edu/~educy520/sec5982/week_2/variable_types.pdf

Isaac, S. & Michael, W. (1995). *Handbook in research and evaluation for education and the behavioral sciences*. San Diego, CA: EdITS.

Kagin, S. L. & Lusebrink, V. B. (1978). The Expressive Therapies Continuum. *The Arts in Psychotherapy, 5*, 171–180. Retrieved from https://doi.org/10.1016/0090-9092(78)90031-5

Kaiser, D. (1996). Indications of attachment security in a drawing task. *The Arts in Psychotherapy, 23*(4), 333–340. Retrieved from https://doi.org/10.1016/0197-4556(96)00003-2

Kaiser, D. & Deaver, S. (2013). Establishing a research agenda for art therapy: A Delphi study. *Art Therapy: Journal of the American Art Therapy Association, 30*(3), 114–121. Retrieved from https://doi.org/10.1080/07421656.2013.819281

Kapitan, L. (2010). *Introduction to art therapy research*. New York, NY: Routledge.

Kapitan, L. (2018). *Introduction to art therapy research* (2nd ed.). New York, NY: Routledge.

Kaplan, F. (1998). Scientific art therapy: An integrative and research-based approach. *Art Therapy: Journal of the American Art Therapy Association, 15*(2), 93–98. Retrieved from https://doi.org/10.1080/07421656.1989.10758719

Kimport, E. & Hartzell, E. (2015). Clay and anxiety reduction: A one-group, pretest/posttest design with patients on a psychiatric unit. *Art Therapy: Journal of the American Art Therapy Association, 32*(4), 184–189. Retrieved from https://doi.org/10.1080/07421656.2015.1092802

Kuo, N. & Plavnick, J. (2015). Using an antecedent art intervention to improve the behavior of a child with autism. *Art Therapy: Journal of the American Art Therapy Association, 32*(2), 54–59. Retrieved from https://doi.org/10.1080/07421656.2015.1028312

Leedy, P. & Ormrod, J. (2005). *Practical research: Planning and design* (8th ed.). Upper Saddle River, NJ: Pearson Merrill Prentice Hall.

Lusebrink, V. (1990). *Imagery and visual expression in therapy*. New York, NY: Plenum Press.

Marshall, J. (2007). Image as insight: Visual images in practice-based research. *Studies in Art Education, 49*(1), 23–41. Retrieved from https://doi.org/10.1080/00393541.2007.11518722

Mayer, J. D. & Gaschke, Y. N. (1988). The experience and meta-experience of mood. *Journal of Personality and Social Psychology, 55*, 102–111. Retrieved from https://doi.org/10.1037/0022-3514.55.1.102

Miller, C. (1993). The effects of art history-enriched art therapy upon anxiety, time on task, and art product quality. *Art Therapy: Journal of the American Art Therapy Association, 10*(4), 194–200. Retrieved from https://doi.org/10.1080/07421656.1993.10759013

Monti, D., Peterson, C., Kunkel, E., Hauck, W., Pequignot, E., Rhodes, L., & Brainard, G. (2006). A randomized, controlled trial of mindfulness-based art therapy (MBAT) for women with cancer. *Psycho-Oncology, 15*, 363–373. Retrieved from https://doi.org/10.1002/pon.988

Nishida, M. & Strobino, J. (2005). Art therapy with a hemodialysis patient: A case analysis. *Art Therapy: Journal of the American Art Therapy Association, 22*(4), 221–226. Retrieved from https://doi.org/10.1080/07421656.1993.10759013

Öster, I., Svensk, A., Magnusson, E., Thyme, K., Sjodin, M., Astrom, S., & Lindh, J. (2006). Art therapy improves coping resources: A randomized, controlled study among women with cancer. *Palliative and Supportive Care, 4*, 57–64. Retrieved from https://doi.org/10.1017/S147895150606007X

Patterson, S., Debate, J., Anju, S., Waller, D., & Crawford, M. (2011). Provision and practice of art therapy for people with schizophrenia: Results of a national survey. *Journal of Mental Health, 20*(4), 328–335. Retrieved from https://doi.org/10.3109/09638237.2011.556163

Patton, M. Q. (2003). *Qualitative research and evaluation methods: Integrating theory and practice* (3rd ed.). Thousand Oaks, CA: Sage.

Pleasant-Metcalf, A. & Rosal, M. (1997). The use of art therapy to improve academic performance. *Art Therapy: Journal of the American Art Therapy Association, 14*(1), 23–29. Retrieved from https://doi.org/10.1080/07421656.1997.10759250

Ponterotto, J. (2005). Qualitative research in counseling psychology: A primer on research paradigms and philosophy of science. *Journal of Counseling Psychology, 52*(2), 126–136. Retrieved from https://doi.org/10.1037/0022 0167.52.2.126

Powers, E. S. (1999). Using historical works of art to decrease anxiety and increase expressivity: Preparing adults to make art (master's thesis, Eastern Virginia Medical School, Norfolk, VA).

Pretorius, G. & Pfeifer, N. (2010). Group art therapy with sexually abused girls. *South African Journal of Psychology, 40*(1), 63–71. Retrieved from https://doi.org/10.1177/008124631004000010

Purswell, K. & Ray, D. (2014). Research with small samples: Considerations for single case and randomized small group experimental designs. *Counseling Outcome Research and Evaluation, 5*(2), 116–126. Retrieved from https://doi.org/10.1177/2150137814552474

Roberts, M. & McChesney, A. (Eds.). (2012). *Art and music therapy curriculum* (State Operated Programs Policy Manual). Richmond, VA: Virginia Department of Education.

Rübeling, H., Schwarzer, S., Keller, H., & Lenk, M. (2011). Young children's non-figurative drawings of themselves and their families in two different cultures. *Journal of Cognitive Education and Psychology, 10*(1), 63–76. Retrieved from https://doi.org/10.1891/1945-8959.10.1.63

Schrade, C., Tronsky, L., & Kaiser, D. (2011). Physiological effects of mandala making in adults with intellectual ability. *The Arts in Psychotherapy, 38*, 109–113. Retrieved from https://doi.org/10.1016/j.aip.2011.01.002

Schreiber, E. & Schreiber, K. (2002). A study of parents of violent children. *Psychological Reports, 20*, 101–104. Retrieved from https://doi.org/10.2466/pr0.2002.90.1.101

Silverman, M. (2009). The effect of single-session psychoeducational music therapy on verbalizations and perceptions in psychiatric patients. *Journal of Music Therapy, 46*(2), 105–131. Retrieved from https://doi.org/10.1093/jmt/46.2.105

Spielberger, C. (1989). *The State-Trait Anxiety Inventory: Bibliography* (2nd Ed.). Palo Alto, CA: Consulting Psychologists Press.

St John, P. (2016). Experimental and control group designs. In D. Gussak & M. Rosal (Eds.), *The Wiley handbook of art therapy* (pp. 793–803). Chichester: Wiley.

Streeter, K. & Deaver, S. (2018). Art therapy with women with infertility. *Art Therapy: Journal of the American Art Therapy Association, 35*(2), 61–67. Retrieved from https://doi.org/10.1080/07421656.2018.1483163

Svensk, A.-C., Oster, I., Thyme, K., Magnusson, E., Sjodin, M., Eisemann, M., Astrom, S., & Lindh, J. (2009). Art therapy improves experienced quality of life among women undergoing treatment for breast cancer: A randomized controlled study. *European Journal of Cancer Care, 18*, 69–77. Retrieved from https://doi.org/10.1111/j.1365-2354.2008.00952.x

Szucs, D. & Ioannidis, J. (2017). When null hypothesis significance testing is unsuitable for research: A reassessment. *Frontiers in Human Neuroscience, 11*. Retrieved from www.frontiersin.org/articles/10.3389/fnhum.2017.00390/full

Vennet, R. van der & Serice, S. (2012). Can coloring mandalas reduce anxiety? A replication study. *Art Therapy: Journal of the American Art Therapy Association, 29*(2), 87–92. Retrieved from https://doi.org/10.1080/07421656.2012.680047

Werner-Reap, B. (1995). The Visual Language Enhancement Prelude: A preparation exercise for art therapy (master's thesis, Eastern Virginia Medical School, Norfolk, VA).

# Chapter 4

# Qualitative Research Methods in Art Therapy

*Theresa Van Lith*

Whereas quantitative studies strive to find out *what* is going on by using numbers to determine a definite result, qualitative studies seek to find out *how* and *why* this is occurring by relying on words and text that represent feelings, expressions, states, and perspectives. Therefore, one might say that qualitative researchers handle the "wicked problems" (Savin-Baden & Howell Major, 2013, p. 5) in the world that cannot be addressed in a concrete fashion as they embrace and even celebrate the unpredictable, ambiguous, multifaceted, but ever-evolving nature of humankind. Further reflecting the richness and diversity that is possible through this methodology, "qualitative research can involve the study of others, but also the self and the complex relationships between, within, and among people and groups, including our entanglements" (Leavy, 2014, p. 1). This requires a deep level of constant questioning, which involves expanding and unpacking the paradoxes of our emotions, attitudes, and behaviors to find understanding about the human experience. In agreement with this view, Brinkmann, Jacobsen, and Kristiansen (2014) explained that, "qualitative research does not represent a monolithic, once-and-for-all, agreed-upon approach to research but is a vibrant and contested field with many contradictions and different perspectives" (p. 17). This chapter has been structured to help navigate the decisions and stages involved in conducting any qualitative study in art therapy. At the same time, it is important to acknowledge the unpredictable nature of qualitative inquiry; constant fine-tuning is required, as is a flexible approach. Therefore, the aim of this chapter is to provide stepping stones to help overcome the 'stuckness' that can occur when embarking on a qualitative study.

This chapter elucidates approaches to qualitative research in art therapy. Beginning with considerations in the development of a study based on qualitative inquiry, factors important to qualitative research questions are explained. This is followed by an overview of philosophical assumptions pertaining to research to augment understanding of where qualitative pursuits fit in, including ontology, epistemology, axiology, and methodology. Similarly, research paradigms essential to comprehension of qualitative research are described: postpositivism, constructivism, transformative, and pragmatism. The emergent and flexible nature of qualitative research is further delineated in the "Bricolage" section, followed by practical information related to recruitment of study participants. Six types of qualitative research designs are presented: case study, grounded theory, phenomenological inquiry, narrative inquiry, ethnography, and participatory action research. Information about methods of data collection is provided, including interviews, focus groups, open-ended questionnaires, Delphi method questionnaires, and field notes. The types of qualitative data analysis – thematic, content, grounded theory, phenomenological, discourse, and narrative – are described. Qualitative research designs in the art therapy literature are referenced to help determine how qualitative findings can help art therapists understand mechanisms effecting change in our clients based on such factors as how clients perceive their experience in art therapy, and what it is about art therapy that leads to change and healing. The chapter concludes with sections delineating strategies for evaluating quality, and ethical and moral responsibilities.

## Considerations in the Development of a Qualitative Study

### Qualitative Research Questions

A qualitative research question is framed using process-oriented language and focuses on understanding the *how* and *why* of a social interaction that the researcher is interested in studying. The researcher phrases the question in such a way that it is clear what type of knowledge she or he is hoping will be revealed by using a particular systematic method (Maxwell, 2013). At the same time, the study parameters also need to be defined within the question, to demonstrate that a satisfactory answer will be provided through the data collection and analysis process. Unlike quantitative research questions that remain fixed from the beginning, a qualitative research question evolves through reflexivity and interaction with the participants. As Agee (2009) clarified, "the ongoing process of questioning is an integral part of understanding the unfolding lives and perspectives of others" (p. 432). Therefore, it can be helpful to start with an overarching question that provides the direction for the study design, data collection, and interpersonal nature of the inquiry. Sub-questions can then be developed to provide details of the sequence of the study and these may be modified as data analysis, scope, or awareness about how transferability takes shape. For example, an investigator may pursue the overarching question, "How do clients use art therapy to improve their wellbeing and decrease their symptoms during an inpatient stay in a psychiatric ward?" The sub-questions might include: "What types of changes to wellbeing and symptom reduction were identified during participants' interviews?"; "How did the participants use their experiences of art therapy to refer to these changes?"; and "What aspects of art therapy did the participants identify as useful and not useful during their inpatient stay?"

## Philosophical Assumptions

Although the researcher's skills, experience, and professional identity are instrumental in informing the design of a study, a number of philosophical assumptions impact how the topic under investigation will be shaped and researched as a qualitative inquiry. These are considered under four main philosophical assumptions: ontology, epistemology, axiology, and methodology (Creswell, 2013).

*Ontology* focuses on examining "What is the nature of reality?" and "Is there a reality?" In qualitative research, the emphasis is on how researchers view the nature of reality and what assumptions they make within their studies about the way in which the world works and how the notion of existence is understood (Denzin & Lincoln, 2013). Therefore, the emphasis within a qualitative study is on how multiple forms of reality can be valued and presented through the sharing of different experiences on the same topic of inquiry (Leavy, 2017). For example, this may take the form of multiple quotes from different participants to illustrate different points of view on the same theme; or a client and an art therapist conveying a similar idea but from their different roles within the art therapy relationship.

*Epistemology* addresses the questions of "What constitutes knowledge?" and "What is the relationship between the researcher and the kind of knowledge being sought?" In qualitative studies, researchers are seen as co-creators of the knowledge; they are not separate from those being researched, nor are they able to remain completely objective (Leavy, 2014). Therefore, researchers need to be transparent about their level of subjectivity by acknowledging relevant personal experiences, how they spent time in the field, and how they used participants' quotes to support the overall findings (Creswell, 2013).

*Axiology* emphasizes the value system within the study and acknowledges the biases present. Therefore, qualitative researchers "position themselves" (p. 20) by including significant biographical information, study motivations, and any details that influenced data collection, analysis, or presentation of the findings.

*Methodology* involves the study procedures, including inductive reasoning and an emerging design within a given context (Creswell,

2013). In order for the study to be replicated, the researcher needs to present a detailed description of the study process, including challenges and considerations that altered the original study plan (Leavy, 2017).

## *Paradigms*

Philosophical and theoretical worldviews (Creswell & Creswell, 2018) or paradigms (Denzin & Lincoln, 2013) are schools of thought and disciplines within which a study is performed (Mertens, 2014). Kuhn (1962) referred to paradigms as a universal set of beliefs that provide a model for how problems can be comprehended and addressed. Nevertheless, while paradigms represent a consensus, the way in which philosophical constructs are clustered still varies. In qualitative research it is paramount to acknowledge the particular paradigm within which a study is conducted as doing so provides a framework and language for how the various philosophical assumptions are valued.

### *Postpositivism*

Whereas positivists and postpositivists both value logic, deduction, and precise empirical (well-known) observations of the behavior of individuals, postpositivists do not see findings as strictly representing a cause and effect relationship with a known probability. Rather, due to the multiple perspectives of participants the probability of the outcome occurring again is seen as dependent on using the exact same study design (Phillips & Burbules, 2000). This is the most traditional and orderly of the paradigms, where themes/codes or concepts are often clustered in a hierarchical order based on how often they appeared, making use of overarching themes and sub-themes. For instance, grounded theory is an application of postpositivism (Spencer, Pryce & Walsh, 2014).

### *Constructivism*

Constructivism is also described as interpretivism because researchers who embrace this paradigm develop interpretations of how their participants make meaning of their experiences (Crotty, 1998). This paradigm focuses more on understanding the *why* through taking a relativist position that respects multiple, attainable, and equally valid realities (Denzin & Lincoln, 2011; Lincoln & Guba, 1985). As the focus is on how individuals construct their reality, the emphasis when using the constructivist paradigm is to bring forward meaningful insights that are derived through researcher-participant dialogue (Creswell & Creswell, 2018). Therefore, findings are regarded as co-constructed because the researcher interprets the participants' responses through the data analysis process. When participants are asked to verify that these findings represent their lived experience, it helps validate the perspective or orientation by which the researcher elicited meanings from the raw data. One method that fits within the constructivist paradigm is phenomenological studies that focus on eliciting lived experiences (Quail & Peavy, 1994).

*Transformative*

Also referred to as the critical-ideological paradigm (Ponterotto, 2005), the transformative paradigm acknowledges power imbalances, seeks social justice, and empowers the marginalized (Denzin & Lincoln, 2011). Therefore, the researcher's proactive values are central to the study in order to collaborate and help change social conditions through working with the participants (Creswell, 2013). A particular philosophy that fits with this paradigm is cooperative or participatory inquiry (Heron, 1996; Heron & Reason, 1997, 2001), where the researcher seeks to conduct research *with* people rather than *on* people. Other philosophies include feminist theory (Burt, 1996; Eastwood, 2012; Hogan, 2001, 2012; Wright & Wright, 2017), critical race (Mayor, 2012), critical race feminism (Sajnani, 2012), indigenous (Dyer & Hunter, 2009; Sweeney, 2009), post-colonialism (Linnell, 2009; Lu & Yuen, 2012; Solomon, 2006; Westwood & Linnell, 2011), queer theory (Zappa, 2017), intersectionality (Kuri, 2017; Talwar, 2010, 2015), and intersectional feminism (Wright & Wright, 2017).

*Pragmatism*

Pragmatism emerged as both a method of inquiry and a device for the settling of battles between research purists and more practically minded scientists (Bryman, 2008; Tashakkori & Teddlie, 2010b). The pragmatic paradigm offers to the researcher permission to study diverse areas of interest and uses findings in a positive manner in harmony with the value system held by the researcher (Creswell, 2013; Tashakkori & Teddlie, 2010a, 2010b; Teddlie & Tashakkori, 2009). This means rejecting traditional dualisms (such as subjectivism versus objectivism, values versus facts), as well as having high regard for the tentative inner world of human experience in action (Johnson, 2008; Johnson, Onwuegbuzie, & Turner, 2007; Onwuegbuzie & Leech, 2005). The pragmatic paradigm is regarded as providing the most freedom in how the researcher determines the best method due to its emphasis on problem solving and utility as manifested in applied research.

## Bricolage

The concept of bricolage was conceived by researchers who recognized the emergent and flexible nature of qualitative research (Hesse-Biber, 2010; Hesse-Biber & Leavy, 2008). Bricoleur refers to the analogy of making a quilt, which requires piecing together different methodological strategies with a do-it-yourself attitude (Denzin, 2010). Bricoleurs use a combination of different historical, philosophical, social, and theoretical lenses (Kincheloe, 2001, 2005) intentionally to develop complementary types of data, while recognizing that this gives rise to contradictory ideas and contested arguments (Greene & Caracelli, 1997, 2003). This piecing together enables development of innovative strategies and can help create a research approach that addresses both the goals of the investigator and the study objectives.

## Sampling, Participants, and Setting

The type of facility (medical, community, educational, correctional, etc.) along with the type of population determines who will participate and where the study will take place. Typically, qualitative researchers use a form of purposeful sampling because the intention is to collect rich and informative accounts that will best address the research question (Patton, 2015). Participants are chosen based on pre-determined selection criteria. The six main types of purposive sampling are:

1. *Convenience*: Participants are selected based primarily on the fact that they are immediately accessible and available.
2. *Snowball*: Participants make recommendations for additional participants throughout the course of the study.
3. *Typical*: Participants are selected based on how well they represent the phenomena that is being studied.
4. *Critical*: Selection is made based on unusual or exceptional circumstances, and is useful especially when resources are limited.
5. *Homogeneous*: When the primary interest is in studying a group in depth, based on the desirability of seeking participants who are all similar in some way.
6. *Maximal variation*: Represents wide variety among the participants, which is desirable when seeking to study range or vast differences within a sample of participants.

Relationship building is a key part of securing participants who are retained through to the completion of the study. The first step in recruiting participants is to meet with the targeted agency/organization face to face to establish the partnership and develop a formal study agreement. The next step is finding out who the "gatekeepers" are so that they can notify and encourage participants. A final step is to build alliances by spending time together, engaging, and becoming a known face at the site. Finally, another important part to maintaining relationships within a study is to convey among stakeholders, staff, and participants how the study findings will be disseminated and if there will be opportunities to discuss the study implications with the participants and site.

## Qualitative Research Designs

### Case Study

Historically, case studies have been art therapists' method of choice (Gussak, 2016) because they enable in-depth examinations of particular clients, encounters, or contexts. Yin (2018) described the case study method as a comprehensive research strategy, given that it enables various forms of data to be sought, while still allowing the researcher to inquire into real-life contexts and real-life cycles, such as engaging in long-term art therapy or examining the recovery trajectory using various approaches to art therapy. As Stake (2005) emphasized, the intention of the case study is to proliferate rather than reduce the data so that one is left with more to pay attention to rather than less. However, McLeod (2010) cautioned that many case studies have been derived from therapist notes and recollections and interpreted solely by the researcher with little client input. Consequently, such studies do not necessarily provide sound evidence about the client's experience.

Case study methods differ depending on the study purpose, discipline, research strategy, and study context. Savin-Baden and Howell-Major (2013) determined six different contexts in which a case study method would be appropriate: exploratory, descriptive, instrumental, interpretive, explanatory, and evaluative. They suggested looking at how the researcher's discipline will then shape how the case is examined. For instance, art therapy case studies most commonly use a psychological lens, where the emphasis is on emotional and behavioral change within the individual client (Eastwood, 2012; Engle, 1997; Greenwood, 2011; Killick, 1996; Lamont, Brunero, & Sutton; 2009). However, they can also draw on sociological methods to examine a particular socially critical issue that requires an in-depth exploration of the interactive systems that are disempowering. For instance, Huss (2016) selected a case of 15 single mothers from the Bedouin community in Israel, out of a larger multiple-case project, to illustrate how the art therapy process and resultant art works elicited experiences of marginalization. Art therapists also use archival records to provide a historical perspective of using art therapy in a particular system or context; however, these types of case studies have not been widely reported in peer-reviewed journals.

## Grounded Theory

Originating from sociology, grounded theory is based on the idea of discovering a theory by scrutinizing concepts that are grounded in the data. Therefore, the focus is on identifying how a basic social process occurs in a particular situation. Theory is generated from participants' experiences (Denzin, 2010). However, the level of flexibility and how close the researcher needs to stay to the data depends on the form of grounded theory that he or she follows (Bryant & Charmaz, 2007). Glasser and Strauss (1967), the pioneers of grounded theory, developed a step-by-step method using inductive and deductive reasoning in order for theory to develop based on a process, action, or interaction generated from the data. This method is considered classic grounded theory, with the intent of staying very close to the data, to derive a theory that could be considered as close to true as possible.

Modified grounded theory as developed by Strauss (1987) and Strauss and Corbin (1998) takes on a more emergent and inductive systematic approach to data analysis through coding. For example, Haeyen, van Hoorven, and Hutschemaekers (2015) used modified grounded theory to generate a theoretical model of the perceived effects of art therapy for patients with personality disorders. First, they interviewed three patients who had just finished their treatment and then five patients who represented diverse descriptive factors, including age, gender, settings, and mode of treatment, for the purpose of theoretical sampling. Next, they interviewed three patients who had completed their treatment at least a month to six years ago as well as a patient who might produce a negative view. They then conducted three focus groups to elicit discussion and interviewed 17 patients from these focus groups to expand on ideas presented among the group. As little research had been conducted on the effects of art therapy with this population, Haeyen et al. were able to develop a theoretical model based on patients' reports of art therapy within a natural setting, without preconceived notions or expectations.

More recently developed approaches to grounded theory include postmodern grounded theory (Clarke, 2005) and discursive grounded theory (McCreaddie & Payne, 2010), which focus on analyzing discourse. Constructivist grounded theory (Charmaz, 2014) has also been a popular method with art therapists because of the flexibility it allows for researchers and participants to be co-constructors of their interactive and iterative realities and subsequently the derived theory. Therefore, the emphasis is more on interpretation than on deriving a "true account." Patterson, Crawford, Ainsworth, and Waller (2011) used Charmaz's method to depict a theory based on interviews, focus groups, and written opinions from 24 art therapists about their practice with people who have schizophrenia. Patterson et al. (2011) then combined these various data sources to demonstrate how art therapists reported client change through the therapeutic use of art materials and the artmaking process within the therapy space. Charmaz would regard the outcome of this study as a social construction that acknowledges the temporal, cultural, and structural contexts within a social dynamic.

## Phenomenological Inquiry

Phenomenology is entrenched in a particular wave of philosophical thinking, tracing back to the work by Husserl ([1936] 1970, [1952] 1980). In stark contrast to his mathematical background, Husserl (1936/1970) became interested in understanding human experience through questioning, "What is this experience like?" Phenomenology, therefore, involves comprehending meanings, the *life world*, of particular phenomena by returning to the essence of pre-reflective understandings (Polkinghorne, 1983). Another important notion in phenomenology is bracketing or reductionism. Husserl (1936/1970) proposed that one must bracket out individual biases and outside distractions to suspend judgment and see the phenomenon clearly. However, Husserl's pupil Heidegger ([1927] 1967) argued that one cannot be fully objective when observing the human experience and therefore researchers should interpret phenomena through the lens of their own backgrounds and experiences. This approach is referred to as hermeneutic phenomenology, which focuses on how one experiences another's life world. For instance, Davis (2010) used hermeneutic phenomenology to investigate "What is the lived experience of a participant in a series of art therapy sessions?" (p. 180) with 19 international students from an Australian university using their art works and accompanying narratives, observations, and follow-up interviews. The concept of the *hermeneutic circle* was used to describe the iterative and interactive relationship between the clients and the researcher's interpretation of their worldview. This involved the researcher using *spiraling* (questions prompted out of responses) as an open-ended form of dialogue to ensure a shared understanding was created out of the participants' experiences. In another example, Rossetto (2012) interviewed eight community artists who engaged in community mural-making to explore worldviews and personal philosophies regarding how art therapy can be used for social action within a Western cultural framework.

Philosophers and writers have modified phenomenology in different ways to reaffirm *being in the world* as an alternative way to access human knowledge (Colaizzi, 1973; Gadamer, trans. 1975; Giorgi, 1994; Merleau-Ponty, 1968; van Manen, 1990, 2007). As a recent art therapy-related illustration, Van Lith (2014a) followed what Crotty (1996) referred to as *new phenomenology*, and what Willis (2001, 2004) re-termed *empathetic phenomenology*, with 12 mental health consumers who were using artmaking for their mental health recovery. In particular, Van Lith (2014a) focused on understanding the nature of the human consciousness of her participants by striving to identify and empathize with their lived experiences.

In his phenomenological approach to interviewing people living with mental illness about their recovery experiences, Davidson (2003) noted that using empathy in research is "a highly disciplined and demanding posture involving an active and artful use of all of one's faculties of memory, imagination, sensitivity and awareness in coming to understand another person's experience from his or her own perspective" (p. 121).

On the other hand, heuristic phenomenology (Moustakas, 1994) emphasizes the personal experiences of the researcher, which inform the process of inquiry either through self-discovery (Fenner, 1996) or through a shared encounter with others (Bloomgarden & Netzer, 1998; Netzer, 2009). Studies by these authors used the following step-by-step process created by Moustakas (1994) to derive findings: initial engagement, immersion, incubation, illumination, explication, and creative synthesis. These steps are elaborated upon in Chapter 5 of this book. As so many different variations of phenomenology exist, it is important that the same school of thought is used within a given study, so that the level by which subjectivity is determined remains consistent.

### Narrative Inquiry

Storytelling has a long history steeped in the oral histories of indigenous peoples (Denzin, Lincoln, & Smith, 2008), and narrative inquiry elicits these life stories relating to social and cultural issues. Conducting a narrative inquiry involves participants providing situated accounts in which they are the protagonists within a particular plot or storyline (Clandinin & Connelly, 2000). Writing up narrative inquiry requires situating the participant as a character, providing a detailed plot line, and describing the context. Then, the participant's own metaphorical and symbolic language is used to convey the magnitude and multitude of the layered meanings within the account. The researcher and participants are seen as collaborators as the accounts get reframed and retold in the form of a reflection that showcases the living and the telling of a person's life (Bruner, 2004). As the researcher also becomes the storyteller, it is important that she or he discloses personal motivations and experiences for both the positionality (Bourke, 2014) and authenticity of the interpretation. Based on her observations and encounters with her students, Kellman (2008) used autobiographical and biographical accounts of facilitating a hospital art class for people with HIV/AIDS. These were written in a series of vignettes structured around a particular incident to illustrate the multilayered components of healing based on the relationships formed, space created, and meanings embedded in the created art works. Narrative inquiry can also take the form of poetry and digital storytelling, where these forms of data become a creative synthesis of the key meanings elicited from the data (Schreibman & Chilton, 2012).

## Ethnography

Stemming from anthropology, ethnography involves documenting or portraying the everyday experiences of individuals to develop an understanding of a particular cultural, social, or political dynamic. Ethnography researchers have taken the stance that their studies cannot remain neutral to the given political, social, and cultural topic and that their work is in fact positioned to effect social change (Horkheimer, [1937] 1972). This approach has been referred to as critical ethnography because these studies tend to examine social justice issues such as disparities and marginalized groups. Therefore, it is important that researchers are highly reflexive and recognize the influence of their values within the study to make clear how interpretations were derived and how biases were considered (Madison, 2012). For instance, Watts, Gilfillan, and de Zárate (2017) used critical ethnography to examine how poverty impacts the emotional wellbeing, educational attainment, and future life chances of children and young people who live in areas of multiple deprivation in West Central Scotland. They were interested in discovering whether art therapists working with these persons adapt their practice to address the practical impact of poverty. Data were collected through interviews conducted at the art therapists' workplace over a three-month period. Watts et al. identified the cultural and structural barriers that make it difficult for art therapists to consistently adapt their practice.

Another common form of ethnography used by art therapists is autoethnography, which uses autobiographical narratives of the art therapist's own experiences. In this way, the researcher is also the participant and a self-narrative is examined through its connection with a social context (Ellis, 2004). This method involves a systematic analysis involving deep self-reflection and self-observation detailing an often life changing or altering circumstance. Autoethnographies can be a way for art therapists to develop self-awareness and empathy (Gray, 2011). For example, Park (2017) conducted an autoethnography on her acculturation process to South Korea after training in England, which brought about awareness of her multicultural identity. Additional examples of the autoethnography method are offered in Chapter 5 of this book.

## Participatory Action Research

This method stems from social sciences and organizational-based research, where the need for change is not just identified but also addressed and then evaluated. One form of action research is participatory action research (PAR), which emphasizes collective and social change among oppressed groups through exploring how power can be balanced (Kemmis & McTaggart, 2005). Participants are regarded as co-researchers and the researcher-participant relationship is much more egalitarian than is the case in other methods. The PAR research design is cyclical and includes the following steps: reflect, plan, decide, and implement. Therefore, change is derived through insights and decision making (Lewin, 1948; Reason & Bradbury, 2006). Strategies are implemented and identified through deliberate intention to develop new insights that improve practice. This might take the form of creating guidelines to create a more streamlined and accountable form of practice. Chataway (2001) described this action research cycle in the following eight steps:

1. *Information gathering*: Immersion in the community.
2. *Problem definition*: Creation of research questions.
3. *Instrument design*: Interview schedule, dialogue group agenda.
4. *Data collection*: Interviews, questionnaires, focus groups, dialogue groups.
5. *Collective interpretation of results*: Written summaries, group discussion, feedback on papers for publication.
6. *Cycling back to earlier steps*: Refine and re-develop research questions, adapt instrument design, return to data collection and collective interpretation.
7. *Action steps*: Individual use of new skills and language, dialogue group.
8. *Cycling back to earlier steps*: Based on the outcomes or goals of the action steps.

Spaniol (2005) used PAR in a two-day conference with art therapists and mental health consumers who had previous experience of making art for therapeutic purposes, with the goal of bringing about shared understanding and new perspectives. Through a series of artmaking workshops, the co-researchers engaged in dialogue and over time art therapists began integrating new perspectives into their professional attitudes and practices. Kapitan, Litell, and Torres (2011) also used PAR to instill change within an oppressive power structure through bringing Nicaraguan communities together and using capacity-building to help members become more empowered. For six years, they conducted an annual three-day retreat with approximately 60 participants, including a core group of 35 Nicaraguan community leaders who participated in all six retreats and went on to share study gains among their own communities. Kapitan et al. (2011) followed Lykes' (2001) criteria for evaluating their study cycle and noted that the implementation of PAR as part of a series of art therapy workshops led to a strengthening of personal, spiritual, and social development among co-researchers, which in turn multiplied broader impacts on their communities. Specific branches that have evolved out of action research, that place more emphasis on democratizing the power between researcher and participants, are known as cooperative or participatory inquiry (Heron & Reason, 1997, 2001; Reason & Heron, 1995). Examples of these collaborative efforts that demonstrate the interactive and evolving process that occurs during analysis include those by Lett, Fox, and von der Borch (2014) and Van Lith (2014a).

## Data Collection

Choosing the most suitable form of data collection depends on a number of factors. One major consideration is the overall research purpose and how the qualitative researcher plans to address the research question (Leavy, 2017). The other major consideration involves deciding upon the paradigm that will inform the study methods. Whereas it can be appealing to choose numerous forms of data collection within one study, qualitative researchers seek deep and rich accounts rather than breadth and vastness. Therefore, the amount of data that can be collected within the allocated timeframe and budget and using the researchers' experience as well as expertise all need to be determining factors in designing a realistic and achievable study.

### Interactive Forms of Data Collection

Interactive forms of data collection involve arranging a social situation, usually an interview or focus group, where participants are asked about their experiences, opinions, beliefs, and attitudes to expand understanding regarding the research topic. The interviews or focus groups are either recorded and transcribed, or involve researchers taking detailed notes that provide an accurate account of participants' responses. Traditionally, the face-to-face format has been most regularly used, but qualitative researchers are also now using telephone, instant messaging, email, computer conferencing, and other web-based formats for both convenience and to access a more diverse sample (Savin-Baden & Howell Major, 2013).

#### Interviews

Interviews allow for qualitative researchers to gather detailed and personalized accounts based on one-to-one engagement. Patton (2015) identified various types of interview questions, including background/demographic questions, knowledge questions, experience/behavior questions, opinion/values questions, feelings questions, and sensory questions. Depending on the focus and length of the interview, one or several of the types may be used. The type of interview conducted is dependent on consideration of researcher style, study focus, and participant variables. Interview types tend to be considered along a continuum between highly structured on one end and unstructured on the other end (Leavy, 2017; Patton, 2015). Highly structured interviews involve creating a specific set of questions that are routinely implemented with each participant (Seidman, 2013). Some art therapy studies involve using a specific set of questions for web-based interviews and then an open-ended style of questioning during face-to-face interviews, relying on the personal connection developed during the interview process to help guide the questions. This orientation is referred to as a semi-structured to unstructured style and lends itself to gathering detailed accounts. For instance, the semi-structured conversational style interviews used by Van Lith (2014b) focused on eliciting experiences of using art making for mental health recovery and were administered three times over a one-year period, in six-month increments, to determine change. Interview questions (p. 7) included:

- Can you tell me about your experience with art making and how you came to use art making in your recovery?
- What kinds of art making have you been doing in the last six months?
- Can you tell me about your art making experience in the last six months?
- What aspects have been the most helpful/unhelpful?
- In what way has art making played a role in your mental health recovery in the last six months? Can you give me examples of some experiences?
- What aspects of the art making context have been most helpful/unhelpful in the last six months?
- What aspects of the art program that you attend have you found to be helpful/unhelpful in the last six months?
- Have there been any significant changes in your life since we last met?
- What are your future plans for art making?

As another example, Wahlbeck, Kvist, and Landgren (2017) conducted semi-structured interviews with 19 women in Sweden who had undergone art therapy treatment for severe fear of childbirth. The interviews were conducted three months after the childbirth experience. The researchers began each interview with the question, "What is your experience of art therapy as a part of the treatment for fear of childbirth?" They then shaped their line of questioning around, "In what way did art therapy help you?" and "What kind of feelings did art therapy evoke?" (p. 3). Each interview took approximately 30–50 minutes.

### Focus Groups

Originating from the 1960s when televisions became a household item, focus groups were implemented to gauge popular opinion on TV programs and advertising campaigns (Savin-Baden & Howell Major, 2013). They are now commonly used for gathering feedback when qualitative researchers are interested in gathering data based on social interactions between participants and researchers. In art therapy research, focus groups are typically used to help evaluate art therapy approaches and provide feedback. For instance, Springham and Camic (2017) were interested in the effect of a specific type of theoretically based art therapy (mentalization-based therapy [MBT]) upon clients diagnosed with personality disorder. They conducted four focus groups with service users (consumers) who were co-researchers, MBT-trained psychologists and art therapists, and art therapy practitioners who videotaped MBT-informed group art therapy sessions. Each focus group lasted approximately three hours. An external focus group moderator provided semi-structured questions to elicit responses about observations of the art therapists' actions, the participants' responses, and noted therapeutic change among the group. To help group members address the questions using examples, the moderator sought clarification when speculative responses were noted.

## Textual-Based Forms of Data Collection

Textual-based forms of data collection involve gathering knowledge on the research topic using written accounts and documents. This format is used when qualitative researchers are focused on the language used by the participants and how they interact within certain health, community, educational, and correctional cultures and systems. Examples include examining journal or log entries, personal documents, client records, social media entries, and responses to written qualitative questionnaires (Creswell & Creswell, 2018). Text-based forms save time because they do not require transcribing, and they can also allow participants to engage in the study in their own time (for instance, through an online questionnaire) (Creswell, 2013).

### Open-Ended Questionnaires

This format involves asking open-ended questions such as "please describe" or "tell us about" to elicit a lengthy response from the participant. The participant can respond using pen and paper or online. For instance, an online questionnaire was developed by Van Lith, Stallings, and Harris (2017) to determine best practices for working with children who have Autism Spectrum Disorder. Their questions were centered on asking for descriptions of theoretical models and examples of certain techniques used, along with details about what does and does not work when using art therapy with children diagnosed with Autism Spectrum Disorder. Alternatively, an open-ended line of questioning may be used alongside a quantitative measure, such as in the study by Zubala, MacIntyre, and Karkou (2014), in which art therapists were asked to provide detailed descriptions of working with people who have depression. Their open-ended questions included asking general information about practice, theoretical principles, and influences as well as assessment and evaluation.

*Delphi Method Questionnaires*

This technique is used when researchers seek consensus on a particular topic of inquiry. The researchers identify a panel of specialists who are diverse, experienced, and can shed light on an otherwise limited knowledge-base in relation to the chosen research area. The panel members' opinions are gathered, organized, and then subsequently fed back to the panel for review during the next stage of questioning. This cycle occurs several times until there is agreement among the panel members' views. Kaiser and Deaver (2013) sought a consensus among American art therapy researchers on research priorities for the field. The following three questions were used as the basis for responses: (a) "What areas are important to research in art therapy and why?"; (b) "What research questions are important to address?"; and (c) "What methods should be used to study the areas and questions you have identified?" (p. 115). Similarly, in the UK, Holttum, Huet, and Wright (2017) conducted a Delphi study to seek consensus about art therapy best practices for people living with a psychotic disorder. They first asked panel members to compile three statements that described their art therapy practice with clients experiencing psychosis. Responses were to be under 15 words and in plain English. This list of responses was then combined with statements from two service user data sets and relevant art therapy literature and sent back to panel members to categorize by level of importance. Finally, those that achieved above 80 percent consensus were confirmed and statements that were categorized as "most important" by 70–80 percent of members were re-rated to ensure that they represented a consensual agreement.

### Naturalistic Forms of Data Collection

Naturalistic forms of data collection involve researchers immersing themselves in the field to understand how the participants construct their realities (Creswell & Creswell, 2018). Peripheral participation occurs when the researcher has no interaction with the participants, such as by observing an art therapy session using a two-way mirror or watching video footage.

Whereas passive participation involves a bystander level of engagement, such as the researcher sitting in on an art therapy session, the researcher's level of involvement with the participants increases through using either a balanced (occasional) or active (full) level of participation, which can involve functioning as both art therapist and researcher during an art therapy session. The most immersed level of participation is referred to as *complete immersion*, when the researcher is also the participant, for example if the researcher records his or her own reactions to the art-making process (Savin-Baden & Howell Major, 2013).

*Field Notes*

Field notes are taken while the researcher observes the social situation under study. There may also be audio- or video-recordings and online data (i.e., chat or email accounts). However, with this form of data collection the researcher is also interested in collecting data specific to being immersed in the setting, such as changes in behavior, social cues, particular events, and the surroundings. While in situ the researcher records observations, often using jottings or short notes that can be expanded upon later (Savin-Baden & Howell Major, 2013). The researcher then immediately writes down observations in a detailed account, just like writing client case notes. It can also be worthwhile to keep a separate log of reflexive notes (Leavy, 2017), which contain the researcher's intuitions and subjective comments. For example, Zago (2008) chronicled observations of infant and adolescent clients making art, based on psychoanalytic principles of holding and seeing the client's internalized world. In particular, Zago noted how art therapists are well-equipped and can enhance their "in-depth capacity for receptivity" (p. 330) by using field notes to strengthen their ability to be with their clients.

## Qualitative Data Analysis

Researchers start out conducting a qualitative form of analysis from either an inductive or deductive standpoint to draw out meaning through an interpretative lens (Bogdan & Biklen, 2007; Creswell, 2013). An inductive lens involves the researcher bracketing out assumptions and approaching the data set with an open mind, to let the emerging findings be the driver. Conversely, a deductive lens focuses on a particular assumption, which is determined through a process of analysis. An evolving and cyclical quality characterizes the qualitative analysis process, wherein findings start to emerge as soon as they are collected (formative) and are then followed by the specific analytical approach chosen (summative) (Ravitch & Mittenfelner, 2016). Therefore, the systematic and detail-oriented attitude that is required to conduct a thorough qualitative analysis is all too frequently underestimated. Although computer-based analysis programs such as NVivo can be used to help fast-track the process, researchers nevertheless need to thoroughly know their data set and be able to provide a record of how the data has been extracted, reduced, synthesized, and abstracted.

The analysis process also requires a high level of intentionality, in which the researcher stays consistently focused on the study topic to become the authority of his or her own interpretation of the data. This means that, when crafting the written account of the findings, researchers must be confident that they have thoroughly vetted and scrutinized the data and that their representation portrays a solid justification for why and how the findings are presented in particular ways. The following section provides the most commonly used data analysis methods used within qualitative art therapy studies. Refer to Box 4.1 at the end of this chapter for an illustrative example of qualitative data analysis as related to the Bringing Research to Life! research simulation experiential (Betts & Potash, 2018).

## *Thematic Analysis*

Although thematic analysis has routinely been used in art therapy research, this form of inductive analysis is rarely thoroughly documented. A thematic analysis does not involve simply extracting themes from the data, but also involves demonstrating the relationships between the themes and how they address the research question(s). Braun and Clarke (2006) advocated the use of visual maps to demonstrate the connections between themes and sub-themes. They also developed a systematic approach to conducting a thematic analysis, which involves the following six stages:

1. Becoming familiar with the data.
2. Generating initial codes or shorthand labels.
3. Searching for themes, which are patterns or re-occurring meaningful constructs.
4. Reviewing potential themes in relation to codes and the rest of the data.
5. Defining and naming themes that have a singular focus, do not overlap, and address the research question(s).

6. Producing the report by providing a rich, yet clear, account that illustrates the themes and accompanying quotes in a logical sequence (Braun & Clarke, 2013; Clarke & Braun, 2013).

Holmqvist, Roxberg, Larsson, and Lundqvist-Persson (2017) implemented an online questionnaire to ask art therapists what they perceive as inner change in their patients and then implemented Braun and Clarke's (2006) thematic analysis method. They identified five themes – therapeutic alliance, creating, affect-consciousness, self-awareness, and ego strength – to illustrate how art therapists use certain language when referring to inner change among their clients. Haeyen, Kleijberg, and Hinz (2018) also used Braun and Clarke's (2006) method to determine the role of the art materials in emotional regulation for patients with personality disorders. They derived the following themes: experiences with the art assignments, material handling/interaction, preferred approach in the art process and the ETC (Expressive Therapies Continuum) level, preferred approach in the art process and emotion regulation, and therapeutic value of the combination of factors.

## *Content Analysis*

Content analysis originated from a need to evaluate mass communication data to develop and apply quantifiable codes derived from written, qualitative sources of data (Neuendorf, 2016). This means seeing the meaning units, categories, and themes as measurable by how many times they appear in the data set, while also looking for the latent meanings and interconnected patterns (Graneheim & Lundman, 2004). Therefore, it is typically used with online content or a large number of written responses. Although at first glance a content analysis may look similar to a thematic analysis, in content analysis, manifested categories (what is written) and latent content (underlying meaning of what is written) are separated to acknowledge both the quantifiable and qualifying data sources. Conversely, in thematic analysis, latent and manifest content are seen as co-dependent and inseparable. According to Elo and Kyngäs (2008), content analysis starts with obtaining a sense of the whole data set, which is reviewed several times. The unit of analysis and the rules for categorizing, such as how to separate manifest and latent content, are decided. Next, the data is coded to create categories that are grouped under higher-order headings. The analysis process and results are then reported through models, maps, and/or descriptions of the emergent story. For instance, Orr (2007) used content analysis with 31 forms of communication focused on using art with children after a disaster, including refereed journal articles, news articles, television interviews, and books. Each source was analyzed for six key areas: design of communication, theoretical basis of art therapy conducted, environment surrounding art therapy practice, the art therapist, the client, and the artwork. Frequencies based on manifest content and themes were both identified, which resulted in the conclusion that semi-structured art interventions are best suited to this population.

### Grounded Theory Analysis

A grounded theory analysis involves a *constant comparative* process to derive theory from the participants' experiences. First described by Glaser and Strauss (1967), there are three main stages of constant comparative analysis: (a) open coding (inspecting, comparing, abstracting, and ordering data); (b) axial coding (reconstructing data into categories based on relationships and patterns within and among the clusters identified in the data) and (c) selective coding (classifying and providing an explanation of the central or core category in the data) (Strauss & Corbin, 1998). Charmaz (2014) referred to these three stages as initial, focused, and theoretical. She also emphasized the iterative nature of the working through each stage and emphasized that the researcher can only move on to the next stage once saturation has been achieved (i.e., nothing new has emerged). Memos can also be used throughout various stages of the analysis process to record speculations about emerging relationships and patterns (ibid.). Springham and Camic (2017) used constructivist grounded theory to derive a theoretical framework that explained how art therapists interact with service users and their artworks. They followed the method outlined by Charmaz (2014), which involved pursuing emergent themes through early analysis, identifying social processes within the data, constructing abstract categories as both explanation and synthesis, sampling and comparing these processes, and then integrating these categories into a theoretical model. As a result, they developed two distinctive types of art therapist interactions with groups: "art therapist demonstrates attention" and "art therapist appears passive" (Springham & Camic, 2017, p. 142) A further eight subordinate conceptual categories were also developed and their interactive nature was clarified to demonstrate the underlying relationships between themes.

### Phenomenological Analysis

There are a number of forms of phenomenological analysis, each of which prioritizes differing ways of eliciting the participants' lived experience. For instance, the descriptive phenomenological method focuses on the essential and rigorous nature of drawing out essences of the participants' lived experience (see Colaizzi, 1978; Giorgi, 1975; Wertz, 2005). The interpretative phenomenological approach, such as used by Eatough and Smith (2017) and van Manen (1990), focuses on unpacking the participants' lived experience by making connections between cognitive, linguistic, affective, and physical states elicited within the data and in turn identifying the relationship between the participants' voices and their emotional and mental states. As a result, the researcher does not focus on the words within the transcript alone; the feelings, physical responses, and silences behind these words are also taken into account (Smith, Flowers, & Larkin, 2009). Regardless of the approach chosen, the type of analysis process used in a phenomenological study needs to be made explicit because the specific guidelines used to extract the emerging patterns and to identify themes differ greatly.

Van Lith (2008) conducted a case study on an adolescent with the provisional diagnosis of borderline personality disorder who was attending art therapy sessions to help transition to a psychosocial residential facility. She used a descriptive phenomenological approach to analyze the client's art-based and written responses within the sessions as well as those contained in a visual journal. The resultant overall themes were: a sense of uncertainty, exploring difficult emotions through art therapy, the emergence of "Lisa" to assist the release of strong emotions, deeper discovery of the inner self, and becoming an individual.

### Narrative Analysis

A narrative form of analysis requires *re-authoring* or *re-storying* dialogue to elicit how participants constructed meaning within a given incident. Although there are various forms of narrative analysis, a widely used approach in art therapy research is that by Riesmann (1993) and Clandinin and Connelly (2000), in which the focus is on examining how the self and identity are expressed through the participant's narrative. Additionally, the work by Polkinghorne (1995) has also been an influential guide to help elicit common storylines across participant accounts. Specific guidelines for using a critical form of analysis were developed by Emerson and Frosh (2004), Keats (2009), and Dutc and Jensen (2011). The narrative analysis used by Collie, Bottorff, and Long (2006) involved examining interviews with women who were using art therapy for psychosocial support as part of their breast cancer treatment. The researchers generated a synthesis of the data by creating meaningful representations based on quotes and information gathered about both the social context of the stories and how they were told. The researchers worked to derive both holistic and categorical levels of content to derive overall meanings and specific topics of focus. On the other hand, Shin, Choi, and Park (2016) focused on a case of dyad art therapy involving a mother and her 10-year-old son. They were particularly interested in conveying storylines evoking the personal psychological dynamics and interactive dynamics between the mother and her child during the art therapy sessions.

## Discourse Analysis

One of the rarer forms of analysis in art therapy research, discourse analysis evolved from the fields of linguistics, literature, and semiotics (Starks & Brown Trindad, 2007). As Gee (1999) emphasized, "Language has a magical property: when we speak or write we craft what we have to say to fit the situation or context in which we are communicating" (p. 11). Therefore, in discourse analysis, the focus is not just on the words themselves but also on how particular words are used to convey actions, feelings, and thoughts within a certain context. Words are also regarded as symbolizing "situated meanings" (p. 41), which refers to assemblies of features that constitute a given time period, relationship, and social/political context. The historical evolution of language practice and how language has been used to shape certain practices is also reviewed. To analyze the contextual and relationship-oriented nature of words, Wood and Kroger (2000) developed a step-by-step inductive process of analysis. They underscored that the in-depth and recursive reading of the data needs to involve an inclusive level of analysis that builds on the evolving meanings of the language. The analysis process continues until the researcher is satisfied that the data have been exhausted and there are no alternatives left for how the research question can be addressed.

## Evaluating Quality

Qualitative researchers strive for understanding through deep engagement with their participants and their world, and thereby derive insights that seek to enhance pre-existing beliefs, attitudes, and perspectives. Therefore, whereas quantitative researchers strive for validity and reliability to verify the extent to which they trust the research procedures and findings, qualitative researchers instead apply *trustworthiness* or *credibility* (Lincoln & Guba, 1985; Lincoln, Lynham, & Guba, 2011). These terms relate to the level of quality in the interpretation of the findings and to the level of confidence that the study was conducted in a rigorous manner (Noble & Smith, 2015). Specifically, qualitative studies must demonstrate the following: that the results are believable and provide an honest account, that the *transferability* of the findings beyond the participants in the study is clearly conveyed, that the findings can be depended upon, that they can be confirmed, and that they have utility (Creswell & Creswell, 2018; Leavy, 2017).

Ellingson (2009) and Richardson and St. Pierre (2008) adopted the metaphor of a crystal to conceptualize the multiple facets involved in evaluating qualitative studies. This reflexive view demonstrates how a text can be turned in many ways; in turning, it reflects and refracts light (multiple meanings) through which we can see whole parts (whole meanings) and particles (feelings, connections, and single elements of the data). Therefore, authenticity and fairness are emphasized through providing a balance of views, while acknowledging any assumptions and clarifying how the embedded relationships informed the presentation of findings (Richardson, 1999; Richardson & St. Pierre, 2008). Many researchers have concurred with this metaphor because it embraces the multiple ways in which reality is constructed and accepts that the constructs being studied are also ever-changing (Ellingson, 2009).

### Strategies for Evaluating Quality

Given the subjective orientation of qualitative research, providing a convincing account of the study requires a high level of critical thinking to portray the truth and benefits of the study. According to Leavy (2017), critical researchers ask the following questions:

- Reality: Whose reality is the research reflecting?
- Communication: Are the findings clearly presented and do important terms have operational definitions?
- Values: What values are prioritized?
- Assumptions: Are aspects of research taken for granted or has creative liberty been used in drawing conclusions?
- Societal consequences: Whose interests are being served and what are the implications?

Practical strategies for ensuring qualitative credibility, as identified by Creswell and Creswell (2018), include the following:

- Triangulating different data sources, methods, investigators, and/or theoretical perspectives.
- Using member checking with participants by asking them to verify that different stages of the analysis process (i.e., individual or common themes) are an accurate reflection of their experiences.
- Providing a rich, thick description that is detailed and clearly portrays the study setting.
- Clarifying any bias through being open and self-reflective.
- Presenting negative or counter information that portrays the reality of the findings.
- Spending prolonged time in the field to learn the culture and establish relationships.
- Using a peer debriefer who looks at the study as an outsider and examines how the study might/might not resonate at a wider level.
- Using an external auditor to review the entire research process to provide an objective assessment of the level of rigor with which the study was conducted.

Creswell and Creswell (ibid., based on the work of Gibbs, 2007) also identified certain criteria for qualitative reliability: checking that the transcript is accurate, operational definitions are consistent, the research team holds documented meetings and shares its analysis, cross-checking occurs regularly, and procedures are developed such as creating an intercoder agreement to establish consensus on coding. Critical appraisal guidelines for evaluating qualitative research were developed by Sandelowski (2015) and Daly et al. (2007). Additional resources were also developed by Fujiura (2015) and Elliott, Fischer, and Rennie (1999), who specify qualitative research standards when preparing studies for publication.

## Ethical and Moral Responsibilities

As qualitative research centers upon relationships between the researcher, the participants, and the setting there are a number of ethical and moral responsibilities to which the researcher must pay attention. Beyond specifying the internal review board (IRB) approvals received, considerations of how the participants and the site are valued need to be made transparent. Of significance here are Bresler's (1996, 2006) key ethical standards of caring for individual participants and for the setting by respecting diversity, maintaining dignity, and caring about the ethics of the message to the scholarly community.

Finlay and Evans' (2009) core values for conducting relational research provide guidance on this challenge. They suggest that the researcher carry out the study with authority, integrity, and reflexivity and regard the participant with acceptance, agency, and empathetic inquiry. Consequently, the established research relationship between participants and researchers ought to be one of mutuality and openness. In turn, the overall outcome should be a study that has transformative impact in a respectful way, while being humble in its resonance with others. Some practical strategies include hosting an information session about the study to ensure participants understand the aims and procedures, seeking consent before each stage of the study to ensure they know what is being asked, emphasizing that consent is a negotiation and not all levels of participation are required to be a participant, seeking feedback about the study, and verifying the findings with the participants (Van Lith, 2014a).

A particular moral concern for art therapy researchers using qualitative methods involves the dual role between art therapist and researcher. Although a dual role requires clear boundary setting, a level of expertise can also be an asset to minimize risks. For instance, art therapists can use their prior experience to help protect the rights, privacy, dignity, and wellbeing of their participants and to gain voluntary informed consent and ensure confidentiality (Wiles, Crow, Heath, & Charles, 2008).

Brinkmann, S., Jacobsen, M. H., & Kristiansen, S. (2014): Historical overview of qualitative research in the social sciences. In P. Leavy (Ed.), *The Oxford handbook of qualitative research* (pp. 17–42). New York, NY: Oxford University Press.

Bruner, J. (2004). Life as narrative. *Social Research, 71*(3), 691–710.

Bryant, A. & Charmaz, K. (Eds.). (2007). *The SAGE handbook of grounded theory*. Thousand Oaks, CA: Sage.

Bryman, A. (2008). Why do researchers integrate/combine/mesh/blend/mix/merge/fuse quantitative and qualitative research? In M. M. Bergman (Ed.), *Advances in mixed methods research: Theories and applications* (pp. 87–100). Thousand Oaks, CA: Sage.

Burt, H. (1996). Beyond practice: A postmodern feminist perspective on art therapy research. *Art Therapy: Journal of the American Art Therapy Association, 13*(1), 12–19.

Bute, J. J. & Jensen, R. E. (2011). Narrative sense-making and time lapse: Interviews with low-income women about sex education. *Communication Monographs, 78*(2), 212–232. Retrieved from https://doi.org/10.1080/03637751.2011.564639

Charmaz, K. (2014). *Constructing grounded theory* (2nd ed.). Thousand Oaks, CA: Sage.

Chataway, C. J. (2001). Negotiating the observer–observed relationship: Participatory action research. In D. L. Tolman & M. Brydon-Miller (Eds.), *From subjects to subjectivities: A handbook of interpretive and participatory methods* (pp. 239–255). New York, NY: New York University Press.

Clandinin, D. J. & Connelly, F. M. (2000). *Narrative inquiry: Experience and story in qualitative research*. San Francisco, CA: Jossey-Bass.

Clarke, A. E. (2005). *Situational analysis: Grounded theory after the postmodern turn*. Thousand Oaks, CA: Sage.

Clarke, V. & Braun, V. (2013). Teaching thematic analysis: Overcoming challenges and developing strategies for effective learning. *The Psychologist, 26*(2), 120–123.

Colaizzi, P. F. (1973) *Reflection and research in psychology: A phenomenological study of learning*. New York, NY: Hunt Publications.

Colaizzi, P. F. (1978). Psychological research as the phenomenologist views it. In K. Valle & M. King (Eds.), *Phenomenological alternatives for psychology* (pp. 48–71). New York, NY: Oxford University Press.

Collie, K., Bottorff, J. L., & Long, B. C. (2006). A narrative view of art therapy and art making by women with breast cancer. *Journal of Health Psychology, 11*(5), 761–775. Retrieved from https://doi.org/10.1177/1359105306066632

Creswell, J. A. (2013). *Qualitative inquiry and research design: Choosing among five approaches* (3rd ed.). Thousand Oaks, CA: Sage.

Creswell, J. W. & Creswell, J. D. (2018). *Research design: Qualitative, quantitative, and mixed methods approaches* (5th ed.). Thousand Oaks, CA: Sage.

Crotty, M. (1996). *Phenomenology and nursing research*. Melbourne, Australia: Churchill Livingstone.

Crotty, M. (1998). *The foundations of social research: Meaning and perspective in the research process*. Thousand Oaks, CA: Sage.

Daly, J., Willis, K., Small, R., Green, J., Welch, N., Kealy, M., & Hughes, E. (2007). A hierarchy of evidence for assessing qualitative health research. *Journal of Clinical Epidemiology, 60*, 43–49.

Davidson, L. (2003). *Living outside mental illness: Qualitative studies of recovery in schizophrenia*. New York, NY: NYU Press.

Davis, B. (2010). Hermeneutic methods in art therapy research with international students. *The Arts in Psychotherapy, 37*(3), 179–189. Retrieved from https://doi.org/10.1016/j.aip.2010.03.003

Denzin, N. K. (2010). Moments, mixed methods, and paradigm dialogs. *Qualitative Inquiry, 16*(6), 419–427. Retrieved from https://doi.org/10.1177/1077800410364608

Denzin, N. K. & Lincoln, Y. S. (Eds.). (2011). *The SAGE handbook of qualitative research* (4th ed.). Thousand Oaks, CA: Sage.

Denzin, N. K. & Lincoln, Y. S. (Eds.). (2013). *The landscape of qualitative research* (4th ed.). Thousand Oaks, CA: Sage.

Denzin, N. K., Lincoln, Y. S., & Smith, L. T. (Eds.). (2008). *Handbook of critical and indigenous methodologies*. Thousand Oaks, CA: Sage.

Dyer, G. & Hunter, E. (2009). Creative recovery: Art for mental health's sake. *Australasian Psychiatry, 17*(S1), S146-S150.

Eastwood, C. (2012). Art therapy with women with borderline personality disorder: A feminist perspective. *International Journal of Art Therapy, 17*(3), 98–114. Retrieved from https://doi.org/10.1080/17454832.2012.734837

Eatough, V. & Smith, J. A. (2017). Interpretative phenomenological analysis. In N. K. Denzin & Y. S. Lincoln (Eds.), *The SAGE handbook of qualitative research in psychology* (pp. 193–211). Thousand Oaks, CA: Sage.

Ellingson L. (2009). *Engaging crystallization in qualitative research: An introduction*. Thousand Oaks, CA: Sage.

Elliott, R., Fischer, C. T., & Rennie, D. L. (1999). Evolving guidelines for publication of qualitative research studies in psychology and related fields. *British Journal of Clinical Psychology, 38*, 215–229. Retrieved from https://doi.org/10.1348/014466599162782

Ellis, C. (2004). *The ethnographic I: A methodological novel about autoethnography*. Walnut Creek, CA: Altamira Press.

Elo, S. & Kyngäs, H. (2008). The qualitative content analysis process. *Journal of Advanced Nursing, 62*(1), 107–115. Retrieved from https://doi.org/10.1111/j.1365-2648.2007.04569.x

Emerson, P. & Frosh, S. (2004). *Critical narrative analysis in psychology*. New York, NY: Palgrave Macmillan.

Engle, P. (1997). Art therapy and dissociative disorders. *Art Therapy: Journal of the American Art Therapy Association, 14*(4), 246–254.

Fenner, P. (1996). Heuristic research study: Self-therapy using the brief image-making experience. *The Arts in Psychotherapy, 23*(1), 37–51.

Finlay, L. & Evans, K. (Eds.). (2009). *Relational-centred research for psychotherapists: Exploring meanings and experience*. Chichester: Wiley-Blackwell.

Fujiura, G. T. (2015). Perspectives on the publication of qualitative research. *Intellectual and Developmental Disabilities, 53*(5), 323–328. Retrieved from https://doi.org/10.1352/1934-9556-53.5.323

Gadamer, H. G. (1975). *Truth and method* (G. Barden & J. Cumming, Trans.). New York, NY: Seabury Press.
Gee, J. P. (1999). *An introduction to discourse analysis: Theory and practice.* New York, NY: Routledge.
Gibbs, G. R. (2007). *Analyzing qualitative data.* Thousand Oaks, CA: Sage.
Giorgi, A. (1975). An application of phenomenological method in psychology. In A. Giorgi, C. Fischer, & E. Murray (Eds.), *Duquesne studies in phenomenological psychology* (Vol. 2, pp. 82–103). Pittsburgh, PA: Duquesne University Press.
Giorgi, A. (1994). A phenomenological perspective on certain qualitative research methods. *Journal of Phenomenological Psychology, 25*(2), 190–220.
Glaser, B. G. & Strauss, A. L. (1967). *Discovery of grounded theory: Strategies for qualitative research.* New York, NY: Routledge.
Graneheim, U. H. & Lundman, B. (2004). Qualitative content analysis in nursing research: Concepts, procedures and measures to achieve trustworthiness. *Nurse Education Today, 24*(2), 105–112. Retrieved from https://doi.org/10.1016/j.nedt.2003.10.001
Gray, B. (2011). Autoethnography and art therapy: The arts meets healing. *Australian and New Zealand Journal of Art Therapy, 6*(1), 67–80.
Greene, J. & Caracelli, V. (Eds.). (1997). Advances in mixed-method evaluation: The challenges and benefits of integrating diverse paradigms. *New Directions for Evaluation, 74.* San Francisco, CA: Jossey-Bass.
Greene, J. & Caracelli, V. (2003). Making paradigmatic sense of mixed methods practice. In A. Tashakkori & C. Teddlie (Eds.), *Handbook of mixed methods in social and behavioral research* (pp. 91–110). Thousand Oaks, CA: Sage.
Greenwood, H. (2011). Long-term individual art psychotherapy. Art for art's sake: The effect of early relational trauma. *International Journal of Art Therapy, 16*(1), 41–51. Retrieved from https://doi.org/10.1080/17454832.2011.570274
Gussak, D. E. (2016). A case for case studies: More than telling a story. In D. E. Gussak & M. L. Rosal (Eds.), *The Wiley handbook of art therapy* (pp. 617–626). Hoboken, NJ: Wiley Blackwell.
Haeyen, S., Kleijberg, M., & Hinz, L. (2018). Art therapy for patients with personality disorders cluster B/C: A thematic analysis of emotion regulation from patient and art therapist perspectives. *International Journal of Art Therapy, 23*(4), 1–13. Retrieved from https://doi.org/10.1080/17454832.2017.1406966
Haeyen, S., van Hooren, S., & Hutschemaekers, G. (2015). Perceived effects of art therapy in the treatment of personality disorders, cluster B/C: A qualitative study. *The Arts in Psychotherapy, 45,* 1–10. Retrieved from https://doi.org/10.1016/j.aip.2015.04.005
Heidegger, M. (1927/1967). *Being and time* (J. Macquarrie & E. Robinson, Trans.). Oxford: Blackwell.
Heron, J. (1996). *Co-operative inquiry: Research into the human condition.* Thousand Oaks, CA: Sage.
Heron, J. & Reason, P. (1997). A participatory inquiry paradigm. *Qualitative Inquiry, 3*(3), 274–294.
Heron, J. & Reason, P. (2001). The practice of co-operative inquiry: Research with rather than on people. In P. Reason & H. Bradbury (Eds.), *Handbook of*

*action research: Participative inquiry and practice* (pp. 179–188). Thousand Oaks, CA: Sage.

Hesse-Biber, S. (Ed.). (2010). *Mixed methods research: Merging theory with practice*. New York, NY: Guilford Press.

Hesse-Biber, S. & Leavy, P. (2008). Introduction: Pushing on the methodological boundaries. In S. N. Hesse-Biber & P. Leavy (Eds.), *Handbook of emergent methods* (pp. 1–15). New York, NY: Guilford.

Hogan, S. (2001). *Gender issues in art therapy*. Philadelphia, PA: Jessica Kingsley.

Hogan, S. (Ed.). (2012). *Revisiting feminist approaches to art therapy*. New York, NY: Berghahn Books.

Holmqvist, G., Roxberg, Å., Larsson, I., & Persson, C. L. (2017). What art therapists consider to be patient's [sic] inner change and how it may appear during art therapy. *The Arts in Psychotherapy, 56*, 45–52. Retrieved from https://doi.org/10.1016/j.aip.2017.07.005

Holttum, S., Huet, V., & Wright, T. (2017). Reaching a UK consensus on art therapy for people with a diagnosis of a psychotic disorder using the Delphi method. *International Journal of Art Therapy, 22*(1), 35–44. Retrieved from https://doi.org/10.1080/17454832.2016.1257647

Horkheimer, M. (Ed.). ([1937] 1972). *Traditional and critical theory: Selected essays* (M. J. O'Conell, Trans.). New York, NY: Herder and Herder.

Huss, E. (2016). Toward a social critical, analytical prism in art therapy: The example of marginalized Bedouin women's images. *The Arts in Psychotherapy, 50*, 84–90. Retrieved from https://doi.org/10.1016/j.aip.2016.05.017

Husserl, E. ([1936] 1970). *The crisis of European sciences and transcendental phenomenology: An introduction to phenomenological philosophy*. (D. Carr, Trans.). Evanston, IL: Northwestern University Press.

Husserl, E. ([1952] 1980). *Ideas pertaining to a pure phenomenology and to a phenomenological philosophy. Third book: phenomenology and the foundations of the sciences*. Dordrecht, Netherlands: Kluwer Academic Publishers.

Johnson, B. (2008). Living with tensions: The dialectic approach. *Journal of Mixed Methods Research, 2*(3), 203–207.

Johnson. B., Onwuegbuzie, J., & Turner, A. (2007). Toward a definition of mixed methods research, *Journal of Mixed Methods Research, 1*(2), 112–133.

Kaiser, D. & Deaver, S. (2013) Establishing a research agenda for art therapy: A Delphi study. *Art Therapy: Journal of the American Art Therapy Association, 30*(3), 114–121. Retrieved from https://doi.org/10.1080/07421656.2013.819281

Kapitan, L., Litell, M., & Torres, A. (2011). Creative art therapy in a community's participatory research and social transformation. *Art Therapy: Journal of the American Art Therapy Association, 28*(2), 64–73. Retrieved from https://doi.org/10.1080/07421656.2011.578238

Keats, P. A. (2009). Multiple text analysis in narrative research: Visual, written, and spoken stories of experience. *Qualitative Research, 9*(2), 181–195. Retrieved from https://doi.org/10.1177/1468794108099320

Kellman, J. (2008). A place for healing: A hospital art class, writing, and a researcher's task. *Journal of Aesthetic Education, 42*(3), 106–121.

Kemmis, S. & McTaggart, R. (2005). Participatory action research: Communicative action and the public sphere. In N. K. Denzin & Y. S.

Daly, J., Willis, K., Small, R., Green, J., Welch, N., Kealy, M., & Hughes, E. (2007). A hierarchy of evidence for assessing qualitative health research. *Journal of Clinical Epidemiology, 60,* 43–49.

Davidson, L. (2003). *Living outside mental illness: Qualitative studies of recovery in schizophrenia.* New York, NY: NYU Press.

Davis, B. (2010). Hermeneutic methods in art therapy research with international students. *The Arts in Psychotherapy, 37*(3), 179–189. Retrieved from https://doi.org/10.1016/j.aip.2010.03.003

Denzin, N. K. (2010). Moments, mixed methods, and paradigm dialogs. *Qualitative Inquiry, 16*(6), 419–427. Retrieved from https://doi.org/10.1177/1077800410364608

Denzin, N. K. & Lincoln, Y. S. (Eds.). (2011). *The SAGE handbook of qualitative research* (4th ed.). Thousand Oaks, CA: Sage.

Denzin, N. K. & Lincoln, Y. S. (Eds.). (2013). *The landscape of qualitative research* (4th ed.). Thousand Oaks, CA: Sage.

Denzin, N. K., Lincoln, Y. S., & Smith, L. T. (Eds.). (2008). *Handbook of critical and indigenous methodologies.* Thousand Oaks, CA: Sage.

Dyer, G. & Hunter, E. (2009). *Creative recovery: Art for mental health's sake. Australasian Psychiatry, 17*(S1), S146-S150.

Eastwood, C. (2012). Art therapy with women with borderline personality disorder: A feminist perspective. *International Journal of Art Therapy, 17*(3), 98–114. Retrieved from https://doi.org/10.1080/17454832.2012.734837

Eatough, V. & Smith, J. A. (2017). Interpretative phenomenological analysis. In N. K. Denzin & Y. S. Lincoln (Eds.), *The SAGE handbook of qualitative research in psychology* (pp. 193–211). Thousand Oaks, CA: Sage.

Ellingson L. (2009). *Engaging crystallization in qualitative research: An introduction.* Thousand Oaks, CA: Sage.

Elliott, R., Fischer, C. T., & Rennie, D. L. (1999). Evolving guidelines for publication of qualitative research studies in psychology and related fields. *British Journal of Clinical Psychology, 38,* 215–229. Retrieved from https://doi.org/10.1348/014466599162782

Ellis, C. (2004). *The ethnographic I: A methodological novel about autoethnography.* Walnut Creek, CA: Altamira Press.

Elo, S. & Kyngäs, H. (2008). The qualitative content analysis process. *Journal of Advanced Nursing, 62*(1), 107–115. Retrieved from https://doi.org/10.1111/j.1365-2648.2007.04569.x

Emerson, P. & Frosh, S. (2004). *Critical narrative analysis in psychology.* New York, NY: Palgrave Macmillan.

Engle, P. (1997). Art therapy and dissociative disorders. *Art Therapy: Journal of the American Art Therapy Association, 14*(4), 246–254.

Fenner, P. (1996). Heuristic research study: Self-therapy using the brief image-making experience. *The Arts in Psychotherapy, 23*(1), 37–51.

Finlay, L. & Evans, K. (Eds.). (2009). *Relational-centred research for psychotherapists: Exploring meanings and experience.* Chichester: Wiley-Blackwell.

Fujiura, G. T. (2015). Perspectives on the publication of qualitative research. *Intellectual and Developmental Disabilities, 53*(5), 323–328. Retrieved from https://doi.org/10.1352/1934-9556-53.5.323

Brinkmann, S., Jacobsen, M. H., & Kristiansen, S. (2014): Historical overview of qualitative research in the social sciences. In P. Leavy (Ed.), *The Oxford handbook of qualitative research* (pp. 17–42). New York, NY: Oxford University Press.

Bruner, J. (2004). Life as narrative. *Social Research, 71*(3), 691–710.

Bryant, A. & Charmaz, K. (Eds.). (2007). *The SAGE handbook of grounded theory.* Thousand Oaks, CA: Sage.

Bryman, A. (2008). Why do researchers integrate/combine/mesh/blend/mix/merge/fuse quantitative and qualitative research? In M. M. Bergman (Ed.), *Advances in mixed methods research: Theories and applications* (pp. 87–100). Thousand Oaks, CA: Sage.

Burt, H. (1996). Beyond practice: A postmodern feminist perspective on art therapy research. *Art Therapy: Journal of the American Art Therapy Association, 13*(1), 12–19.

Bute, J. J. & Jensen, R. E. (2011). Narrative sense-making and time lapse: Interviews with low-income women about sex education. *Communication Monographs, 78*(2), 212–232. Retrieved from https://doi.org/10.1080/03637751.2011.564639

Charmaz, K. (2014). *Constructing grounded theory* (2nd ed.). Thousand Oaks, CA: Sage.

Chataway, C. J. (2001). Negotiating the observer–observed relationship: Participatory action research. In D. L. Tolman & M. Brydon-Miller (Eds.), *From subjects to subjectivities: A handbook of interpretive and participatory methods* (pp. 239–255). New York, NY: New York University Press.

Clandinin, D. J. & Connelly, F. M. (2000). *Narrative inquiry: Experience and story in qualitative research.* San Francisco, CA: Jossey-Bass.

Clarke, A. E. (2005). *Situational analysis: Grounded theory after the postmodern turn.* Thousand Oaks, CA: Sage.

Clarke, V. & Braun, V. (2013). Teaching thematic analysis: Overcoming challenges and developing strategies for effective learning. *The Psychologist, 26*(2), 120–123.

Colaizzi, P. F. (1973) *Reflection and research in psychology: A phenomenological study of learning.* New York, NY: Hunt Publications.

Colaizzi, P. F. (1978). Psychological research as the phenomenologist views it. In K. Valle & M. King (Eds.), *Phenomenological alternatives for psychology* (pp. 48–71). New York, NY: Oxford University Press.

Collie, K., Bottorff, J. L., & Long, B. C. (2006). A narrative view of art therapy and art making by women with breast cancer. *Journal of Health Psychology, 11*(5), 761–775. Retrieved from https://doi.org/10.1177/1359105306066632

Creswell, J. A. (2013). *Qualitative inquiry and research design: Choosing among five approaches* (3rd ed.). Thousand Oaks, CA: Sage.

Creswell, J. W. & Creswell, J. D. (2018). *Research design: Qualitative, quantitative, and mixed methods approaches* (5th ed.). Thousand Oaks, CA: Sage.

Crotty, M. (1996). *Phenomenology and nursing research.* Melbourne, Australia: Churchill Livingstone.

Crotty, M. (1998). *The foundations of social research: Meaning and perspective in the research process.* Thousand Oaks, CA: Sage.

| Research Method | Experiential "Data" | "Findings" |
|---|---|---|
| **Qualitative**<br>Research question: *What is the lived experience of graduate art therapy students' engagement in an immersive art experience?* | Content analysis of reflective writing on why the selected art is meaningful. | In-depth understanding of how exhibit attendees understand art that is meaningful. |
| **Program Development/ Action Research** | Content analysis of relational aesthetics questionnaire and reflective writing. | How to design more meaningful exhibits in the future. |
| **Case Study/Ethnography** | Thematic analysis of facilitator notes on one participant during his or her time in the exhibit. | In-depth description of process. |

Source: Betts and Potash (2018).

## References

Agee, J. (2009). Developing qualitative research questions: A reflective process. *International Journal of Qualitative Studies in Education, 22*(4), 431–447. Retrieved from https://doi.org/10.1080/09518390902736512

Betts, D. J. & Potash, J. (2018). Research simulation experiential: Bringing research to life! (personal collection of D. Betts and J. Potash, the George Washington University, Washington, DC).

Bloomgarden, J. & Netzer, D. (1998). Validating art therapists' tacit knowing: The heuristic experience. *Art Therapy: Journal of the American Art Therapy Association, 15*(1), 51–54.

Bogdan, R. C. & Biklen, S. K. (2007). *Qualitative research for education: An introduction to theory and methods* (5th ed.). Boston, MA: Pearson Allyn & Bacon.

Bourke, B. (2014). Positionality: Reflecting on the research process. *The Qualitative Report, 19*(33), 1–9. Retrieved from http://nsuworks.nova.edu/tqr/vol19/iss33/3

Braun, V. & Clarke, V. (2006). Using thematic analysis in psychology. *Qualitative Research in Psychology, 3*(2), 77–101.

Braun, V. & Clarke, V. (2013). *Successful qualitative research: A practical guide for beginners*. Thousand Oaks, CA: Sage.

Bresler, L. (1996). Towards the creation of a new ethical code in qualitative research. *Bulletin of the Council for Research in Music Education, 130*, 17–29.

Bresler, L. (2006). Toward connectedness: Aesthetically based research. *Studies in Art Education: A Journal of Issues and Research, 48*(1), 52–69.

Additionally, participants should be informed of the extent to which anonymity and confidentiality can be assured in publication and dissemination of the findings and in potential re-use of data.

## Summary

This chapter elucidated approaches to qualitative research in art therapy. Beginning with considerations in the development of a study based on qualitative inquiry, factors important to qualitative research questions were explained. This was followed by an overview of philosophical assumptions pertaining to research to augment understanding of where qualitative pursuits fit in, including ontology, epistemology, axiology, and methodology. Similarly, research paradigms essential to comprehension of qualitative research were described: postpositivism, constructivism, transformative, and pragmatism. The emergent and flexible nature of qualitative research was further delineated in the section on bricolage, followed by practical information related to recruitment of study participants. Six types of qualitative research designs were presented: case study, grounded theory, phenomenological inquiry, narrative inquiry, ethnography, and participatory action research. Information about data collection was provided, including on interviews, focus groups, open-ended questionnaires, Delphi method questionnaires, and field notes. The types of qualitative data analysis – thematic, content, grounded theory, phenomenological, discourse, and narrative – were described. Finally, strategies for evaluating quality, and ethical and moral responsibilities were delineated.

This chapter shed light on the increase in the use of qualitative approaches in art therapy research and the ways in which this methodology is congruent with the work of art therapists, given our natural inclination to help others through facilitation of the creative process as healing and life-enhancing. In Chapter 5, another research approach that is highly compatible with the worldview of art therapists is presented – that of arts-based research.

---

**Box 4.1 Bringing Research to Life!Qualitative Data Analysis Example**

**Objective:** Please refer to Box 1.1 (Chapter 1) and Appendix A for the purpose, set-up, and materials to guide the application of this experiential. The following provides information on the *qualitative* data analysis portion of the Bringing Research to Life! experiential (after the mock experiment and data collection has been completed):

Lincoln (Eds.), *The SAGE handbook of qualitative research* (pp. 559–603). Thousand Oaks, CA: Sage.

Killick, K. (1996). Un-integration and containment in acute psychosis. *British Journal of Psychotherapy, 13*(2), 232–242.

Kincheloe, J. L. (2001). Describing the bricolage: Conceptualizing a new rigor in qualitative research. *Qualitative Inquiry, 7*(6), 679–692.

Kincheloe, J. L. (2005). On to the next level: Continuing the conceptualisation of the bricolage. *Qualitative Inquiry, 11*(3), 323–350.

Kuhn, T. (1962). *The structure of scientific revolutions*. Chicago, IL: University of Chicago Press.

Kuri, E. (2017). Toward an ethical application of intersectionality in art therapy. *Art Therapy: Journal of the American Art Therapy Association, 34*(3), 118–122. Retrieved from https://doi.org/10.1080/07421656.2017.1358023

Lamont, S., Brunero, S., & Sutton, D. (2009). Art psychotherapy in a consumer diagnosed with borderline personality disorder: A case study. *International Journal of Mental Health Nursing, 18*(3), 164–172. Retrieved from https://doi.org/10.1111/j.1447-0349.2009.00594

Leavy, P. (2014). *The Oxford handbook of qualitative research*. Oxford: Oxford University Press.

Leavy, P. (2017). *Research design: Quantitative, qualitative, mixed methods, arts-based, and community-based participatory research approaches*. New York, NY: Guilford Press.

Lett, W., Fox, K., & von der Borch, D. (2014). Process as value in collaborative arts-based inquiry. *Journal of Applied Arts & Health, 5*(2), 209–217. Retrieved from https://doi.org/10.1386/jaah.5.2.209_1

Lewin, K. (1948). *Resolving social conflicts*. New York, NY: Harper Collins.

Lincoln, Y. S. & Guba, E. G. (1985). *Naturalistic inquiry*. Thousand Oaks, CA: Sage.

Lincoln, Y. S., Lynham, S. A., & Guba, E. G. (2011). Paradigmatic controversies, contradictions, and emerging confluences, revisited. In N. K. Denzin & Y. S. Lincoln (Eds.), *The SAGE handbook of qualitative research* (4th ed.) (pp. 97–128). Thousand Oaks, CA: Sage.

Linnell, S. (2009). Becoming "otherwise": A story of a collaborative and narrative approach to art therapy with indigenous kids "in care." *Australian and New Zealand Journal of Art Therapy, 41*(1), 15–26.

Lu, L. & Yuen, F. (2012). Journey women: Art therapy in a decolonizing framework of practice. *The Arts in Psychotherapy, 39*(3), 192–200. Retrieved from https://doi.org/10.1016/j.aip.2011.12.007

Lykes, M. B. (2001). Activist participatory research and the arts with rural Mayan women: Interculturality and situated meaning making. In D. L. Tolman & M. Brydon-Miller (Eds.), *Qualitative studies in psychology. From subjects to subjectivities: A handbook of interpretive and participatory methods* (pp. 183–199). New York, NY: New York University Press.

Madison, D. S. (2012). *Critical ethnography: Method, ethics, and performance* (Vol. 2, 2nd ed.). Thousand Oaks, CA: Sage.

Manen, M. van. (1990). *Researching lived experience: Human science for an action sensitive pedagogy*. Albany, NY: State University of New York Press.

Manen, M. van. (2007). Reflectivity and the pedagogical moment: The practical ethical nature of pedagogical thinking and acting. In I. Westbury & G. Milburn (Eds.), *Rethinking schooling* (pp. 81–114). New York, NY: Routledge.

Maxwell, J. A. (2013). *Qualitative research design: An interactive approach* (3rd ed.). Thousand Oaks, CA: Sage.

Mayor, C. (2012). Playing with race: A theoretical framework and approach for creative arts therapists. *The Arts in Psychotherapy, 39*(3), 214–219. Retrieved from https://doi.org/10.1016/j.aip.2011.12.008.

McCreaddie, M. & Payne, S. (2010). Evolving grounded theory methodology: Towards a discursive approach. *International Journal of Nursing Studies, 47*(6), 781–793.

McLeod, J. (2010). *Case study research in counselling and psychotherapy.* Thousand Oaks, CA: Sage.

Merleau-Ponty, M. (1968). *The visible and the invisible.* (A. Lingus, Trans.). Evanston, IL: Northwestern University Press.

Mertens, D. M. (2014). *Research and evaluation in education and psychology: Integrating diversity with quantitative, qualitative, and mixed methods.* Thousand Oaks, CA: Sage.

Moustakas, C. (1994). *Phenomenological research methods.* Thousand Oaks, CA: Sage.

Netzer, D. (2009). From linear to imaginal: Choosing research methods to inform art therapy practice. *Art Therapy: Journal of the American Art Therapy Association, 26*(1), 38–41. Retrieved from https://doi.org/10.1080/07421656.2009.10129314

Neuendorf, K. A. (2016). *The content analysis guidebook* (2nd ed.). Thousand Oaks, CA: Sage.

Noble, H. & Smith, J. (2015). Issues of validity and reliability in qualitative research. *Evidence-Based Nursing, 18*, 34–35. Retrieved from https://doi.org/10.1136/eb-2015-102054

Onwuegbuzie, A. & Leech, N. (2005). On becoming a pragmatic researcher: Importance of combining quantitative and qualitative research methodologies. *International Journal of Social Research Methodology, 8*(5), 375–387.

Orr, P. (2007). Art therapy with children after a disaster: A content analysis. *The Arts in Psychotherapy, 34*(4), 350–361. Retrieved from https://doi.org/10.1016/j.aip.2007.07.002

Park, B. (2017). A Korean art therapist's autoethnography concerning re-acculturation to the motherland following training in the UK. *International Journal of Art Therapy, 22*(4), 154–161. Retrieved from https://doi.org/10.1080/17454832.2017.1296008

Patterson, S., Crawford, M. J., Ainsworth, E., & Waller, D. (2011). Art therapy for people diagnosed with schizophrenia: Therapists' views about what changes, how and for whom. *International Journal of Art Therapy, 16*(2), 70–80. Retrieved from https://doi.org/10.1080/17454832.2011.604038

Patton, M. (2015). *Qualitative evaluation and research methods* (4th ed.). Thousand Oaks, CA: Sage.

Phillips, D. C. & Burbules, N. C. (2000). *Postpositivism and educational research.* Lanham, MD: Rowman & Littlefield.

Polkinghorne, D. (1983). *Methodology for the human sciences: Systems of inquiry.* Albany, NY: State University of New York.

Polkinghorne, D. (1995). Narrative configuration in qualitative analysis. *International Journal of Qualitative Studies in Education, 8*(1), 5–23. Retrieved from https://doi.org/10.1080/0951839950080103

Ponterotto, J. G. (2005). Qualitative research in counseling psychology: A primer on research paradigms and philosophy of science. *Journal of Counseling Psychology, 52*(2), 126–136.

Quail, J. M. & Peavy, R. V. (1994). The phenomenologic research study of a client's experience in art therapy. *The Arts in Psychotherapy, 21*(1), 45–57.

Ravitch, S. M. & Mittenfelner, C. N. (2016). *Qualitative research: Bridging the conceptual, theoretical and methodological.* Thousand Oaks, CA: Sage.

Reason, P. & Bradbury, H. (Eds.). (2006). *Handbook of action research: Concise paperback edition.* Thousand Oaks, CA: Sage.

Reason, P. & Heron, J. (1995). Co-operative inquiry. In J., Smith, R., Harre, & L. Van Langenhove (Eds.), *Rethinking methods in psychology* (pp. 122–142). Thousand Oaks, CA: Sage.

Richardson, L. (1999). Feathers in our cap. *Journal of Contemporary Ethnography, 28*(6), 660–668.

Richardson, L. & St. Pierre, E. (2008). A method of inquiry. In N. Denzin & Y. Lincoln (Eds.), *The SAGE handbook of qualitative research* (pp. 959–978). Thousand Oaks, CA: Sage.

Riesmann, C. (1993). *Narrative analysis.* Thousand Oaks, CA: Sage.

Rossetto, E. (2012). A hermeneutic phenomenological study of community mural making and social action art therapy. *Art Therapy: Journal of the American Art Therapy Association, 29*(1), 19–26. Retrieved from https://doi.org/10.1080/07421656.2012.648105

Sajnani, N. (2012). Response/ability: Imagining a critical race feminist paradigm for the creative arts therapies. *The Arts in Psychotherapy, 39*(3), 186–191. Retrieved from https://doi.org/10.1016/j.aip.2011.12.009

Sandelowski, M. (2015). A matter of taste: Evaluating the quality of qualitative research. *Nursing inquiry, 22*(2), 86–94. Retrieved from https://doi.org/10.1111/nin.12 080

Savin-Baden, M. & Howell Major, C. (2013). *Qualitative research: The essential guide to theory and practice.* New York, NY: Routledge.

Schreibman, R. & Chilton, G. (2012). Small waterfalls in art therapy supervision: A poetic appreciative inquiry. *Art Therapy: Journal of the American Art Therapy Association, 29*(4), 188–191. Retrieved from https://doi.org/10.1080/07421656.2012.730924

Seidman, I. (2013). *Interviewing as qualitative research: A guide for researchers in education and the social sciences* (3rd ed.). New York, NY: Teachers College Press.

Shin, S. K., Choi, S. N., & Park, S. W. (2016). A narrative inquiry into a mother–child art therapy experience: A self-exploration of the therapist and the mother. *The Arts in Psychotherapy, 47,* 23–30. Retrieved from https://doi.org/10.1016/j.aip.2015.09.001

Smith, J., Flowers, P., & Larkin, M. (2009). *Interpretative phenomenological analysis: Theory, method, and research.* Thousand Oaks, CA: Sage.

Solomon, G. (2006). Development of art therapy in South Africa: Dominant narratives and marginalized stories. *Canadian Art Therapy Association Journal, 19*(1), 17–32. Retrieved from https://doi.org/10.1080/17454830500112318

Spaniol, S. (2005). "Learned hopefulness": An arts-based approach to participatory action research. *Art Therapy: Journal of the American Art Therapy Association, 22*(2), 86–91.

Spencer, R., Pryce, J. M., & Walsh, J. (2014). Philosophical approaches to qualitative research. In P. Leavy (Ed.), *The Oxford handbook of qualitative research* (pp. 81–98). Oxford: Oxford University Press.

Springham, N. & Camic, P. M. (2017). Observing mentalizing art therapy groups for people diagnosed with borderline personality disorder. *International Journal of Art Therapy, 22*(3), 138–152. Retrieved from https://doi.org/10.1080/17454832.2017.1288753

Stake, R. E. (2005). Qualitative case studies. In N. Denzin & Y. Lincoln (Eds.), *The SAGE handbook of qualitative research* (3rd ed., pp. 443–466). Thousand Oaks, CA: Sage.

Starks, H. & Brown Trinidad, S. (2007). Choose your method: A comparison of phenomenology, discourse analysis, and grounded theory. *Qualitative Health Research, 17*(10), 1372–1380. Retrieved from https://doi.org/10.1177/1049732307307031

Strauss, A. L. (1987). *Qualitative analysis for social scientists.* Cambridge: Cambridge University Press.

Strauss, A. & Corbin, J. (1998). *Basics of qualitative research: Techniques and procedures for developing grounded theory* (2nd ed.). Thousand Oaks, CA: Sage.

Sweeney, S. (2009). Art therapy: Promoting wellbeing in rural and remote communities. *Australasian Psychiatry, 17*(Suppl. 1), S151–S154.

Talwar, S. (2010). An intersectional framework for race, class, gender, and sexuality in art therapy. *Art Therapy: Journal of the American Art Therapy Association, 27*(1), 11–17. Retrieved from https://doi.org/10.1080/07421656.2010.10129567

Talwar, S. (2015). Culture, diversity, and identity: From margins to center. *Art Therapy: Journal of the American Art Therapy Association, 32*(3), 100–103. Retrieved from https://doi.org/10.1080/07421656.2015.1060563

Tashakkori, A. & Teddlie, C. (2010a). Putting the human back in "human research methodology": The researcher in mixed methods research. *Journal of Mixed Methods Research, 4*(4), 271–277.

Tashakkori, A. & Teddlie, C. (2010b). *SAGE handbook of mixed methods in social & behavioral research.* Thousand Oaks, CA: Sage.

Teddlie, C. & Tashakkori, A. (2009). *Foundations of mixed methods research: Integrating quantitative and qualitative techniques in the social and behavioral sciences.* Thousand Oaks, CA: Sage.

Van Lith, T. (2008). A phenomenological investigation using art therapy processes in assisting transition to a psychosocial residential setting. *Art Therapy: Journal of the American Art Therapy Association, 25*(1), 24–31. Retrieved from https://doi.org/10.1080/07421656.2008.10129357

Van Lith, T. (2014a). A meeting with "I–Thou": Exploring the intersection between mental health recovery and art making through a co-operative inquiry.

Action Research Journal, 12(3), 254–272. Retrieved from https://doi.org/10.1177/1476750314529599

Van Lith, T. (2014b). "Painting to find my spirit": Art making as the vehicle to find meaning and connection in the mental health recovery process. Journal of Spirituality in Mental Health, 16(1), 19–36. Retrieved from https://doi.org/10.1080/19349637.2013

Van Lith, T., Stallings, J., & Harris, C. (2017). Discovering good practice for art therapy with children who have Autism Spectrum Disorder: The results of a small-scale survey. The Arts in Psychotherapy, 54, 78–84. Retrieved from https://doi.org/10.1016/j.aip.2017.01.00

Wahlbeck, H., Kvist, L. J., & Landgren, K. (2017). Gaining hope and self-confidence: An interview study of women's experience of treatment by art therapy for severe fear of childbirth. Women and Birth, 1–8. Retrieved from https://doi.org/10.1016/j.wombi.2017.10.008

Watts, P., Gilfillan, P., & de Zárate, M. H. (2017). Art therapy and poverty: Examining practitioners' experiences of working with children and young people in areas of multiple deprivation in West Central Scotland. International Journal of Art Therapy, 1–10. Retrieved from https://doi.org/10.1080/17454832.2017.1399920

Wertz, F. J. (2005). Phenomenological research methods for counseling psychology. Journal of Counseling Psychology, 52(2), 167–177. Retrieved from https://doi.org/10.1037/0022-0167.52.2.167

Westwood, J. & Linnell, S. (2011). The emergence of Australian art therapies: Colonial legacies and hybrid practices. ATOL: Art Therapy Online, 2(2), 1–19.

Wiles, R., Crow, G., Heath, S., & Charles, V. (2008). The management of confidentiality and anonymity in social research. International Journal of Social Research Methodology, 11(5), 417–428. Retrieved from https://doi.org/10.1080/13645570701622231

Willis, P. (2001). The "things themselves" in phenomenology. Indo-Pacific Journal of Phenomenology, 1(1), 1–14.

Willis, P. (2004). From the things themselves to a feeling of understanding: Finding different voices in phenomenological research. Indo-Pacific Journal of Phenomenology, 4(1), 1–13.

Wood, L. A. & Kroger, R. O. (2000). Doing discourse analysis: Methods for studying action in talk and text. Thousand Oaks, CA: Sage.

Wright, T. & Wright, K. (2017). Exploring the benefits of intersectional feminist social justice approaches in art psychotherapy. The Arts in Psychotherapy, 54, 7–14. Retrieved from https://doi.org/10.1016/j.aip.2017.02.008

Yin, R. K. (2018). Case study research and applications: Design and methods (6th ed.). Thousand Oaks, CA: Sage.

Zago, C. (2008). Coming into being through being seen: An exploration of how experiences of psychoanalytic observations of infants and young children can enhance ways of "seeing" young people in art therapy. Infant Observation, 11(3), 315–332.

Zappa, A. (2017). Beyond erasure: The ethics of art therapy research with trans and gender-independent people. Art Therapy: Journal of the American Art

*Therapy Association, 34*(3), 129–134. Retrieved from https://doi.org/10.1080/07421656.2017.1343074

Zubala, A., MacIntyre, D. J., & Karkou, V. (2014). Art psychotherapy practice with adults who suffer from depression in the UK: Qualitative findings from a depression-specific questionnaire. *The Arts in Psychotherapy, 41*(5), 563–569. Retrieved from https://doi.org/10.1016/j.aip.2014.10.007

Chapter 5

# Arts-Based Research in Art Therapy

*Jordan S. Potash*

Art therapists' unique contributions to research pursuits are those "born out of direct engagement with what connects us to our deepest selves" (Allen, 2012, p. 16). This linkage is the intentional creation of and reflection on art as a means towards increasing awareness. In other words, "Open your eyes, open your mind. Art is a way of knowing" (Allen, 1995, p. 194). Appreciating arts-based research necessitates accepting art making as a tool for revealing ideas, understanding the world, and enabling us to know something that cannot be known in any other way. Even if images are at first obscure, ambiguous, or confusing, ultimately they offer symbols and metaphors that guide us, as well as point to further questions. McNiff (1998; 2011; 2013; 2018) translated these concepts into research by harnessing these discoveries for improving oneself, inspiring others, furthering professional practice, and satisfying the need for knowledge for its own sake.

In this chapter, I describe arts-based research by drawing on my experiences as a researcher and advisor to master's and doctoral students. Even though arts-based research extends beyond art therapy, I demonstrate how this methodology fits into the overall profession. Leavy (2015) credited the creative arts therapies as having a significant influence on this research method as both emphasize "meaning-making, empowerment, identity exploration, emotional expression, multisensory communication, consciousness-raising, healing, self-reflection and personal growth, relational connections, intersubjectivity, and expressive power (G. Chilton, personal communication, 2013)" (p. 16). Gaining inspiration from other arts-based research scholars (Chilton, 2013; Rumbold, Fenner, & Brophy-Dixon, 2012), I employed an arts-based approach to fuel my ideas for authoring this chapter. As I began to formulate ideas and establish the major headings for the chapter, I created artworks and wrote a haiku in response to each one to inform my own understanding. I intentionally selected black, white, and gray oil pastel to mirror the black and white text and page of this volume.

## Definition

Arts-based research can be complex, and this can be addressed by gaining understanding of its parameters. Chilton and Leavy (2014) provided an excellent summary of the various terms and history as originating from diverse fields such as education, anthropology, archeology, and creative arts therapies. Some of the more commonly used terms include *arts-based research* (Barone & Eisner, 2011; Leavy, 2015; 2018; McNiff, 2012), *arts-informed research* (Knowles & Cole, 2008), *artistic inquiry* (Wadsworth Hervey, 2000), and *a/r/tography* (Irwin & de Cosson, 2004). From these various conceptions, I came to see the emergence of an essence and core (Figure 5.1). As such, in this chapter I use the term *arts-based research* to honor the work of McNiff, a pioneer of this approach in the creative arts therapies professions. Despite his more recent and succinct definition (McNiff, 2014), I appreciate the features of his original description, "a method of inquiry which uses the elements of the creative arts therapy experience, including the making of art by the researcher, as a means of understanding the significance of what we do within our practice" (McNiff, 1998, p. 12). Further exploration into the components of this definition helps to augment understanding of this methodology.

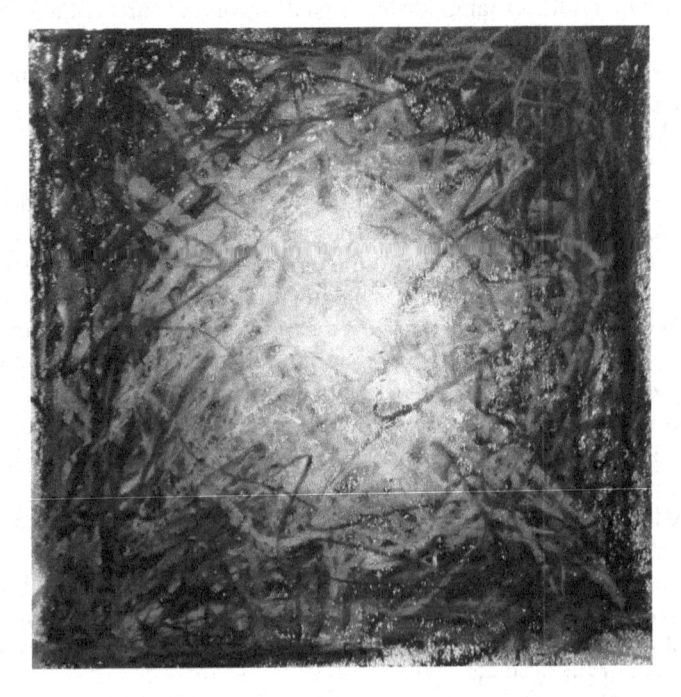

*Figure 5.1 Definition. Naming for Knowing. Blurred Edges? Yes, But Yet, Certainty Emerges*

### Elements of the Creative Arts Therapy Experience

Arts-based research can build on the practices that art therapists engage in with their clients to facilitate their own search for meaning and expression. This implies that the creative process is rooted in the arts but necessitates a focus on specifics to the profession such as meaning making, insight orientation, awareness raising, and behavioral change. Eisner's (2008) "emphasis on inquiry, a tolerance of ambiguity, a preference for what is open-ended, a desire for what is fluid rather than what is rigid" parallels art therapy (p. 22). Irwin's (2013) description of *a/r/tography* embraces an artist's necessity to maintain his or her artistic process while being willing to investigate his or her art productions to further experimentation and curiosity. The emphasis on *arts* rather than *art* indicates the importance of researchers using a range of creative media (visual, music, performance, movement, poetry, creative writing) depending on researcher capabilities and situational demands (Cahnmann-Taylor, 2008; McNiff, 2011; 2018).

### Making of Art by the Researcher

The distinguishing feature of arts-based research is that researchers create art as a central method of investigation and discovery (McNiff, 2011). Furthermore, the research can include collaborators rather than being viewed as a solo effort (McNiff, 2014). The acronym component of *a/r/tography* (artist/researcher/teacher) emphasizes the integration of these roles and therefore the importance of researchers creating art (Irwin & de Cosson, 2004). By engaging in one's own creative process, researchers trust the significance of their own imagination and artwork as a source of wisdom (Eisner, 2008).

Several studies use the phrase *arts-based research* but describe procedures in which art is created by participants or subjects. Kapitan (2018) referred to this as the difference between arts-based research (researcher-created art) and *arts-informed research* (participant-created art). Similarly, McNiff (2011) emphasized "first-hand artistic experimentation as the domain of art-based research" as differentiated from "examination of artistic expressions made by others" (p. 386).

### Significance of What We Do Within our Practice

Arts-based researchers create art that informs audiences, uncovers problems, and elucidates solutions. Researchers simultaneously think like an artist and "like a public intellectual ... to make one's research relevant and accessible to the public" (Leavy, 2015, p. 30). According to Barone (2008), arts-based research intends to "*both* find its inspiration in the arts *and* leads to progressive forms of social awareness" (pp. 34–35). McNiff (2011) recommended studies that help art therapists to better understand and apply theories and practices. Even when arts-based research does not result in specific answers and applications, the methodology is committed to remain in a state of engaged reflection (Barone, 2001; Barone & Eisner, 2012; Eisner, 2008; Irwin, 2013).

## Arts-Based Research Traditions

Perhaps due to interdisciplinary influences, arts-based researchers vary in their approach. Archibald and Gerber (2018) identified four ways in which arts-based research intersects with mixed methods studies: (a) *communicative integration* (arts to share findings), (b) *data source integration* (arts as data), (c) *analytical integration* (arts to explicate data), and (d) *conceptual integration* (arts as integral to all stages of research). These ideas parallel those of other scholars in that some place more emphasis on interpreting participant experiences through researcher generated art, whereas others prioritize creating art based on their own experiences. To bring clarity to this subject, I have found it helpful to conceptualize arts-based research according to two main traditions: explication and self-inquiry. In my early drafts of this chapter, I saw these traditions as distinct, but through my art making realized these distinctions are useful for articulating theory, even if they blend, merge, and inform each other in practice (Figure 5.2).

### *Explication*

Arts-based research as a means of explication emphasizes art making by the researcher in all stages of research to present a new perspective of a phenomenon, raise more questions than it answers, and use findings to make changes in the world. Researchers may choose to engage arts-based research for formulating questions as well as gathering, analyzing, and presenting data (Cahnmann-Taylor, 2008; Kaiser & Kay, 2015; Kapitan, 2018; Leavy, 2015; McNiff, 1998).

#### *Research Question*

Sometimes, we are aware of a problem, but have difficulty putting it into words. Art making can help a researcher explore the world to uncover what questions exist. Chilton (2013) used altered books to learn about arts-based research by immersing herself in it. The various pages offer images and poems to convey ideas and insights regarding her understanding of theory and evolution of her changing ideas. In the end, she arrived at an understanding of arts-based research as a unique paradigm but identified questions to form the basis of further research.

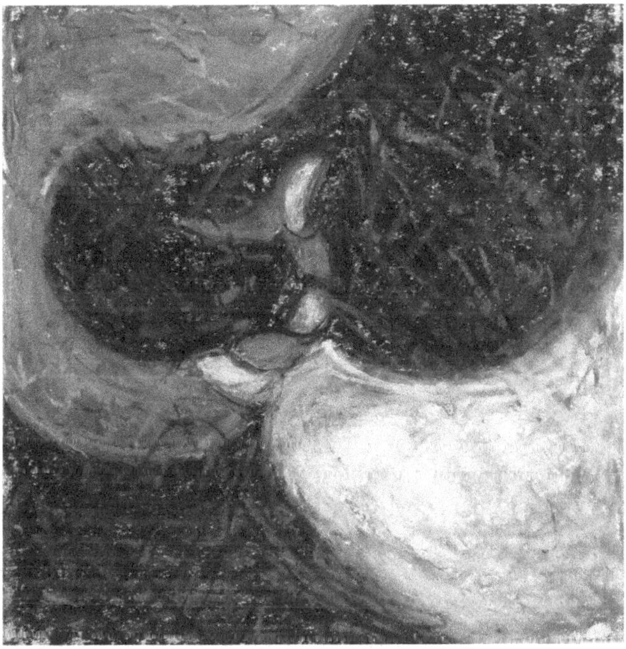

*Figure 5.2 Traditions.* Separate Streams Intertwine, But Stay Distinct. Which Informs? Why, Both

*Data Enhancement*

After amassing data through quantitative or qualitative means, researchers create art inspired by what they collected to enhance, expand, illuminate, and ascertain its essence. Maintaining a strict focus on the research phenomenon and the participants' experiences prevents researchers from delving into their own projections, thereby guarding against subjective bias (Boydell, Hodgins, Gladstone, & Stasiulis, 2017).

*Field Notes and Memo-Writing*

Maintaining a journal of reflections throughout data collection is an important component of qualitative and ethnographic research (Leavy 2015). To honor the practice of field notes, researchers generate "a series of artistic expressions as a means of personal introspection and the process of inquiry generates empirical data which are systematically reviewed" (McNiff, 1998, p. 57). Such art making helps researchers document experiences and bracket biases.

*Analysis*

Researchers can engage the arts to find relationships among data to generate themes and to find connections with theory (Leavy, 2015). Hunter, Lusardi, Zucker, Jacelon, and Chandler (2002) described the liminal space of analysis as ripe for creative and imaginative modes for making meaning of data. Among the strategies they endorsed, Zucker's description of "thematic maps or models" (p. 390), Hunter's use of metaphor, and Jacelon's playwriting all provide examples. Thematic and concept maps may appear as static flow charts, but they represent a "causal network" of "data showing their inter-relationship" (Williamson & Long, 2005, p. 14). The arts envision such connections and thematic categories (Manders & Chilton, 2013).

*Dissemination*

Rather than remain restricted to tables, graphs, and charts, arts-based researchers disseminate data by creating artistic renderings, staging performances, and mounting exhibits to metaphorically represent findings. Such ways of presenting data are particularly useful for non-academic audiences. Two doctoral dissertations offer examples of researcher-generated videos to present findings. Albert-Proos (2015) conducted a qualitative investigation of immigrant expressive arts therapists' conceptions of home to understand how the migration experience impacts their sense of sense and professional identity. She selected direct quotations to create a poem to express the themes. She offered the poetry as the script of her video combined with the metaphor of a flower removed from the ground and set in a vase as a way to convey the emotional essence of her participants' reflections. Dejkameh (2016) created a video that combined documentary-style videos of her clients, shots of her driving between the three art therapy agencies in which she worked, and her own generated art. In explaining her concept of the art therapist as nomad, the video conveys the dynamic of moving through spaces, as well as shifting among theories and practices. Although each of these videos is a stand-alone work of art, together they complement the written dissertation with an expression that offers viewers an authentic and direct approximation of the participants' emotions and lived experiences.

**Self-Inquiry**

Arts-based research for the purpose of "psychological inquiry" (McNiff, 2011, p. 389) encourages researchers to identify a topic of personal interest and then to pursue it in the art studio/laboratory. As a predecessor to this tradition, Jung's seminal ideas are rooted in his own arts-based process and exploration contained in the *Liber Novus* (*The Red*

*Book*; 2009) (Allen, 2012). By undertaking an arts-based approach of his own psychological state, Jung was able to arrive at insights that he generated into theories and practices (McNiff, 2011). Similarly, a well-constructed and interpreted arts-based self-inquiry allows a researcher to make use of personal experiences to understand more general ones. Heuristic and autoethnographic research traditions parallel this process.

### Heuristic Research

Heuristic research describes a process of discovering the human condition within an autobiographical framework. Moustakas (1990) wrote, "the qualitatively heuristic scientist seeks to discover the nature and meaning of the phenomenon itself and to illuminate it from direct first-person accounts" (p. 38). By retaining a strict inward focus, the researcher uncovers answers to questions, but also transforms the self. Combining the researchers' personal investigation with the "essences of universally unique experiences" authorizes them to extend their findings to others and for others to find resonance with their discoveries as inspiration for their own situations (p. 13). Rather than subsume the individual experience within a larger narrative, the universal reveals itself through intensive focus on the individual (Kenny, 2012).

Heuristic research aims to have researchers investigate matters through self-dialectical means or with others who share the same phenomenological experience. To achieve this goal, Moustakas (1990) identified six phases of research. Artists and art therapists will notice parallels with the creative process, particularly Allen's (2005) Open Studio Process, which is based on Jungian active imagination (Table 5.1). Although arts-based research has heuristic components, not all heuristic research involves art making. The similarities between arts-based research and heuristic inquiry are rooted in introspection (Barone & Eisner, 2012; McNiff, 2018). However, McNiff (2018) cautioned that arts-based research is more empirical due to the presence of the arts as physical artifacts for investigation.

As an example, Muldoon (2015) reviewed art making from earlier in her life following the death of her parents and created new art to reflect on how her grief had changed in the present moment. She identified themes in relation to the meaning-reconstruction theory. As a result, she was able to determine in which ways theory could help her make sense of her own bereavement, while also offering a personal perspective on the advantages and limitations of the model.

### Autoethnographic Research

Autoethnography approximates heuristic inquiry, but it intentionally places the subject in a social-cultural context to comment on how these

Table 5.1 Parallels between heuristic research phases and the open studio process

| Open studio process (Allen, 2005) | | Phases of Heuristic Research (Moustakas, 1990) | |
|---|---|---|---|
| Intention | "focusing awareness, it also has the function of creating boundaries ... In its boundary-creating capacity, intention limits and helps gives shape to what we receive" (p. 22) | Initial Engagement | "discover an intense interest, a passionate concern that calls out to the researcher, one that holds important social meanings and personal, compelling implications" (p. 27) |
| Art Making | "under the surface of our fixed ideas, is everything, all possibilities" (p. 28) | Immersion | "be on intimate terms with the question – to live it and grow in knowledge and understanding of it" (p. 28) |
| | | Incubation | "retreats from the intense, concentrated focus on the question ... on another level expansion of knowledge is taking place" (p. 28) |
| | | Illumination | "breakthrough into conscious awareness ... corrections of distorted understandings or disclosure of hidden meanings" (p. 29) |
| Witness | "The intention of writing is to extend the creative act, to promote the relationship between the artist and image, and to mediate the separation of the artist from the image as the art making time comes to a close" (p. 66) | Explication | "fully examine what has awakened in consciousness, to understand its various layers of meaning" (p. 31) |
| | | Creative Synthesis | "put the components and core themes into ... narrative ... or some other creative form" (p. 32) |

systemic forces impact the researcher's lived experiences (Denzin, 2014). The purpose is to present a narrative in a relational context that takes into account multiple facets of identity and how those facets are informed and impacted by historical and contemporary contexts pertaining to, but not limited to, conceptions of gender, race, sexuality, nationality, and ability.

The following examples describe arts-based research with an autoethnographic focus. Klorer's (2014) Guardhouse Project forced her to confront her neighborhood's discriminatory past to authentically present the stories of those who lived in her area. Her historical research and use of primary documents (letters, journals, meeting minutes) were combined through her own modern interpretation. Burrell (2016) initiated a focus group in which she and others could create art and discuss conceptions of belongingness as African American students in predominantly White art therapy programs to identify the racial dynamics that informed their educational experiences. In reviewing her clinical process notes and personal journals to note social identity factors, Linde (2017) created paintings and reflective writing that she coded according to White racial identity development theories to more fully understand cross-racial and cultural therapeutic interactions.

## Arts-Based Research Characteristics

Many scholars (i.e., Chilton & Leavy, 2014; Leavy 2015; McNiff, 2018) view arts-based research as its own unique methodology. Kapitan (2018) explained, "The outcomes of ABR [arts-based research] are grounded neither in the mathematical language of quantitative research nor in the words of qualitative research but in the symbolic language and forms of arts practices" (p. 213). Moreover, according to McNiff (2011),

> it is grounded in a common commitment to artistic knowing via the endlessly variable conditions of an artist's style, materials, process of expression and the structure of a particular project. Art is also a thoroughly physical activity that generates empirical data which in certain cases can be counted, measured and analysed, and so it cannot be exclusively called qualitative, in spite of its highly introspective features. Thus art-based inquiries are always empirical and can be quantitative and/or qualitative, as well as historical, philosophical, heuristic, phenomenological, hermeneutic, ethnographic and experimental.
>
> (p. 388)

In my own work as an arts-based researcher, I have at times struggled to define this methodology as truly separate from qualitative inquiry. However, this position risks diluting what arts-based research has to offer

128  Arts-Based Research

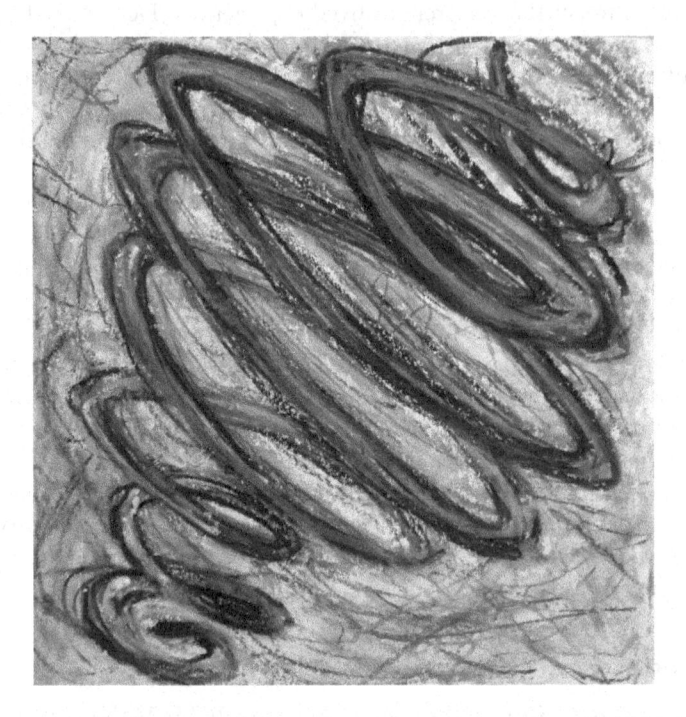

*Figure 5.3 Characteristics.* Secure Foundation Unencumbered, Unleashed Moves Knowledge Forward

and compels it to justify itself in relation to other research methods rather than viewing it from its own standard of truth (Smith, 2013). Reflecting on my art (Figure 5.3), I can see that my hesitation derives from a desire to maintain arts-based research within a secure base, but that I also understand its unique contributions that are unencumbered by traditional reductions of data into numbers or prosaic words. Whether entrenched in other research traditions or serving as its own, arts-based research has distinctive characteristics. In a similar manner, Kramer (1975) was a staunch voice for art therapists to maintain their own artistic practices and define aesthetics exclusive to our profession. Her conceptions of quality parallel important characteristics of arts-based research. By pairing them, I aim to help art therapists identify how arts-based research fits within our paradigms of working.

### *Evocative Power*

Kramer (1975) encouraged clients to create art with "evocative power" (p. 54), which can translate to basing one's art on one's lived experiences, emotions, memories, dreams, and impulses. McNiff (2011) recognized great value in researchers using their own art as a means to avoid exploiting the art of others to tell the researcher's own story, and limiting the tendency to reduce others' art to single dimensions informed by the research question. By reflecting on their own art, researchers are constantly reminded of intricacies, complexities, and tensions. Similarly, Carolan (2001) put forth:

> The image is what leads us and facilitates our moving beyond what we know toward the possible, or seemingly impossible. Art and art-based research can bridge the mystery in healing; they can facilitate the freeing and the holding of tacit knowledge that expands beyond the cognitive, linear ways of understanding. It is not science that we must move beyond, it is the concept that all that is real is that which can be confirmed through our senses.
>
> (p. 203)

Kramer's insistence on evocative quality was intended to not only ensure that the art is emotionally invested for the creator but is also provocative to the viewer. Compared to standard academic reporting, the arts stimulate the audience's emotional and political sensibilities (Leavy, 2015). Rather than presenting results that force a singular worldview, arts-based research encourages *conspiratorial conversations*; on-going discussions about prevailing worldviews (Barone, 2001).

## *Inner Consistency*

Kramer (1975) insisted that clients find the best match between the experience they intend to communicate and the image that can best convey it – a characteristic she identified as "inner consistency" (p. 54). Arts-based research values the use of vernacular rather than overly academic language to assure that it is understandable to a wide range of audiences. The focus is often on identifying metaphors that can transmit the essence of the experience, while still ensuring "a heightened degree of ambiguity" to evoke audience curiosity (Barone, 2001, p. 25). Metaphors have the advantage of employing images that allow for expression and a way for audiences to enter into another's worldview that transcends strictly literal portrayals (Boydell, Hodgins, Gladstone, & Stasiulis, 2017). The resulting art should give a sense that it is rooted in the researcher's personal style, voice, and "fingerprint" (Leavy, 2015, p. 280).

## *Economy of Means*

Kramer's (1975) final criteria of "economy of artistic means" (p. 54) pertains to artistic skill. Although many characterize art therapy as focused on process over product, Kramer saw an important role for artistry and technique. The importance of skill was to ensure that clients had the ability to adequately translate their images into physical form. Although Kramer was interested in how this would further sublimation, the parallel in arts-based research is the accuracy of transmitting the research findings. To honor the value of art, Chilton and Leavy (2014) argued that the resulting artworks need to be completed with enough skill so as to be able to effectively communicate and inspire.

Cahnmann-Taylor (2008) addressed the concern over skill by distinguishing between two types of aesthetics prevalent in arts-based research: *hybrid forms* and *art for scholarship's sake*. Hybrid forms blend art and social sciences in such a way that the distinction of where one ends and the other begins is difficult to discern. Audiences are aware that the presented art is based on the artist's experience of the data, but the art is not expected to prescribe solutions. The goal is to create an artifact that is recognized as art, but whose main function is to spread research findings. Similar to expressive arts therapist Knill's (2005) concept of *low skill/high sensitivity*, researchers are expected to have minimal artistic training, but a strong ability to use the artistic accomplishments to express meaningful ideas. In contrast, "art for scholarship's sake is grounded in extensive artistic training and aims to imbue art with socially engaged meaning from research and imbue socially engaged research with art" (Cahnmann-Taylor, 2008, pp. 10–11). Art skills are employed to convey findings in an engaged manner.

## Advantages of Arts-Based Research

Researchers should be aware of the advantages of arts-based research when making their choice to use it as a means of investigation. I noted how arts-based research offers energy and excitement as a means of furthering both introspection and changing the world (Figure 5.4).

### Honors Artistic Knowing

When studying a phenomenon firmly grounded in the arts, arts-based researchers use artistic engagement rather than interpreting image experiences into verbal expressions. McNiff (1998) wrote, "it may not be possible to transfer what we experience and know within the framework of painting to a verbal or spoken text" (p. 44). Arts-based research methods legitimize art therapy by using its own tools of inquiry. The arts are recognized for being able to express and communicate those experiences that are both non-verbal and outside certain levels of awareness (Chilton & Leavy, 2014).

Chilton and Scotti (2014) undertook collage making to investigate how this art form can inform research and function as a means

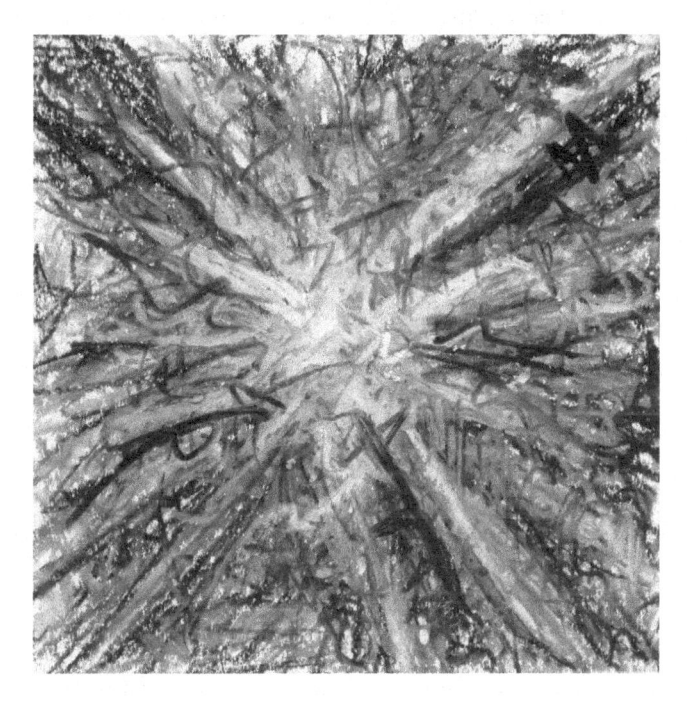

*Figure 5.4 Advantages.* Radiance All Around! Enlightening to Reach Inwards and Transcend Beyond!

of data-gathering and analysis. Their study demonstrated how collage furthered theoretical and practical layering and synthesis, enhanced their understanding of themselves as arts-based researchers, and kept them in constant contact with the creative process that was the source of their inquiry. Studying collage through collage allowed them to maintain focus on the material and process.

### Expands Knowledge

Arts-based research expands knowledge in a given area by illuminating what was formerly unknown to enable the imagining of new possibilities. By openly admitting that there are multiple perspectives to consider, arts-based researchers declare adherence to the notion that there are different ways to view a situation (Eisner, 2008; Sullivan, 2006). At the same time, art making provides additional means for data collection and triangulation.

Dickson (2017) committed to visual journaling to determine how it affected her stress, anxiety, and pain due to living with sickle cell disease.

Although some of her findings were expected, others were not. She discovered a persistent fear of death that she had not allowed herself to consciously confess, even though the mortality rate for the disorder is well documented. She also found that there were days when the art making was either not helpful or exacerbated her pain. The findings helped her to see the ways in which the process could lead to insights, but also to come to terms with the risks of art making pertaining to her unique lived experience.

### Encourages Creative Inquiry

A general criticism of an overly scientific approach to research is that it can lose its ability to honor "[u]ncertainty and mystery" (McNiff, 1998, p. 43), "creative enchantment," "magic in illuminating the scene" (Eisner, 2008, p. 20), and "imaginative insight" (Sullivan, 2006, p. 19). Research questions and hypotheses provide direction for a line of inquiry, but often reveal expected outcomes. Conversely, immersion in the creative process invites acceptance of the unknown, which transforms the nature of research as well as the researcher. Although there is always the possibility of failed experiments, creative engagement reminds us to be open to the infinite range of interpretations and outcomes.

Garlock and I explored the Jungian concepts of compensation (how the psyche generates images) and integration (how the significance becomes conscious) as central to the function of creativity for achieving wholeness (Potash & Garlock, 2016). Every day for 14 days, we each created art individually and engaged in reflective writing. In our analysis, we discovered shared outcomes related to structuring art making, invoking aesthetics to further meaning, experiencing uncertainty, and appreciating commonalities. Even though we were familiar with Jungian notions, through the research we were able to better appreciate them and develop empathy with clients' experiences of wonder, frustration, and insight.

### Extends Audience Reach

By presenting research results artistically, investigators open new platforms for sharing. Reaching beyond a limited academic audience engages the general public by inviting their participation through "dialogues of meaning" (Barone, 2008, p. 43). This stance considers research as a community act by bringing research into public spaces and engaging audiences in questions and searches for meaning (Cahnmann-Taylor, 2008; Leavy, 2015, 2018; Sanders, 2006).

Klorer (2014) presented the art from her Guardhouse Story as an exhibit titled *Art in Archives; Archives in the Art*. It was staged in a public library to share the findings within the community. Rather than simply offer the pieces, she hid them throughout the library to encourage viewers to seek out the information. The exhibition was followed by several art making workshops in which families brought their own memorabilia to combine with historical records to document their own ancestral story of the neighborhood.

### Raises Social Awareness

Arts-based research gives voice to those who otherwise may not be heard. Researcher-generated art can be a catalyst for sharing what was learned about the particular phenomenon or group of participants. One of the profound benefits of arts-based research is the way in which it aims to challenge stereotypes and promote empathy (Chilton & Leavy, 2014; Leavy, 2015). The resulting art is meant to disturb preconceptions to serve as an emancipatory catalyst by shifting mindsets through questions, rather than defining a singular worldview (Barone, 2001; 2008).

Fish's (2018) investigation of her clinical work led her to increased activism. She utilized response art to document her reactions and transference to her social welfare clients. Through drawing and painting, dialoguing with images, and reflective writing, Fish identified her own emotions as well as gaining valuable insight into how her clients experienced their situations and ways in which she viewed them. In addition to helping her keep her focus on her clients' well-being, she generated metaphors to inform colleagues. She also used the art pieces in her advocacy efforts to improve agency systems.

## Credibility of Arts-Based Research

In describing the challenges to arts-based research, Boydell, Hodgins, Gladstone, and Stasiulis (2017) summarized "the delicate balance ... to ensure both rigour and creativity" (p. 195). This delicate balance can be achieved through adherence to criteria for evaluating arts-based research, such as was offered by Leavy (2018): *methodology* (appropriateness of methods to answer research question), *usefulness, significance, or substantive contribution* (value of findings), *public scholarship* (accessibility), *audience response* (effect, encourage multiple interpretations), *aesthetics or artfulness* (quality and authenticity), *personal fingerprint or creativity* (researcher style), and *ethical practice* (multidimensional portrayals). Figure 5.5 revealed to me that there is importance in setting boundaries for evaluation, but that these boundaries may be better conceived as semipermeable rather than rigid. This position is reflected in Eisner (2008), whose ideas replace strict definitions of suitability with a continuum of considerations that "can also be motivating" and "evoke a sense of vitality" (p. 17). Approaching evaluation of arts-based research

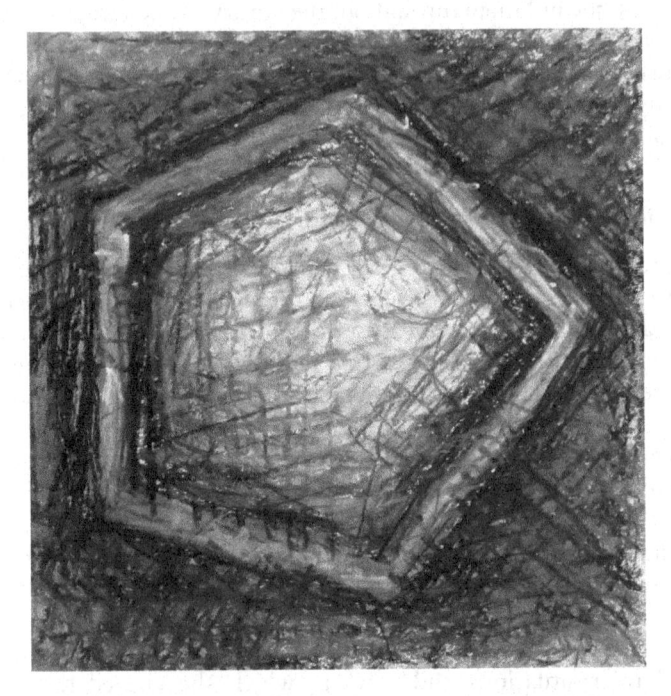

*Figure 5.5 Credibility.* A Demarcation of In and Out, Right and Wrong? Yes? No? Assurance

as a semipermeable process is further anchored in Eisner's model of credibility as appraised through five tensions: "work imaginatively" – "referential clarity" (p. 19); "particular" – "general" (p. 20); "aesthetics" – "verisimilitude" (p. 21); "better questions" (p. 22) – "better answers" (p. 23); and "objectivity" – "projection" (p. 24). Each of these is subsequently elucidated.

### Work Imaginatively – Referential Clarity

Art can be inspirational and expressive but should also contribute to knowledge. Too much expression without satisfactory communication makes the research inaccessible. One of the challenges to presenting clear findings is that arts-based researchers remain faithful to their experience within their comfort for self-disclosure (Manders & Chilton, 2013). Such research is biographical and personal, but it is not the same as an autobiography or memoir. There needs to be enough information for the results to be coherent and transparent, while also allowing researchers to determine how much they share personal experiences. To minimize this tension, Eisner (2006) recommended testing research by *referential adequacy*, "the extent to which we can locate what the critic claims is there" (p. 15).

## Particular – General

All research is concerned with the ability to generalize or transfer findings beyond the specific situation. Transferability in arts-based research should be approached as preventing the bias imposed by egocentrism to advance knowledge (McNiff, 2011). Furthermore:

> Suggestions of narcissism and the more general lack of understanding of how personal inquiry can generate objective and universally valid knowledge may be the most daunting obstacles to expanding the practice and acceptance of art-based research.... The creation of individualised methods and contents is the essential element of imaginative inquiry, and art-based researchers must have the freedom to do this while dealing with the inevitable need to establish a structure and useful outcomes.
>
> (p. 394)

Even when transferability is limited, researchers' insights into their study can inspire others in similar circumstances. Understanding how fiction yields truths (Kalmanowitz, 2013), Eisner (2008) compared literature to statistics to demonstrate how the arts promote complex connections that are lost in numbers alone.

## Aesthetics – Verisimilitude

Focusing too much on producing quality art can obscure the truth. Whereas attention to creative representation may overly accentuate the artwork, Eisner (2008) referenced how drama intentionally overplays scenes compared to real life for emphasis. Researchers need to be careful to focus on the art while maintaining a focus on the subject of inquiry. Leavy (2015) reframed this concern by replacing the question "'Is this a good piece of art?'" with "'What is this piece of art good for?' (Leavy, 2010, 2011a)" (p. 30). Ultimately, audience reaction can be an arbiter of the art's success in whether it conveyed its intended meaning (Franklin, 2012).

The tension pertaining to aesthetics revolves around a question of authenticity. Moustakas' (1990) guidelines for assessing heuristic research call attention to the degree to which the researcher asserts findings within "exhaustive self-searching" (p. 33) and rich descriptions of the process. Similarly, Kapitan (2018) offered three points of advice: (a) ensure a clear question, (b) maintain focus on the objective, and (c) articulate a clear plan.

## Better Questions – Better Answers

Academics may be willing to entertain theories and tolerate ambiguity, but frontline workers and policy makers often need direct answers for how research translates into practice. Arts-based research can unsettle preconceptions but should contribute to raising the quality of existing theories and services (Eisner, 2008). Chilton and Leavy (2014) insisted that researchers invest in the art making but retain focus on the study's aims as a test of success. Given the nature of the process, findings can maintain an open-endedness to encourage further exploration and curiosity.

## Objectivity – Projection

The crux of this argument entails the legitimacy of the arts in the research process given their subjective nature. Building in sufficient checks for rigor can include verifying results compared to existing literature, triangulating findings by other means, and providing a sufficient audit trail to document the process from data to results. At the same time, arts-based researchers need not be pulled into defending their objectivity as the methodology aims to heighten subjectivity. In my arts-based research into my feelings of apathy and frustration amid a socially engaged project, I discovered that the subjective nature of arts-based research granted me greater flexibility to move between objective and subjective stances depending on which was needed in any given moment (Potash, 2013).

## Steps for Conducting Arts-Based Research

Having outlined the basic tenets of arts-based research, I now introduce a pragmatic framework for employing this methodology. My artwork (Figure 5.6) reminded me of the importance of identifying these steps, while still allowing for a specific path to emerge for each individual study. As such, I articulate a process, but do not prescribe a particular approach.

### Researcher Stance

Undertaking arts-based research requires investigators to embrace and integrate several roles that combine to inform this unique mode of inquiry. I have come to see the importance of embracing various roles. The *artist* requires an ability to follow imagination and remain spontaneous, but to also engage craft and skill to bring art expression to its most polished form (Barone & Eisner, 2012; Leavy, 2015). The *scientist* invokes discipline, strategy, and methodology to hone a critical mindset (Franklin, 2012; Leavy, 2015; McNiff, 2011). The *adventurer*

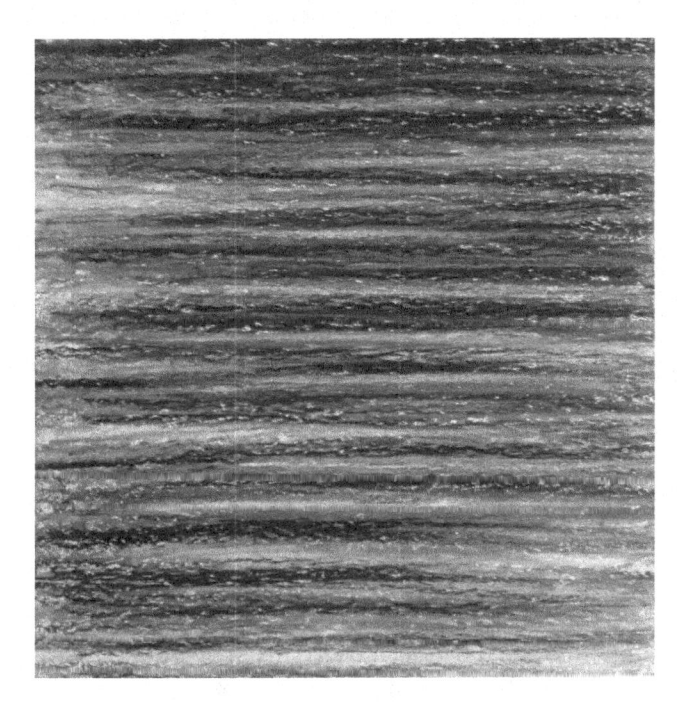

*Figure 5.6 Steps.* Layers Built upon a Groundwork Set to Reveal Steps along the Path

embraces the unknown while remaining committed to the journey or as Leavy (2015) wrote, "Worry less about being 'good' and focus on being engaged" (p. 31). The *witness* maintains a contemplative outlook that honors shifting thoughts and feelings, as well as bodily sensations and felt sense (Franklin, 2012; Rappaport, 2013).

### Research Question

Like all research, arts-based researchers begin with a focused research question or objective. McNiff (2011) recommended maintaining focus on simple questions to explain processes by answering "what, why, and how is this useful?" (p. 391). The basic characteristics of such research questions generally aim to reveal the essence of a situation and retain an exploratory qualitative nature, rather than predicting or searching for causal relationships among variables. In keeping with the focus on professional practice, research questions should have a clear connection to art therapy theories, practices, and circumstances. As examples, Fish (2013) explored response art, Chilton and Scotti (2014) investigated collage, and Kalmanowitz (2013) surveyed the studio environment. Leavy (2015) highlighted questions of identity for personal storytelling and intersections of social-cultural-political contexts. Einstein and Forinash (2013) demonstrated the intersections of personal and social contexts in relation to the Arab-Israeli conflict.

### Literature Review

Prior to initiating the study, arts-based researchers conduct a preliminary review of the literature. This does not need to be exhaustive at first but should ground the researcher to contextualize the work. This permits a secure footing, while also being able to be open to new interpretations that the investigation will unearth (McNiff, 2011). The review does not need to be limited to one's own field of study, but can embrace interdisciplinary sources (Kenny, 2012). Art therapists would benefit from infusing their own literature and that from related health professions with contributions from anthropology and artists. After the conclusion of the study, and either concurrent with or after the data analysis, researchers return to the literature as new ideas typically emerge.

### Procedures

The procedures are structured but open-ended to allow for the researcher to be guided by the creative encounter. McNiff (2011) identified the benefits of clearly outlined procedures for providing certainty, much as Rubin (2005) described how a *framework for freedom* can enhance creativity in striving for balance between freedom and structure as requisite for creative growth. As Barone (2001) explained, "the research of artists may not involve inquiry that is rigidly systematic, but neither is it merely 'intuitive' (an unfortunate adjective that serves to perpetuate a myth about how artists work)" (p. 26).

The created art should be accompanied by reflective writing and/or audio- or video-recordings as a means of documenting the process. Manders and Chilton (2013) referred to the conversion of art into narrative as *translation*. This important step is not intended to diminish the produced art as a communication unto itself but is intended to provide further reflection and eventually pave the way for data analysis. They recommended several strategies derived from the creative arts therapies. *Spill writing (free writing)* documents through continuous writing without attention to form. *Free association* mines the imagery and process for immediate symbols to delve beneath the surface of the artwork. *Creative dialogue* initiates a discussion with the art by setting it as a partner for conversation. *Poetry* allows for a creative interpretation that makes use of phrases that arise from the creative process and descriptive lines to describe elements of the artwork. *Story or fairytale* encourages researchers to engage fiction writing to stoke imagination. In addition to these written forms of translation, they also recommended creative arts strategies such as using another art media or form (music, movement, ...). Gerber and Myers-Coffman (2018) articulated three successive phases of translation: (a) *formative* (documenting immediate reactions and responses), (b) *assemblage, construction, an interpretation* (amplifying fragments with narrative and structure), and (c) *final synthesis – interpretation, representation, and dissemination* (aesthetically reconfigured).

Even though external ethical oversight from an institutional review board may not be required, researchers need to maintain responsibility for their procedural choices. Chief among these is attention to how researchers take care of themselves given the personal and intimate nature of both the phenomenon and the processes. It is important to keep in mind, however, that a certain amount of "angst" and "turmoil" is expected and necessary to usher "the breaking of forms to create anew" (McNiff, 2011, p. 392). Rumbold, Fenner, and Brophy-Dixon (2012) identified the risks of arts-based research as having the potential for feeling shame, causing the emergence of distressing ideas, revising unpleasant experiences, revealing family histories, upsetting relationships, disrupting worldviews, and rejecting of one's artistic choices or style. Researchers build in procedures to avoid dissociation and unnecessary pain or discomfort. Although there are risks in representing experiences in art, the authors concluded that the process ultimately yields the rewards of knowledge, power in vulnerability, and increased intimacy, as well as establishes both intrapersonal and interpersonal connections.

### Documentation

Researchers determine the best procedures for documenting their process throughout the study. These may include maintaining the actual art or retaining photographs and/or videos of procedures that are ephemeral or that do not leave a record (such as movement or improvisation). Each piece should be carefully documented with the date and other relevant contextual factors.

### Credibility

Ensuring credibility by giving attention to the five tensions throughout the process is key to maintaining authenticity in the process (Eisner, 2008). Often, it is helpful to employ a trusted adviser or work with colleagues (Rumbold, Fenner, & Brophy-Dixon, 2012). Ramanathan's (2004) study on visual journaling included weekly review of her art, reflections, and preliminary ideas with a peer reviewer. Similarly, Gibson (2018) shared her response art with a supervisor to identify themes pertinent to compassion fatigue and professional burnout to ensure authentic expressions and meaning making.

## Analysis

Even though researchers may have tacit understanding of what their art means to them, these claims need to be as explicit as possible. In many ways, this process may follow standard qualitative thematic analysis whereby researchers identify relevant themes, group them into categorical representations, and order them into a logical story (Braun & Clarke, 2006). When developing themes, researchers can use emergent methods to discover patterns within the data or search their art for predetermined themes based on established theories. For example, Weishaar (2017) studied his reactions to child inpatient psychiatric clients and analyzed his productions according to theories that pertain to countertransference reactions, as well as models of male therapist roles.

To honor the methodology, researchers maintain focus on both the art and written reflections or translations. Analyzing art considers both coding for objective features, often referred to as formal elements (composition, color, subject matter, ...), as well as semiotic analysis intended to ascertain the significance of the art (Creswell, 2016). The latter part is aided by the aforementioned translation procedures, whereas attention to the formal elements necessitates careful attention to the image.

Revisiting the data to distill it into significant findings may also invoke anguish. Qualitative researchers have long recognized the emotional toll of listening to others' stories of suffering (Creswell, 2016). Woodby, Williams, Wittich, and Burgio (2011) described this as "cumulative distress" that results from repeatedly engaging stories to uncover the underlying patterns of significance (p. 833). Whereas they are careful to distinguish this from vicarious traumatization reported in health professions, this type of emotional distress presents a potential complication for researchers being challenged by their own art (Manders & Chilton, 2013). In addition to building in self-care processes, researchers can allow for a period of incubation or time away from the data to come back to it with fresh eyes (Moustakas, 1990). This step is akin to the painter who walks away from her painting to come back to it another day. Refer to Box 5.1 at the end of this chapter for an illustrative example of arts-based data analysis as related to the Bringing Research to Life! research simulation experiential (Betts & Potash, 2018).

## Presentation

Arts-based researchers have several choices for presenting findings that range from scientific-style papers to exhibitions or performances. When writing, researchers follow the expectations set by dissertation committees or journal editorial boards. Arts-based researchers may not necessarily be tied to the standard scientific reporting format (introduction, methods, results, discussion) as often they need to include an abundance of art, the flexibility to make organic connections to describe their process, and a structure that adheres to the creative process (Atkins, 2012; McNiff, 2018; Smith, 2013). However, if this is required, researchers should privilege documentation of the artistic processes and derived significance, while carefully tending to standards of professional writing.

Outside the realm of thesis or article-style publications, arts-based researchers can disseminate their research through exhibitions, performances, and videos. Moon and Hoffman (2014) described a six-phase process of conducting and disseminating arts-based research that culminates in a performance, exhibition, or community-engaged project along with a contextual essay that documents the process and grounds it in relevant literature, theory, and practice. Just as essays go through several drafts and faculty review, performances are also presented in a series of rehearsals and critique workshops to assure that the researcher's meaning is sufficiently conveyed to the audience.

Guillemin and Cox (2017) warned that researchers need to consider the ethics of presenting. When arts-based research is based on participant data, then a research review board must approve the study. Even when participants provide their consent for the use of their information to be turned into art, researchers must be mindful of the degree to which the created art can identify participants. They must also consider who the audiences will be and how they may be affected. The idea of arts-based research is to stimulate questions and maybe even discomfort, but it should stop short of harming viewers. Prior to presenting the research, it can be helpful to prepare audiences by alerting them to the motivations for the art and aesthetic expectations, as well as providing them with an opportunity to reflect on their own reactions (Barone & Eisner, 2012; Boydell, Hodgins, Gladstone, & Stasiulis, 2017).

## Conclusion

For my final art piece, I surveyed the six artworks together as a montage and selected a phrase from each of the haikus to create an integrative poem (Figure 5.7). The image reinforced that, although arts-based research may at first appear to be nebulous, it offers exciting opportunities for investigators to make use of their own experiences and artistic endeavors to contribute new knowledge. Artists have long understood how their art making generates new awareness. Art therapists recognize this potential and infuse it with the health traditions to transform insights into meaningful actions that enhance one's self, relationships, and community. By relocating the creative process from personal and therapeutic practices to acts of scholarship, arts-based researchers harness artistic prowess within systematic inquiry to generate theory and practice.

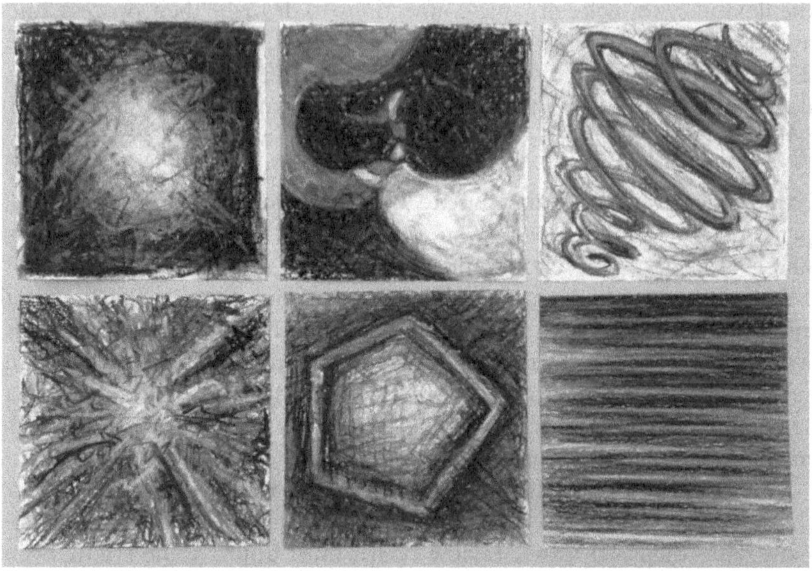

142  Arts-Based Research

*Figure 5.7 Conclusion.* Blurred Edges and Separate Streams Move Knowledge Forward, All Around. Assurance to Reveal Steps along the Path

---

**Box 5.1  Bringing Research to Life! Arts-Based Data Analysis Example**

**Objective:** Please refer to Box 1.1 (Chapter 1) and Appendix A for the purpose, set-up, and materials to guide the application of this experiential. (The online course cartridge materials for the instructor include a downloadable PowerPoint presentation that can be modified for use in the classroom.) The following provides information on the *arts-based* data analysis portion of the Bringing Research to Life! research simulation experiential (after the mock experiment and data collection has been completed):

| *Research Method* | *Experiential "Data"* | *"Findings"* |
|---|---|---|
| **Arts-Based/Heuristic** Research question: *What is the lived experience of graduate art therapy students' engagement in an immersive art experience?* | Thematic analysis of response art and content analysis of accompanying reflective writing. | In-depth understanding of one's own experiences, thoughts, and emotions. |

Source: Betts and Potash (2018).

# References

Albert-Proos, D. (2015). Separation from and reconstruction of home: A study of immigrant expressive arts therapists (doctoral dissertation, Lesley University, Cambridge, MA).

Allen, P. B. (1995). *Art is a way of knowing*. Boston, MA: Shambhala.

Allen, P. B. (2005). *Art is a spiritual path*. Boston, MA: Shambhala.

Allen, P. B. (2012). Art as enquiry: Towards a research method that holds soul truth. *Journal of Applied Arts & Health, 3*(1), 13–20. Retrieved from https://doi.org/10.1386/jaah.3.1.13_1

Archibald, M. M. & Gerber, N. (2018). Arts and mixed methods research: An innovative methodological merger. *American Behavioral Scientist, 62*(7), 956–977. Retrieved from https://doi.org/10.1177/0002764218772672

Atkins, S. (2012). Where are the five chapters? Challenges and opportunities in mentoring students with art-based dissertations. *Journal of Applied Arts & Health, 3*(1), 59–66. Retrieved from https://doi.org/10.1386/jaah.3.1.59_1

Barone, T. (2001). Science, art, and the predispositions of educational researchers. *Educational Researcher, 30*(7), 24–28.

Barone, T. (2008). How arts-based research can change minds. In M. Cahnmann-Taylor & R. Siegesmund (Eds.), *Arts-based research in education: Foundations for practice* (pp. 28–49). New York, NY: Routledge.

Barone, T. & Eisner, E. (2012). *Arts based research*. Thousand Oaks, CA: Sage.

Betts, D. J. & Potash, J. (2018). Research simulation experiential: Bringing research to life! (personal collection of D. Betts and J. Potash, the George Washington University, Washington, DC).

Boydell, K. M., Hodgins, M. J., Gladstone, B. M., & Stasiulis, E. (2017). Ineffable knowledge: Tensions (and solutions) in art-based research representation and dissemination. *Journal of Applied Arts & Health, 8*(2), 193–207. Retrieved from https://doi.org/10.1386/jaah.8.2.193_1

Braun, V. & Clarke, V. (2006). Using thematic analysis in psychology. *Qualitative Research in Psychology, 3*(2), 77–101. Retrieved from https://doi.org/10.1191/1478088706qp063oa

Burrell, S. S. (2016). Increasing racial diversity in the field of art therapy: Recruitment and retention of African American students (master's culminating project, the George Washington University, Washington, DC).

Cahnmann-Taylor, M. (2008). Arts-based research: Histories and new directions. In M. Cahnmann-Taylor & R. Siegesmund (Eds.), *Arts-based research in education: Foundations for practice* (pp. 3–15). New York, NY: Routledge.

Chilton, G. (2013). Altered inquiry: Discovering arts-based research through an altered book. *International Journal of Qualitative Methods, 12*(1), 457–477. Retrieved from https://doi.org/10.1177/160940691301200123

Chilton, G. & Leavy, P. (2014). Arts-based research practice: Merging social research and the creative arts. In P. Leavy (Ed.), *The Oxford handbook of qualitative research* (pp. 403–422), Oxford: Oxford University Press.

Chilton, G. & Scotti, V. (2014). Snipping, gluing, writing: The properties of collage as an arts-based research practice in art therapy. *Art Therapy: Journal of the American Art Therapy Association, 31*(4), 163–171. Retrieved from https://doi.org/10.1080/07421656.2015.963484

Creswell, J. W. (2016). *30 essential skills for the qualitative researcher.* Los Angeles, CA: Sage

Dejkameh, M. (2016). The art therapist as a nomadic force: A proposition for contemporary practice (doctoral thesis, Mount Mary University, Milwaukee, WI).

Denzin, N. K. (2014). *Interpretive autoethnography.* Thousand Oaks, CA: Sage.

Dickson, R. (2017). Finding ways to cope with sickle cell disease using mandalas and art journaling: An arts-based heuristic study (master's culminating project, the George Washington University, Washington, DC).

Einstein, T. & Forinash, M. (2013). Art as a mother tongue: Staying true to an innate language of knowing. *Journal of Applied Arts & Health, 4*(1), 77–85. Retrieved from https://doi.org/10.1386/jaah.4.1.77_1

Eisner, E. (2006). Does arts-based research have a future? *Studies in Art Education, 48*(1), 9–18.

Eisner, E. (2008). Persistent tensions in arts-based research. In M. Cahnmann-Taylor & R. Siegesmund (Eds.), *Arts-based research in education: Foundations for practice* (pp. 16–27). New York, NY: Routledge.

Fish, B. J. (2013). Painting research: Challenges and opportunities of intimacy and depth. *Journal of Applied Arts & Health, 4*(1), 105–115. Retrieved from https://doi.org/10.1386/jaah.4.1.105_1

Fish, B. J. (2018). Drawing and painting research. In P. Leavy (Ed.), *Handbook of arts-based research* (pp. 336–354). New York, NY: Guilford Press.

Franklin, M. A. (2012). Know thyself: Awakening self-referential awareness through art-based research. *Journal of Applied Arts & Health, 3*(1), 87–96. Retrieved from https://doi.org/10.1386/jaah.3.1.87_1

Gerber, N. & Myers-Coffman, K. (2018). Translation in arts-based research. In P. Leavy (Ed.), *Handbook of arts-based research*, (pp. 587–607). New York, NY: Guilford Press.

Gibson, D. (2018). A visual conversation with trauma: The use of visual journaling in art therapy to combat vicarious trauma. *Art Therapy: Journal of the American Art Therapy Association, 35*(2), 99–103. Retrieved from https://doi.org/10.1080/07421656.2018.1483166

Guillemin, M. & Cox, S. (2017). Audience engagement and impact: Ethical considerations in art-based health research. *Journal of Applied Arts and Health, 8*(2), 141–153. Retrieved from https://doi.org/10.1386/jaah.8.2.141_1

Hunter, A., Lusardi, P., Zucker, D., Jacelon, C., & Chandler, G. (2002). Making meaning: The creative component in qualitative research. *Qualitative Health Research, 12*(3), 388–398. Retrieved from https://doi.org/10.1177/104973202129119964

Irwin, R. L. (2013). Becoming a/r/tography. *Studies in Art Education, 54*(3), 198–215.

Irwin, R. L. & de Cosson, A. (Eds.). (2004). *A/r/tography: Rendering self through arts-based living inquiry.* Vancouver, BC: Pacific Educational Press.

Jung, K. G. (2009). *The red book: Liber novus* (S. Shamdasani, Ed.). New York, NY: W.W. Norton.

Kaiser, D. H. & Kay, L. (2015). Arts-based research: The basics for art therapists. In D. E. Gussak & M. L. Rosal (Eds.), *The Wiley handbook of art therapy* (pp. 663–672). New York: NY: Wiley.

Kalmanowitz, D. (2013). On the seam: Fiction as truth. What can art do? *Journal of Applied Arts & Health, 4*(1), 37–47. Retrieved from https://doi.org/10.1386/jaah.4.1.37_1

Kapitan, L. (2018). *Introduction to art therapy research* (2nd ed.). New York, NY: Routledge.

Kenny, G. (2012). An introduction to Moustakas's heuristic method. *Nurse Researcher, 19*(3), 6–11.

Klorer, P. G. (2014). My story, your story, our stories: A community art-based research project. *Art Therapy: Journal of the American Art Therapy Association, 31*(4), 146–154. Retrieved from https://doi.org/10.1080/07421656.2015.963486

Knill, P. (2005). Foundation for a theory of practice. In P. Knill, E. Levine & S. Levine (Eds.), *Principles and practice of expressive therapy: Toward a therapeutic aesthetic* (pp. 75–170). London: Jessica Kingsley.

Knowles, J. G. & Cole, A. L. (Eds.). (2008). *Handbook of the arts in qualitative research: Perspectives, methodologies, examples, and issues*. Thousand Oaks, CA: Sage.

Kramer, E. (1975). The problem of quality in art. In E. Ulman & P. Dachinger (Eds.), *Art therapy in theory and practice* (pp. 43–59). Chicago, IL: Magnolia Street Publishers.

Leavy, P. (2015). *Method meets art: Arts-based research practice* (2nd ed.). New York, NY: Guilford Press.

Leavy, P. (2018). Criteria for evaluating arts-based research. In P. Leavy (Ed.), *Handbook of arts-based research* (pp. 575–586). New York, NY: Guilford Press.

Linde, H. (2017). Experiencing differences: A heuristic study using art making and reflective journaling to aid in cultural competency (master's culminating project, the George Washington University, Washington, DC).

Manders, E. & Chilton, G. (2013). Translating the essence of dance: Rendering meaning in artistic inquiry of the creative arts therapies. *International Journal of Education & the Arts, 14*(16). Retrieved from www.ijea.org/v14n16/

McNiff, S. (1998). *Art-based research*. Philadelphia, PA: Jessica Kingsley.

McNiff, S. (2011). Artistic expressions as primary modes of inquiry. *British Journal of Guidance & Counselling, 39*(5), 385–396.

McNiff, S. (Ed.). (2013). *Art as research: Opportunities and challenges*. Chicago, IL: Intellect.

McNiff, S. (2014). Art speaking for itself: Evidence that inspires and convinces. *Journal of Applied Arts and Health, 5*(2), 255–262.

McNiff, S. (2018). Philosophical and practical foundations of artistic inquiry: Creating paradigms, methods, and presentations based in art. In P. Leavy (Ed.), *Handbook of arts based research* (pp. 22–36). New York, NY: Guilford Press.

Moon, B. L. & Hoffman, N. (2014). Performing art-based research: Innovation in graduate art therapy education. *Art Therapy: Journal of the American Art Therapy Association, 31*(4), 172–178. Retrieved from https://doi.org/10.1080/07421656.2015.963485

Moustakas, C. (1990). *Heuristic research: Design, methodology, and applications*. Newbury Park, CA: Sage.

Muldoon, K. (2015). The exploration of post-loss art through the lens of meaning-reconstruction and art therapy: A heuristic study (master's culminating project, the George Washington University, Washington, DC).
Potash, J. S. (2013). A more complete knowing: The subjective objective partnership. *Journal of Applied Arts and Health, 4*(1), 49–56. Retrieved from https://doi.org/10.1386/jaah.4.1.49_1
Potash, J. S. & Garlock, L. R. (2016). Unconscious compensation and integration: Art making for wholeness and balance. In K. Madden (Ed.), *The unconscious roots of creativity* (pp. 189–216). Asheville, NC: Chiron.
Ramanathan, D. (2004). A mirror and more: An art therapist researcher's heuristic exploration of the drawing journal as a tool for reflection and well-being. *Qualitative Research Journal, 4*(1), 26–51.
Rappaport, L. (2013). Trusting the felt sense in art-based research. *Journal of Applied Arts & Health, 4*(1), 97–104. Retrieved from https://doi.org/10.1386/jaah.4.1.97_1
Rubin, J. A. (2005). *Child art therapy* (25th anniversary ed.). Hoboken, NJ: Wiley.
Rumbold, J., Fenner, P., & Brophy-Dixon, J. (2012). The risks of representation: Dilemmas and opportunities in art-based research. *Journal of Applied Arts & Health, 3*(1), 67–78. Retrieved from https://doi.org/10.1386/jaah.3.1.67_1
Sanders, J. H. III. (2006). Performing arts-based education research: An epic drama of practice, precursors problems and possibilities. *Studies in Art Education, 48*(1), 89–107.
Smith, T. D. (2013). Shall I hide an art-based study within a recognized qualitative framework? Negotiating the spaces between research traditions at a research university. *Journal of Applied Arts & Health, 4*(1), 87–95. Retrieved from https://doi.org/10.1386/jaah.4.1.87_1
Sullivan, G. (2006). Research acts in art practice. *Studies in Art Education, 48*(1), 19–35.
Wadsworth Hervey, L. (2000). *Artistic inquiry in dance/movement therapy*. Springfield, IL: Charles C Thomas.
Weishaar, M. (2017). Understanding empathy and countertransference through art making (master's culminating project, the George Washington University, Washington, DC).
Williamson, T. & Long, A. F. (2005). Qualitative data analysis using data displays. *Nurse Researcher, 12*(3), 7–19.
Woodby, L. L., Williams, B. R., Wittich, A. R., & Burgio, K. L. (2011). Expanding the notion of researcher distress: The cumulative effects of coding. *Qualitative Health Research, 21*(6), 830–838. Retrieved from https://doi.org/10.1177/1049732311402095

Chapter 6

# Mixed Methods Research in Art Therapy

Mixed methods research (MMR) consists of just what the phrase sounds like: combining quantitative and qualitative research approaches in specific ways using rigorous, epistemologically sound methods. Researchers have long combined quantitative and qualitative methods but only in the last 25 years or so has MMR emerged as a distinct methodology in and of itself (Creswell, 2015). During those 25 years, hundreds of pages of journal articles and book chapters have been devoted to debating and puzzling out the definitions, methods, and philosophies underlying MMR. Thus, MMR can be considered an emerging methodology, with more developments surely to come in the future. Johnson and Onwuegbuzi (2004) defined MMR as "the class of research where the researcher mixes or combines quantitative and qualitative research techniques, approaches, concepts or language into a single study" (p. 17) and called MMR the "third research movement" (p. 17) beyond quantitative and qualitative research. Creswell (2015) provided this succinct definition of MMR as:

> [a]n approach to research in the social, behavioral, and health sciences in which the investigator gathers both quantitative (closed-ended) and qualitative (open-ended) data, integrates the two, and draws interpretations based on the combined strengths of both sets of data to understand research problems.
>
> (p. 2)

Key to Creswell's definition is the notion of integration of quantitative data (which provides breadth in understanding a researched phenomenon) and qualitative data (which provides depth in understanding a researched phenomenon). The integration of data is thought to provide deeper and more complete answers to research questions than either type of data could by itself; this is the primary rationale for conducting MMR. However, debate continues regarding how to clearly define MMR; whether two divergent stances on research, postpositivism and constructivism, can be logically combined into a single methodology;

whether MMR favors quantitative methods over qualitative methods; specifics on research designs; and the like (Creswell, 2011; Johnson, Onwuegbuzie, & Turner, 2007). This chapter introduces basic concepts associated with MMR.

A rationale for using MMR must be clarified before proceeding with a study. In addition to the primary rationale of obtaining both qualitative and quantitative data to provide comprehensive answers to research questions, "mixed methods present the best of both worlds in that they can strengthen a study's validity and compensate for the limitations or weaknesses of any one method" (Kapitan, 2018, p. 103). MMR appears to be growing in the art therapy field, with many art therapy researchers combining quantitative and qualitative data in studies; however, only a few have described in depth the rationale for doing so or the MMR design they have employed, and interestingly, no MMR studies were included in Slayton, D'Archer, and Kaplan's (2010) analysis of art therapy outcome studies, although quantitative studies and qualitative studies were. The results of Kaiser and Deaver's 2013 Delphi study of art therapy research identified researching "the processes that occur in art therapy treatment and contribute to its effectiveness" (p. 119) as a priority, and MMR was identified as among the preferred approaches to use. Indeed, the "processes and mechanisms of art therapy" (p. 116) are elusive, although there is promising research on art and neuroscience that may eventually yield insights into the mechanisms of change in art therapy (King, 2016; King et al., 2017). However, currently MMR presents the opportunity to learn through qualitative inquiry research participants' thoughts about and responses to art therapy interventions, processes, and experiences, thus illuminating aspects of the quantitative results that would otherwise remain obscure. Conversely, adding quantitative methods, which are designed to test hypotheses, to a qualitative investigation may provide "hard data" that could lead to much needed theory development in the field.

## Underlying Philosophy

A paradigm is a worldview or philosophical position on the nature of social or behavioral phenomena, and when applied to research, the researcher's embrace of a particular paradigm informs her or his choice of methodological approach. In the introductory chapter of this book, we discussed research paradigms associated with the differing research approaches. Quantitative research, with its pillars of objectivity, generalization, and replication, is philosophically associated with the positivist and postpositivist paradigms whereas qualitative research, emphasizing context and collaborative generation of knowledge, is associated with the constructivist paradigm. The paradigm of *pragmatism* is most often associated with MMR (Biesta, 2010; Greene, 2007; Feilzer, 2010;

Johnson & Grey, 2010; Johnson & Onwuegbuzie, 2004). Pragmatism simply means doing what makes the most sense; in the case of MMR, pragmatism is related to both philosophy and methods and suggests applying the most logical combination of quantitative and qualitative approaches and methods to answer research questions.

Taking into account the tensions that exist between postpositivist and constructivist paradigms, Greene (2007) advocated for a *dialectic* paradigm for MMR, declaring:

> I view the mixing of methods overall as a methodological strategy that can yield better understanding of the phenomena being studied than can a single method, as all methods each offer but one perspective, one partial view. And I believe that better understanding takes its most important form as generative insights, which are in turn best attained through a respectful conversation among … many different ways of seeing and knowing.
>
> (p. 79)

Johnson and Grey (2010) integrated Greene's position on dialecticism into their advocacy of *dialectical pragmatism* as the paradigm most philosophically akin to MMR since it requires the researcher's careful consideration of multiple perspectives throughout the research process, rejects an "either/or" stance in favor of philosophical and methodological integration, and permits the creative construction of innovative research approaches to answer an array of research questions in the social, behavioral, and health sciences. Gerber (2016) asserted that, because art therapy's origins are diverse – including psychoanalysis and psychology; humanism; art history, art, and aesthetics; and science – and embrace and include both postpositivist, constructivist, and transformational worldviews, MMR is a synergetic philosophical match for art therapy research. She declared that, "the dynamic aesthetic, intersubjective, and dialectical nature of art therapy parallels the philosophical assumptions and methodologies of mixed methods research, which embraces creativity, pluralism, eclecticism, dynamism, and dialecticism in pursuit of truth and knowledge" (p. 804). Thus, MMR provides an approach to art therapy research that is congruent with art therapists' ways of knowing, and holds great promise for moving the field forward.

## Required Skills

Art therapists who wish to conduct MMR must have both qualitative and quantitative research skills (Creswell, 2015; Fraenkel, Wallen, & Hyun, 2012). This suggests that mixed methods researchers must be able to integrate the two different paradigms involved – constructivist and postpositivist – into a coherent study design that provides a strong rationale for combining the two types of data. This integration of paradigms requires an appreciation that there are "multiple ways of seeing and hearing, multiple ways of making sense of the social world, and multiple standpoints on what is important and to be valued" (Greene, 2007, p. 20). Thus, an ability to embrace this "mixed methods way of thinking" (p. 20) is a basic requirement in addition to an aptitude for both types of research. This includes the ability to formulate both research hypotheses and research questions to focus and drive a study.

Executing certain MMR designs requires not only these skills but also considerable time and energy. For example, in a program evaluation MMR study, data would need to be gathered before, during, and after the program of interest, from multiple stakeholders, with analysis occurring simultaneously for some data and after the study for other data. Such a study would benefit from a research team, which consists of individuals with a range of theoretical orientations and professional skills, such as the principal investigator (optimally an art therapist); other investigators from other fields such as neuroscientists or psychologists; a psychometrician involved in design and quantitative data analysis; and a group of research assistants who would assist in consent procedures, data collection, and qualitative data analysis. Crucial to the success of such studies is how effectively the research team interacts to achieve the study aims (Creswell, 2015). Interdisciplinary research has been encouraged and supported in art therapy (Kaiser & Deaver, 2013; Knowles & Cole, 2008), and has been carried out, particularly in medical settings [see, for example, Monti et al. (2006) and Nainis et al. (2006)], but these have not often been identified as using mixed methods designs.

In MMR, formulating research questions is an additional necessary and unique skill because it is important to have three types of research questions to guide a study: (a) quantitative questions, (b) qualitative questions, and (c) mixed methods questions (Creswell, 2015; Watkins & Gioia, 2015). Although it would be possible to substitute a hypothesis for the quantitative questions, it is more common for mixed methods researchers to use "quantitative questions" that are constructed to be answered through the quantitative strand(s) of the MMR study. Examples of quantitative questions would include, "Is there a statistically significant difference between the pretest and posttest depression scores of older adults participating in group art therapy?" or "Is there a relationship between number of art therapy sessions attended and improvement in participants' depression scores?" Qualitative research questions typically focus on the *how* and *why* of participants' experiences; an example would be "How did participants experience the various art therapy processes and materials that were utilized in the intervention?" Mixed methods research questions are not simply a compilation of quantitative and qualitative questions. Instead, mixed methods questions address the integration or merging of quantitative and qualitative data. For example, a mixed methods question might be "How do the qualitative results amplify or explain the quantitative results?" (Creswell & Plano Clark, 2011).

## Mixed Methods Research Designs

Scholars have presented a range of typologies for combining qualitative and quantitative data in MMR designs. For example, Fraenkel et al. (2012) described three: exploratory, explanatory, and triangulation designs, and Hanson, Creswell, Plano Clark, Petska, and Creswell (2005) described two broad typologies: sequential and concurrent. Sequential designs are those in which the collection of the two different types of data occurs one after the other, and concurrent designs are those in which both types of data are collected simultaneously throughout a study. The typologies described by Creswell (2015) and Creswell and Plano Clark (2011) are most commonly referred to in the literature (Caruth, 2013; Greene, 2007; Guest, 2012; Watkins & Gioia, 2015). Creswell's most recent typology (2015) of six designs is presented here. He classified the first three designs as basic, and the final three as advanced, and clarified that basic designs are common to all MMR, whereas advanced designs are basic designs with particular additions. The designs are described below; all figures illustrating the designs are adapted from the following sources: Creswell (2015), Creswell and Plano Clark (2011), and Watkins and Gioia (2015).

### Convergent Parallel (Basic)

In this design, illustrated in Figure 6.1, quantitative and qualitative data are collected separately, and then analyzed and merged (Creswell, 2015). According to Creswell and Plano Clark (2011), the purpose of the convergent parallel design is to optimally understand the research problem through collecting "different but complementary data on the same topic" (Morse, 1991, p. 122). The approach includes triangulation of the two types of data for purposes of comparison, validation, and

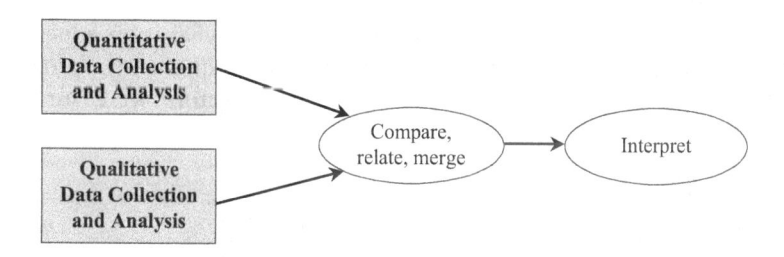

*Figure 6.1* Convergent parallel design

synthesis. The convergent parallel design typifies the pragmatic philosophical and methodological paradigm discussed above.

Kaimal, Rattigan, Miller, and Haddy (2016) studied the findings from a 2012 national Survey of Public Participation in the Arts (SPPA), which was administered by the US National Endowment for the Arts, in order to understand the applicability of specific data from the survey to art therapy practice. The SPPA, which is conducted periodically in conjunction with the US Census Bureau, seeks information from a large random sample of adult American citizens regarding their involvement in a diverse range of artistic and cultural endeavors (ibid.). To yield quantitative data, Kaimal et al. conducted a secondary analysis of the SPPA results by analyzing select data pertaining to participant demographics and to their use of digital media including art making and art sharing. Statistical analysis yielded descriptive data on participants' use of digital media to access, make, or share visual art. Qualitative data consisted of the authors' written reflections on the results of the secondary analysis. Although the method for analyzing the qualitative data in this study is unclear, the integration/merging of data in the research report is illuminating. It consists of a discussion of the secondary survey results along with individual authors' personal reflections in narrative form, and specific implications of the study for art therapy research, practice, education, and for art therapists' personal art making.

### *Explanatory Sequential (Basic)*

In this design, illustrated in Figure 6.2, first quantitative data are collected and then qualitative data are collected. The qualitative data collection follows logically based upon the quantitative results. The purpose of this approach is to use qualitative data to amplify or explain quantitative results. Philosophically, the design moves from postpositivist to constructivist so the researcher must be able to embrace both paradigms (Creswell & Plano Clark, 2011). Deaver's 2012 study of art-based learning in art therapy education is an example of an explanatory sequential MMR design.

There were two phases of the study, which was designed to answer questions regarding what sort of art-based learning techniques were used in master's level art therapy education, and what were educators' and recent graduates' experiences with these techniques and approaches (Deaver, 2012). First, art therapy program directors were surveyed

Quantitative Data Collection and Analysis — Followed by → Qualitative Data Collection and Analysis → Interpret

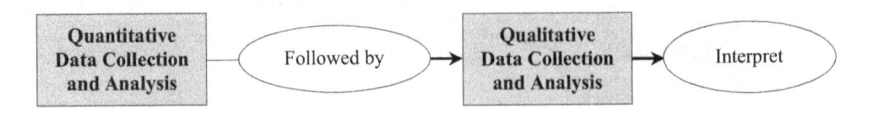

*Figure 6.2* Explanatory sequential design

electronically regarding which courses and which art-based learning strategies were implemented in their programs. Then, both program directors and recent graduates were contacted electronically with requests to participate in semi-structured interviews, and the interviews were conducted. Thus the study yielded two data sets: quantitative data from the survey and qualitative data from the interviews. The electronic survey software calculated frequency counts of the responses to survey questions, and a thematic analysis of the transcribed interviews was conducted.

The results were presented separately and then merged in the discussion section of the research report. The survey results were displayed in bar graphs that illustrated in which courses and at what frequency specific art-based learning approaches were implemented. The thematic analysis results were explicated through verbatim quotes from participant interviews, and illuminated the survey results through six themes: the integrative function of art-based learning; personal growth and development resulting from such strategies; documentation of experience in classes and internship; transfer to clinical work from classroom and personal art making; privacy concerns regarding art making in the classroom setting; and ambivalence regarding grading student artwork on the part of both program directors and recent graduates (Deaver, 2012). The results suggested that "using art-based learning strategies in art therapy graduate education supports broad educational goals such as knowledge of specific course content, clinical sensitivity and skill, and self-awareness" (p. 164). The use of mixed methods deepened understanding of the topic studied, as the interview data enhanced the survey results.

### Exploratory Sequential (Basic)

The exploratory sequential design (see Figure 6.3) utilizes three phases of research to develop instruments, measures, or intervention strategies that emerge from the experiences of research participants in the study (Creswell, 2015). The three phases consist of the first qualitative phase, then a quantitative phase, followed by the final, qualitative, phase. Onwuegbuzie, Bustamante, and Nelson (2010) described an elaborate process, consisting of ten phases, of quantitative and qualitative data collection, field testing, revisions, and analyses for the purpose of instrument development and construct validation of the instrument.

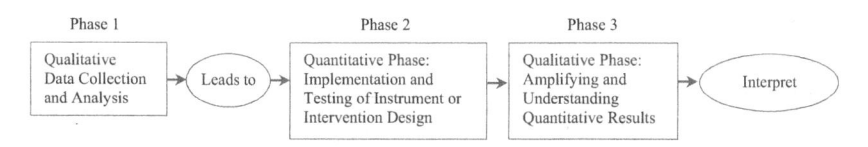

*Figure 6.3* Exploratory sequential design

Onwuegbuzie et al. asserted that this method yields more in-depth information for instrument development than do traditional, solely quantitative test development methods. It is likely that, with the exception of Gantt's Formal Elements Art Therapy Scale (1990), no art therapy instrument or assessment has undergone such rigorous development. In fact, it appears that no art therapy or music therapy research has employed the exploratory sequential design (Bradt, Burns, & Creswell, 2013).

In addition to instrument development, the exploratory sequential design is useful for developing effective interventions (Creswell, 2015). In designing and executing such a study, an art therapist would first engage in a qualitative inquiry of participants regarding, for example, their responses to the art therapy processes and materials implemented in six sessions of group art therapy. The inquiry, in the form of semi-structured interviews designed to understand the participants' experiences in group art therapy, could focus on art therapy processes and materials considered by the participants to be most effective in meeting specific treatment goals such as reduced symptoms of depression. Based upon the results of the first phase thematic analysis of the interviews, the researcher would then implement the art therapy processes and materials judged most successful by the first phase participants in a quantitative phase. There would be another six weeks of group art therapy with different participants, and pre and post standardized measures would be used to test the effectiveness of the identified art therapy processes and materials in meeting treatment goals. Then, based upon the results of statistical analysis of the difference between scores on the pre and post measures, the final, qualitative, phase could involve semi-structured interviews of participants as in the first phase, perhaps enhanced by qualitative analysis of art produced by participants. Using this design, art therapy researchers could discover implications for more effective practice, including data relevant to understanding the mechanisms underlying change that occurs through engagement in art therapy.

### *Intervention or Embedded Design (Advanced)*

This design, illustrated in Figure 6.4, entails collecting and embedding either quantitative or qualitative data within either a traditional quantitative design or a traditional qualitative design in a single study or a series of related studies. If the major part of the study is qualitative, the embedded part would be quantitative, and vice versa. For example, a researcher designing a primarily qualitative study such as a case study could embed some quantitative data collection within the design. Creswell and Plano Clark (2011) referred to this as the embedded design, whereas Creswell (2015) subsequently limited the approach to combining a randomized controlled trial with qualitative data and called it the intervention design. This shifting and refining of definitions is characteristic of the emergent nature of MMR, as noted above.

```
┌─────────────────────────────────────┐
│    Randomized Controlled Trial       │
│                                      │
│    Quantitative Data Collection      │         ┌──────────┐
│   (pretests and posttests) and Analysis │ ──> │ Interpret │
│                                      │         └──────────┘
│   ┌──────────────────────────────┐  │
│   │  Qualitative Data Collection │  │
│   │  and Analysis (before, during,│  │
│   │          and after)          │  │
│   └──────────────────────────────┘  │
└─────────────────────────────────────┘
```

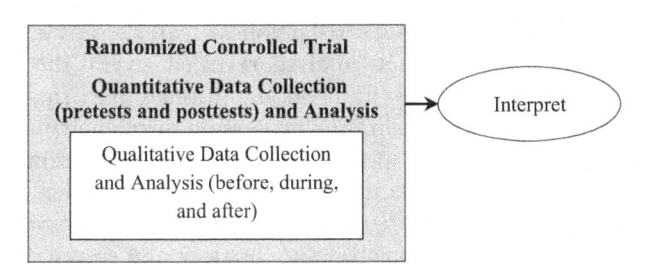

*Figure 6.4* Embedded/intervention design

In discussing the advantages of mixed methods approaches in trauma research, Creswell and Zhang (2009) noted that, in an embedded intervention design, "the quantitative data provide only a rough indicator of why the intervention worked or did not work" (p. 618) and that qualitative interviews provide a "fine-grained understanding" (p. 618) that standardized measures cannot. Along these lines, Boeije, Drabble, and O'Cathain (2015) noted that, "the need to address questions related to the how and why interventions work through understanding mechanisms of action and the transferability of the evidence has led to the inclusion of qualitative methods within [RTCs]" (p. 120).

The research on art therapy with veterans with posttraumatic stress disorder (PTSD) that has emerged from Campbell's (2014) thesis is an example of an art therapy study that used an embedded design, with qualitative data collection embedded within a randomized controlled experiment. The study compared the effect upon veterans with combat PTSD of eight sessions of individual Cognitive Processing Therapy (CPT) and eight additional individual verbal therapy sessions to eight sessions of CPT with an additional eight sessions of individual art therapy (Campbell, Decker, Kruk, & Deaver, 2016). The mixed methods design included quantitative measures of PTSD symptoms and depression as well as subjective ratings of participants' satisfaction with treatment. In addition, semi-structured interviews were administered individually before and after the intervention to provide qualitative data for analysis. Participants were randomized to either the experimental condition of CPT + art therapy, or the control condition of CPT + additional verbal therapy sessions; five completed the experimental intervention and six completed the control intervention. Data collected on pre and post valid and reliable standardized depression and PTSD outcome measures were analyzed statistically, and treatment satisfaction was measured with a Likert scale. Thematic analysis methods were used to analyze the individual interviews as well as participant artwork. The results were promising, as both groups improved statistically significantly on both the

PTSD and depression outcome measures, and experimental participants rated satisfaction with CPT at 3.2 and satisfaction with art therapy at 4.6 on a five-point Likert scale. Interview analysis revealed several themes, such as art therapy's effectiveness in breaking through participants' avoidance of trauma symptoms, facilitating expression through artwork, and understanding trauma's effect upon their psychological functioning. Themes noted in participant artwork included aspects of formal elements such as prominent colors and theorized graphic equivalents to psychological phenomena such as containment, safety, anxiety, and emptiness.

Decker, Deaver, Abbey, Campbell, and Turpin (in press) built upon Campbell's work (Campbell, 2014; Campbell et al., 2016) by continuing to collect both quantitative and qualitative data, using the same mixed methods design as did Campbell. Increased numbers of participants allowed greater confidence in the statistical analysis of quantitative measures, which revealed that all participants improved on the PTSD and depression measures, but the experimental group demonstrated statistically significantly greater improvement on both measures than did the control group. The subjective ratings of treatment satisfaction indicated that experimental participants rated art therapy higher than CPT. Interview data indicated that art therapy provided safe distancing from past trauma and facilitated trauma recall and processing.

Finally, Pierce and Decker (2017) and co-researchers conducted a thematic analysis of interview data collected in the study, from which emerged four overarching patterns and ten themes and sub-themes; these ranged from depth descriptions of participants' experiences with combat, depression, and PTSD, to their experiences engaging in art therapy. Participants identified the mechanisms underlying the art therapy process as nonverbal, action-oriented processes, uncovering memories, and meaning making. The graphic trauma narrative and mask making were identified as the most effective art therapy processes for working with PTSD and depression symptoms. The analysis of the qualitative data enriched understanding of the study's benefits beyond the statistical results, providing clues as to how the art therapy experience contributed to decreased symptomology and improved trauma processing. Thus, this mixed methods study that consisted of several stages succeeded in generating, analyzing, and integrating quantitative and qualitative data that provided deeper and more complete answers about art therapy for veterans with combat PTSD than either type of data could have alone.

### *Social Justice Design (Advanced)*

Whereas Creswell and Plano Clark (2011) referred to this as the transformative design, Creswell (2015) subsequently referred to the same design as the social justice design. The purpose of such research is to examine problems and phenomena using a social justice or transformative philosophical lens that informs every stage of the study. Topics addressed through these studies relate to injustices experienced due to colonization, sexism, racism, and other societal ills imposed by those privileged and in power upon marginalized or disenfranchised persons. Often the researcher is motivated to advocate for improved conditions for persons in the communities studied (Fraenkel et al., 2012; Mertens, Bledsoe, Sullivan, & Wilson, 2010). In the design, data collection may occur in multiple phases and may be concurrent or sequential within each phase so long as quantitative and qualitative data are weighted equally and that every stage of the study is informed by the transformative/social justice lens (Creswell & Plano Clark, 2011). This research design is illustrated in Figure 6.5.

Mertens (2007) advocated for mixed methods informed by transformative philosophy because such an approach to research recognizes that, historically, those in power have not used research methods that adequately and accurately address the problems of marginalized communities, and thus the communities' needs have not been met and human rights have not been furthered. Transformative MMR addresses the power issues inherent in postpositivist research approaches by emphasizing the importance of involving members of the communities of interest in all steps of a research project. Mertens asserted:

> The transformative paradigm holds that reality is socially constructed, but it does so with a conscious awareness that certain individuals occupy a position of greater power and that individuals with other characteristics may be associated with a higher likelihood of exclusion from decisions about the definition of the research focus, questions, and other methodological aspects of the inquiry.
>
> (p. 216)

She described a researcher who embraces the transformative paradigm as "one who recognizes inequalities and injustices in society and strives to challenge the status quo, who is a bit of a provocateur with overtones

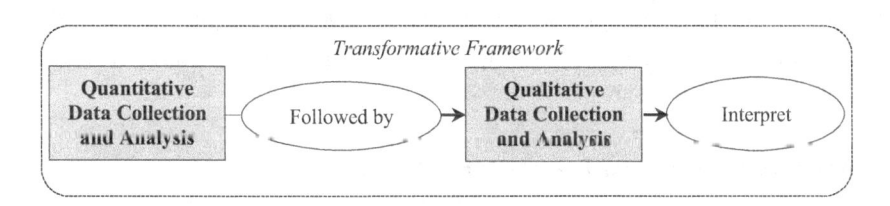

*Figure 6.5* Social justice/transformative design

of humility, and who possesses a shared sense of responsibility" (p. 212). This description is congruent with the American Art Therapy Association's Values Statement (AATA, 2017) and suggests that art therapy researchers who embrace it are prepared in terms of values and ethics to embark upon transformative and social justice MMR.

Sweetman, Badiee, and Creswell (2010) conducted an extensive literature search to locate MMR studies that utilized a transformative/advocacy stance that exemplified best practices in this research approach; they found only 13 studies from various fields that met their criteria, suggesting that such a design is not frequently implemented. It is not surprising that none of these were art therapy studies. However, there are many recent art therapy studies that are informed by a transformative, social justice lens, but none have been identified as using a mixed methods design. For example, Kapitan, Litell, and Torres (2011) conducted an art-based multiyear participatory action research (PAR) study in which creative arts therapies facilitators (outsiders) and members of collectively traumatized communities in Nicaragua (insiders) worked together as co-researchers with the goal of creating positive social change in the community. In a report on the project, Kapitan et al. identified empowerment, capacity building in the community participants, equity of benefits, and sustainability as results, and acknowledged the social transformation that occurred as a result of the facilitator-community collaboration. Art therapist Timm-Bottos (2011) reported on a project that aimed to "reduce clothing fabric waste" and "document the social justice and ecological issues involved in clothing production and distribution" (p. 57). This project involved stewardship of the earth in the form of an art studio in a thrift store that evolved into community action coalescing around art making, repurposing donated clothing into art materials, and significantly reducing the amount of clothing items going to the landfill. Other, art-based but non-art therapist researchers have advocated for the transformative power of art making in conflict resolution and building peace (Shank & Schirch, 2008) and for addressing the problems faced by immigrants and asylum seekers in the UK (O'Neill, 2008). Recent art therapy literature urges art therapists to incorporate an intersectional mindset and embrace a social justice framework in their practice (Karcher, 2017; Kuri, 2017; Talwar, 2010). Transformative MMR studies of art therapy practices that are informed by a social justice lens would likely yield results that would inform value driven and culturally competent practice, enriching the field and benefiting those we serve.

### Multiphase Program Evaluations (Advanced)

The multiphase design is associated with program evaluation and is comprised of both concurrent (parallel) and sequential data collection;

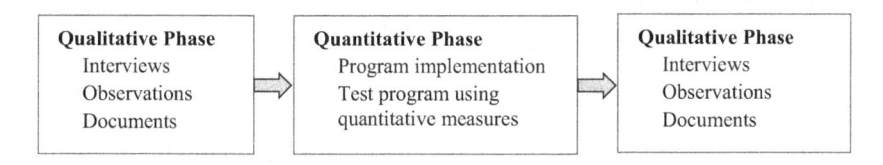

| Qualitative Phase | Quantitative Phase | Qualitative Phase |
| --- | --- | --- |
| Interviews | Program implementation | Interviews |
| Observations | Test program using | Observations |
| Documents | quantitative measures | Documents |

*Figure 6.6* Multiphase program evaluation design

the purpose of the design is to "address a program objective, such as for program development and evaluation" (Creswell & Plano Clark, 2011, p. 73). This design is typically utilized in grant-funded multiyear projects that involve a series of interrelated individual studies, all aimed at achieving an overarching program objective. Usually such studies require research teams rather than individual researchers, because of the amount of data that is collected, analyzed, mixed, and interpreted, and the time involved. Often these designs are implemented for evaluating large state or national government programs (ibid.). This design is illustrated in Figure 6.6.

Although the field of art therapy would benefit from such large scale multisite studies (Kaiser & Deaver, 2013), no such studies have been found in the literature. An art therapy example that was not as complex as those described by Creswell and Plano Clark (2011) but that illustrates the basics of mixed methods program evaluation is Allan, Barford, Horwood, Stevens, and Tanti's (2015) study of an art therapy program in the UK that was designed to support and assist severely mentally ill adults' transition from acute care to mental health recovery in a community setting. The "philosophy of recovery" (p. 14) pertains to the notion that psychiatric patients improve more readily while living in their own homes rather than in extended hospitalization; this philosophy has impacted the National Health Service in the UK by closing inpatient settings and increasing community-based care centers for individuals who have been discharged from inpatient settings but who may remain symptomatic. These are the individuals for whom Allan et al. designed their Art Therapy in the Community (ATIC) program. Congruent with the philosophy of recovery, the program is located in a studio space in a community arts center rather than at a clinical site, and offers participants adequate space for interaction with others or for being alone. The program encourages, through weekly group art therapy, development of an "artistic identity" (p. 17) and collaboration among consumers; the program has employed a former group member as a peer arts facilitator. The program's aims include improving consumers' well-being, reducing their distress, and increasing their social interaction.

From the conceptualization stage of the ATIC, Allan et al. integrated an MMR evaluation design into the program. Qualitative data were collected through interviews with consumers before and after attending a series of group sessions, and through a focus group after data analysis. Quantitative data consisted of consumers' scores on pre and post standardized measures of psychological distress, well-being, and social inclusion. Scores on outcome measures were analyzed statistically; psychological distress lessened and well-being increased significantly but pre to post differences in social isolation scores did not reach significance. Thematic analysis of interview data revealed five overarching themes and several sub-themes that amplified the results of the quantitative analysis, such as factors related to improved well-being, social interaction, discovery of artistic identity, feelings of safety, and meaning making. An interesting part of the design was the use of a focus group, after data analysis, that was comprised of consumers who had not been involved in any data collection and were unaware of the results of the evaluation. The focus group discussion, with no prompting, spontaneously confirmed the themes that had emerged from the qualitative analysis. The focus group functioned as a triangulation method for corroborating the results of the thematic analysis, thus increasing the credibility and confirmability of the findings.

## Evaluating MMR Studies

There are existing ways to evaluate the scientific integrity of quantitative research, such as statistical analyses that include measures of reliability, validity, and significance of results (Isaac & Michaels, 1995); additionally, there are existing schema for evaluating the credibility, trustworthiness, and transferability of the results of qualitative research (Creswell & Creswell, 2018). Only recently have scholars begun to explore systematic methods for evaluating MMR studies (Leech, Dellinger, Brannagan, & Tanaka, 2010). Leech et al. developed a system for evaluating the quality of data, including inferences drawn from them, in MMR, which involves five "elements" that cover all aspects of a study. The first, *foundational*, element pertains to evaluating the quality of the theoretical basis for a study as seen through the literature review. The second, *construct validation*, element refers to assessing the quality of the design, and the rigor of the interpretations made about results; this element also considers existing criteria for both quantitative (validity) and qualitative (credibility) studies. The third, *translation/inferential consistency*, element pertains to how "inferences from a study are logically consistent with other elements of the study" (p. 21). This element has to do with situating a study within a historical, theoretical, and literature based framework and whether the design and methods adequately address the purpose of the study. According to Leech et al., the fourth, *historic utilization*, element relates to whether the researchers administered appropriate, reliable, and valid measures in the study design. The fifth, *consequential*, element relates to whether and how study results were used in subsequent studies, thus lending validity and credibility to the study.

O'Cathain (2010) developed a framework that integrates the work of other MMR scholars, which includes eight domains of quality to use as guides throughout the design, implementation, and aftermath of a mixed methods study. Her framework is integrated, specific, and practical and can be used throughout all stages of a study as a set of standards to be met in MMR. In it, each stage of an MMR study is evaluated separately using differing quality standards. O'Cathain's "Quality Framework for Mixed Methods Research" (pp. 541–544) is presented here.

The first stage of an MMR study consists of comprehensive planning. This stage of the study can be evaluated by assessing the "planning quality" (p. 541) by considering the depth and comprehensiveness of a literature review that leads to appropriate research questions and methods. The study must have a clear rationale for using mixed methods, based upon the paradigm(s) embraced by the researcher, and explicit detail about design, data collection, and data analysis. Furthermore, the study can be accomplished using available resources, such as time, research team, and funding. In actually executing an MMR study, "design quality" (p. 542) can be evaluated through considering the suitability and rigor of the design, and "data quality" can be assessed through the quality of data collected and adequacy of analyses. O'Cathain included two approaches to evaluating the quality of interpretations in an MMR study. The first is "interpretive rigor" (p. 543), which refers to the extent to which study conclusions are transparent and based upon its findings, and to the consistency of interpretations with theory, as well as how effectively integrated/mixed are the quantitative and qualitative results. An additional domain for interpreting results is "inference transferability" (p. 543), which pertains to the possible application of study results to populations and contexts other than those studied.

Three final domains of quality are included in O'Cathain's evaluation scheme for MMR studies. Assessing "reporting quality" (p. 544) can be accomplished during the dissemination stage of a study by considering whether all important aspects of the study are included in the research report and how available that report is (published in peer-reviewed journals, in digital databases, etc.). Evaluating a study's "synthesizability" (inclusion in systematic reviews) and "utility quality" (use by service users and in policy making) (p. 544) are the final aspects of O'Cathain's system. Applying these criteria to the design, implementation, interpretation, and dissemination of art therapy MMR studies will improve the quality of art therapy research overall, increase translation of research into practice, and enhance the credibility of the field.

## Strengths and Weaknesses of MMR

A particular strength of MMR for art therapist researchers is that its underlying paradigm of dialectical pragmatism and its openness to eclecticism and creativity are philosophically compatible with art therapy and provide an approach that can move art therapy research forward with integrity (Gerber, 2016). MMR is an inclusive and creative form of research that allows researchers freedom in the design and conduct of studies. Reflecting the dialectical pragmatism philosophy underlying MMR, research questions facilitate methods that yield the most useful results (Johnson & Onwuegbuzie, 2004). The principal strength of MMR is that mixing qualitative and quantitative methods yields study results that answer research questions with both depth and breadth, which could not have occurred with just one method. Such studies explore relationships between variables in specific ways, primarily through insights regarding the interplay between the qualitative and quantitative data. Furthermore, when qualitative and quantitative results merge into a single interpretation, researchers are in a position to confirm relationships among variables or disconfirm a relationship if there is no convergence (Fraenkel et al., 2012).

Johnson and Onweugbuzie (2004) described in detail the strengths and weaknesses of MMR. Among the strengths is the complementary nature of the data; words and imagery can enhance numbers, and numbers can structure and organize words and imagery. Research questions are not confined to one method and thus can be broader and deeper than if restricted to one approach. The various research designs each have specific strengths in terms of weighting and mixing quantitative and qualitative methodologies. Furthermore, the weaknesses in one MMR approach can be compensated for by including an additional approach in the same study.

However, MMR can be difficult for a researcher to execute due to the significant amount of time required to implement two types of data collection, particularly if it is sequential; a research team may be needed. In addition, the requirement of knowing both quantitative and qualitative methods is not easily met. Finally, the field of MMR is continually evolving, and keeping up with current theoretical and methodological innovations may be difficult (Johnson & Onweugbuzie, 2004).

## Summary

This chapter began with a definition of mixed methods research (MMR) describing MMR as a methodology that combines quantitative and qualitative data in the same study, integrates them, and interprets the results. MMR is an emerging methodology that capitalizes on the strengths of both quantitative and qualitative methods; the primary rationale for MMR is that the integration of the two types of data provides both depth and breadth in answering research questions, more so than either type of data could alone. The underlying paradigm of MMR is pragmatism, which involves thoughtful and logical combinations of methodological approaches to best answer specific questions. MMR, since it is grounded in diverse philosophies, is a good fit for art therapy researchers, because of the diverse and eclectic philosophical origins of art therapy and art therapy's embrace of postpositivist, constructivist, and transformational world views.

Art therapists considering pursuit of MMR studies must have skills in both quantitative and qualitative methods, value the differing perspectives of postpositivism and constructivism, and be able to formulate quantitative, qualitative, and mixed methods research questions. The chapter described six MMR designs: convergent parallel, explanatory sequential, exploratory sequential, intervention/embedded, social justice/transformative, and multiphase program evaluation. Sequential designs involve collecting the different types of data one after the other, and in concurrent designs the different types of data are collected simultaneously. Depending on the design chosen, MMR can be time and energy consuming, and often is difficult to complete without a research team. Two systems for evaluating the quality of MMR studies were described, both of which emphasize the requirement that there must be a clear rationale for conducting the study using mixed methods, and the suitability and rigor of the chosen design.

The chapter ended with a brief discussion of the strengths and weaknesses of MMR, including the strength of the complementary nature of the data that can provide both depth and breadth in answering research questions. Weaknesses include the amount of time involved in MMR studies, the necessity of a research team in some cases, and the requirement to know both quantitative and qualitative research methods.

## References

Allan, J., Barford, H., Horwood, F., Stevens, J., & Tanti, G. (2015). ATIC: Developing a recovery-based art therapy practice. *International Journal of Art Therapy, 20*(1), 14–27. Retrieved from https://doi.org/10.1080/17454832.2014.968597

American Art Therapy Association (AATA). (2017). *Values statement.* Retrieved from https://arttherapy.org/values-statement/

Biesta, G. (2010). Pragmatism and the philosophical foundations of mixed methods research. In A. Tashakkori & C. Teddlie (Eds.), *SAGE handbook of mixed methods in social and behavioral research* (2nd ed., pp. 95–117). Thousand Oaks, CA: Sage.

Boeije, H., Drabble, S., & O'Cathain, A. (2015). Methodological challenges of mixed methods intervention evaluations. *Methodology, 11*(4), 119–125. Retrieved from https://doi.org/10.1027/1614-2241/a000101

Bradt, J., Burns, D., & Creswell, J. (2013). Mixed methods research in music therapy research. *Journal of Music Therapy, 50*(2), 123–148. Retrieved from https://doi.org/10.1093/jmt/50.2.123

Campbell, M. (2014). Art therapy and cognitive processing therapy for combat PTSD: A randomized, controlled trial (master's thesis, Eastern Virginia Medical School, Norfolk, VA).

Campbell, M., Decker, K. P., Kruk, K., & Deaver, S. P. (2016). Art therapy and cognitive processing therapy for combat-related PTSD: A randomized controlled trial. *Art Therapy: Journal of the American Art Therapy Association, 33*(4), 169–177. Retrieved from https://doi.org/10.1080/07421656.2016.1226643

Caruth, G. (2013). Demystifying mixed methods research design: A review of the literature. *Mevlana International Journal of Education, 3*(2), 112–122. Retrieved from https://doi.org/10.13054/mije.13.35.3.2

Creswell, J. W. (2011). Controversies in mixed methods research. In N. Denzin & Y. Guba (eds.), *The SAGE handbook of qualitative research*. Thousand Oaks, CA: Sage.

Creswell, J. W. (2015). *A concise introduction to mixed methods research*. Los Angeles, CA: Sage.

Creswell, J. W. & Creswell, J. D. (2018). *Research design: Qualitative, quantitative, and mixed methods approaches* (5th ed.). Thousand Oaks, CA: Sage.

Creswell, J. W. & Plano Clark, V. (2011). *Designing and conducting mixed methods research* (2nd ed.). Los Angeles, CA: Sage.

Creswell, J. W. & Zhang, W. (2009). The application of mixed methods designs to trauma research. *Journal of Traumatic Stress, 22*(6), 612–621. Retrieved from https://doi.org/10.1002/jts.20479

Deaver, S. (2012). Art-based learning strategies in art therapy graduate education. *Art Therapy: Journal of the American Art Therapy Association, 29*(4), 158–165. Retrieved from https://doi.org/10.1080/07421656.2012.730029

Decker, K., Deaver, S., Abbey, V., Campbell, M., & Turpin, C. (in press). Quantitatively improved treatment outcomes for combat-associated PTSD with adjunctive art therapy: Randomized controlled trial. *Art Therapy: Journal of the American Art Therapy Association*.

Feilzer, M. (2010). Doing mixed methods research pragmatically: Implications for the rediscovery of pragmatism as a research paradigm. *Journal of Mixed Methods Research, 4*(1), 6–16. Retrieved from https://doi.org/10.1177/1558689809349691

Frankel, J., Wallen, N., & Hyun, H. (2012). *How to design and evaluate research in education* (8th ed.). New York, NY: McGraw-Hill.

Gantt, L. M. (1990). A validity study of the Formal Elements Art Therapy Scale (FEATS) for diagnostic information in patients' drawings (doctoral dissertation, University of Pittsburgh, Pittsburgh, PA).

Gerber, N. (2016). Mixed methods in art therapy research. In D. Gussak & M. Rosal (Eds.), *The Wiley handbook of art therapy* (pp. 804–813). Chichester: Wiley.

Greene, J. (2007). *Mixed methods in social inquiry*. San Francisco, CA: Wiley.

Guest, G. (2012). Describing mixed methods research: An alternative to typologies. *Journal of Mixed Methods Research, 7*(2), 141–151. Retrieved from https://doi.org/10.1177/1558689812461179

Hanson, W., Creswell, J. W., Plano Clark, V., Petska, K., & Creswell, J. D. (2005). Mixed methods research designs in counseling psychology. *Journal of Counseling Psychology, 52*(2), 224–235. Retrieved from https://doi.org/10.1037/0022-0167.52.2.224

Isaac, S. & Michaels, W. (1995). *Handbook in research and evaluation* (3rd ed.). San Diego, CA: Educational and Industrial Testing Services.

Johnson, B. & Gray, R. (2010). A history of philosophical and theoretical issues for mixed methods research. In A. Tashakkori & C. Teddlie, (Eds.), *SAGE handbook of mixed methods in social and behavioral research* (2nd ed., pp. 69–94). Thousand Oaks, CA: Sage.

Johnson, R. B. & Onwuegbuzie, A. (2004). Mixed methods research: A research paradigm whose time has come. *Educational Researcher, 33*(7), 14–26. Retrieved from http://www.jstor.org/stable/3700093

Johnson, R. B., Onwuegbuzie, A., & Turner, L. (2007). Toward a definition of mixed methods research. *Journal of Mixed Methods Research, 1*(2), 112–133. Retrieved from https://doi.org/10.1177/1558689806298224

Kaimal, G., Rattigan, M., Miller, G., & Haddy, J. (2016). Implications of national trends in digital media use for art therapy practice. *Journal of Clinical Art Therapy, 3*(1). Retrieved from http://digitalcommons.lmu.edu/jcat/vol3/iss1/6

Kaiser, D. & Deaver, S. (2013). Establishing a research agenda for art therapy: A Delphi study. *Art Therapy: Journal of the American Art Therapy Association, 30*(3), 114–121. Retrieved from https://doi.org/10.1080/07421656.2013.819281

Kapitan, L. (2018). *Introduction to art therapy research* (2nd ed.). New York, NY: Routledge.

Kapitan, L., Litell, M., & Torres, A. (2011). Creative art therapy in a community's participatory research and social transformation. *Art Therapy: Journal of the American Art Therapy Association, 28*(2), 64–73. Retrieved from https://doi.org/10.1080/07421656.2011.578238

Karcher, O. (2017). Sociopolitical oppression, trauma, and healing: Moving toward a social justice art therapy framework. *Art Therapy: Journal of the American Art Therapy Association, 34*(3), 108–117. Retrieved from https://doi.org/10.1080/07421656.2017.1358024

King, J. (Ed.). (2016). *Art therapy, trauma, and neuroscience: Theoretical and practical perspectives*. New York, NY: Routledge.

King, J., Knapp, K., Shaikh, A., Fang Li, F., Sabau, D., Pascuzzi, R., & Osburn, L. (2017). Cortical activity changes after art making and rote motor movement as measured by EEG: A preliminary study. *Biomedical Journal of Science & Technical Research, 1*(4). Retrieved from https://doi.org/10.26717/BJSTR.2017.01.000366

Knowles, J. G. & Coles, A. (2008). *Handbook of the arts in qualitative research: Perspectives, methodologies, examples, and issues*. Thousand Oaks, CA: Sage.

Kuri, E. (2017). Toward an ethical application of intersectionality in art therapy. *Art Therapy: Journal of the American Art Therapy Association, 34*(3), 118–122. Retrieved from https://doi.org/10.1080/07421656.2017.1358023

Leech, N., Dellinger, A., Brannagan, K., & Tanaka, H. (2010). Evaluating mixed research studies: A mixed methods approach. *Journal of Mixed Methods Research, 4*(1), 17–31. Retrieved from https://doi.org/10.1177/1558689809345262

Mertens, D. (2007). Transformative paradigm: Mixed methods and social justice. *Journal of Mixed Methods Research, 1*(3), 212–225. Retrieved from https://doi.org/10.1177/1558689807302811

Mertens, D., Bledsoe, K., Sullivan, M., & Wilson, A. (2010). Utilization of mixed methods for transformative purposes. In A. Tashakkori & C. Teddlie, (Eds.), *SAGE handbook of mixed methods in social and behavioral research* (2nd ed., pp. 193–214). Thousand Oaks, CA: Sage.

Monti, D., Peterson, C., Kunkel, E., Hauck, W., Pequignot, E., Rhodes, L., & Brainard, G. (2006). A randomized, controlled trial of mindfulness-based art therapy (MBAT) for women with cancer. *Psycho-Oncology, 15*, 363–373. Retrieved from https://doi.org/10.1002/pon.988

Morse, J. (1991). Approaches to qualitative–quantitative methodological triangulation. *Nursing Research, 40*(2), 120–123. Retrieved from https://doi.org/10.1097/00006199-199103000-00014

Nainis, N., Paice, J., Ratner, J., Wirth, J., Lai, J., & Shott, S. (2006). Relieving symptoms in cancer: Innovative use of art therapy. *Journal of Pain Management, 31*(2), 162–169. Retrieved from https://doi.org/10.1016/j.jpainsymman.2005.07.006

O'Cathain, A. (2010). Assessing the quality of mixed methods research: Toward a comprehensive framework. In A. Tashakkori & C. Teddlie, (Eds.), *SAGE handbook of mixed methods in social and behavioral research* (2nd ed., pp. 531–555). Thousand Oaks, CA: Sage.

O'Neill, M. (2008). Transnational refugees: The transformative role of art? *Forum: Qualitative Social Research, 9*(2). Retrieved from https://doi.org/10.17169/fqs-9.2.403

Onwuegbuzie, A., Bustamante, R., & Nelson, J. (2010). Mixed research as a tool for developing quantitative instruments. *Journal of Mixed Methods Research, 4*(1), 56–78. Retrieved from https://doi.org/10.1177/1558689809355805

Pierce, V. & Decker, K. (2017, November). Veterans' experiences of adjunctive art therapy during cognitive processing therapy for PTSD. Paper presented at the meeting of the American Art Therapy Association, Albuquerque, NM.

Shank, M. & Schirch, L. (2008). Strategic arts-based peacebuilding. *Peace & Change: A Journal of Peace Research, 33*(2), 217–242. Retrieved from https://doi.org/10.1111/j.1468-0130.2008.00490.x

Slayton, S., D'Archer, J., & Kaplan, F. (2010). Outcome studies on the efficacy of art therapy: A review of findings. *Art Therapy: Journal of the American Art Therapy Association, 27*(3), 108–118. Retrieved from https://doi.org/10.1080/07421656.2010.10129660

Sweetman, D., Badiee, M., & Creswell, J. W. (2010). Use of the transformative framework in mixed methods studies. *Qualitative Inquiry, 16*(6), 441–454. Retrieved from https://doi.org/10.1177/1077800410364610

Talwar, S. (2010). An intersectional framework for race, class, gender, and sexuality in art therapy. *Art Therapy: Journal of the American Art Therapy Association, 27*(1), 11–17. Retrieved from https://doi.org/10.1080/07421656.2010.10129567

Timm-Bottos, J. (2011). Endangered threads: Socially committed community art action. *Art Therapy: Journal of the American Art Therapy Association, 28*(2), 57–63. Retrieved from https://doi.org/10.1080/07421656.2011.578234

Watkins, D. & Gioia, D. (2015). *Mixed methods research*. New York, NY: Oxford University Press.

# Chapter 7

# Assessment Research in Art Therapy

Graduate art therapy students and art therapists must understand the context of clinical assessment and the role of the art therapist in the assessment process. In addition, the standards and guidelines for US-based accredited art therapy graduate programs stipulates that:

> The curriculum must provide students with the opportunity to become familiar with a variety of specific art therapy instruments and procedures used in appraisal and evaluation. Additional areas of coverage include the selection of assessments with clients/patients as the basis for treatment planning, establishing treatment effects, evaluating assessment validity and reliability, documentation of assessment results and ethical, cultural, and legal considerations in their use.
>
> (CAAHEP, 2016, p. 21)

According to the *Ethical Principles* of the American Art Therapy Association (2013), "art therapists use only those assessment methods in which they have acquired competence through appropriate training and supervised experience" (principle 3.2, p. 5). Similarly, it behooves art therapists to recognize how assessments are developed, in order to make clinically sound decisions about assessment selection and application. This chapter provides instruction on the development of assessments through research, and how art therapists can continue to improve assessment strategies through further investigations of existing instruments and approaches. The development and application of art therapy assessments and scoring and evaluation procedures are presented through examples from previous research. Pertinent concepts such as validity and reliability for the assessments used with a range of clients are detailed for the purposes of teaching and learning.

A word on phraseology used in this chapter: Art therapy assessments are referred to as process-based, "constructive," or "performance-based" measures. These terms more accurately reflect the current terminology used in psychological assessment. Bornstein (2007) is credited with contextualizing personality tests based on the psychological processes that occur as people respond to test stimuli, known as the "process-based" approach. This emphasis on process and how it is measured during a testing situation dovetails with approaches in art therapy assessment, in terms of the recognized imperative to examine clients' verbalizations and behaviors as they engage in the process of art making (refer to Betts [2017] for a table linking art therapy assessments to Bornstein's process-based framework).

The advantages of process-based testing are well established in the psychological assessment literature. The process-based approach is promoted by Bornstein (2011) as a means to not only improve psychological assessment procedures but also increase understanding of test score misuse and test bias by revealing the inter- and intra-personal factors that lead to differential performance across patient groups. Schore's (2011) work lends further support to the use of assessments that are classified as process- and performance-based. Citing Finn (2011), Schore (2011) agreed that neuroimaging studies support the use of assessments such as the Adult Attachment Projective Picture System (AAP; George & West, 2012) and the Rorschach (Exner, 2003) as "sensitive to limbic functioning and right hemisphere disorganization and therefore to implicit deficits of early attachment trauma" (Schore, 2011, p. 11) as contrasted with verbal self-report tests such as the Minnesota Multiphasic Personality Inventory, second edition (MMPI-2, Butcher et al., 2001) and the Beck Depression Inventory (BDI; Beck, Ward, Mendelson, Mock, & Erbaugh, 1961), which tend to tap "left hemisphere cortical functions and explicit models of self and other" (Schore, 2011, p. 11). Process- and performance-based assessments (like those developed by art therapists), therefore, "are very useful in part because they tap right-hemisphere and subcortical brain functioning and provide information that clients cannot directly report" (Finn, 2012, p. 440). Furthermore, according to Kaiser (1996), presenting problems can appear more distinctly in artwork than through verbal explanation alone, particularly when triangulated with narrative data, and can aid in fostering the therapeutic alliance.

## Art Therapy Assessment Research: Background

When a client is referred for treatment, the person will typically be evaluated via multiple means, often under the direction of a psychologist. This approach enables clinicians to gain a broader understanding of the client's presenting problems. The clinical interview is the most common form of assessment, and can include information that the person self-reports, and insight that the clinician gains from behavioral observations (Mihura, Meyer, Dumitrascu, & Bombel, 2012). Interviews also enable the clinician to assess a range of neurophysiological processes, ascertain hidden mental states, observe changes in symptoms and traits over time, and evaluate dyadic and intergroup dynamics (Bornstein, 2011).

To augment understanding of complex psychological problems, well-established tests that assess an array of characteristics are often used by psychologists, such as the MMPI-2 (Butcher et al., 2001), performance tasks (e.g., an intelligence test or the Rorschach), and observations based on an outside source (e.g., teacher, parent, and/or spouse ratings). In settings that include an art therapist, the clinical evaluation process can be augmented through the inclusion of an art therapy assessment because of the rich and diverse information that can be gleaned from artwork and viewing the process of art making (Betts & Groth-Marnat, 2014). In 2002, Deaver observed that the profession of art therapy was a long way from where it should be "in terms of realizing art's potential to accurately and objectively measure a range of attributes" (p. 25). Due to the subsequent contributions of Deaver and a number of others, art therapy assessment research has advanced considerably, yielding more successful applications for deriving clinically useful information about clients based on their art products and artistic processes. For instance, art therapy assessments that are under development have been used to evaluate numerous variables, such as specific psychiatric symptoms, as well as issues salient to successful treatment outcomes, such as clients' acceptance of diagnosis, extent and course of illness, and prognosis.

### Art Therapy Assessment Research: The Integrative Approach

Although research in the field has helped to demonstrate the validity and reliability of some art therapy assessments, much more work is needed. Specific guidelines pertinent to art therapy assessment research are based on strategic objective 3.2 of the National Institute of Mental Health (NIMH, 2016) strategic plan for research: "Develop ways to tailor existing and new interventions to optimize outcomes." The NIMH further underscored the development and application of assessments that yield objective, quantitative data in keeping with its Research Domain Criteria (RDoC). In other words, in order for art therapy assessments to demonstrate viability in the scientific community, our assessment instruments must be psychometrically sound and should abide by current guidelines put forth by the NIMH. Doing so could also increase the likelihood of art therapy assessment researchers' ability to gain federal grant monies and other support to conduct the kind of research that is needed to develop our tools. Thus, art therapists should continue to build the research base on assessments that can be validated in a quantitative and objective manner, particularly in relation to aspects of cognition, emotion, and social behavior that predict clinical responses. Indeed, the purpose of assessment research is to "discover the predictive ability of a variable or a set of variables to assess or diagnose a particular disorder or problem profile" (Rosal, 1992, p. 59). To do this, we can follow the NIMH (2016) specifications to develop and validate objective approaches for differentiating subjects so that we can make well-informed treatment recommendations for clients. Notably, however, this emphasis on the quantitative approach to assessment research does not exclude the importance of qualitative data generated during the assessment process (Betts, 2012; Elliott, Fischer, & Rennie, 1999; Yoon, Betts, & Holttum, submitted).

Qualitative methods should be equally mandated in the development of assessments, because such methods provide vital information related to the details of people's experiences. Support for the combining of qualitative and mixed methods approaches to validating assessment – the *integrative* approach – are available in the psychology literature, particularly in the realm of positive psychology (Betts, 2012).

Qualitative information-seeking is considered to be a more humanistically oriented means of data collection as it enables consideration of cultural context (see Betts, 2013), history, and other elements essential to an in-depth appreciation of an individual's condition. Qualitative methods provide vital information related to "the particulars of human experience and social life (including discourse) by taking into account matters such as history, language and context that relativize the knowledge gained to the individuals and situations studied and to those doing the inquiry" (Elliott et al., 1999, p. 217). Indeed, as is described by Betts (2012), strict reliance upon quantitative and completely objective methods for assessment research provides a narrow understanding of client symptoms given the complexities of the human condition.

The psychology literature lends further support to the integration of qualitative and mixed methods approaches to validating assessment approaches, specifically collaborative assessment (Fischer, 2000, 2001) and therapeutic assessment (Finn, 2007). As Finn (2012) observed, "we have grossly underestimated the importance of the assessor-client relationship, as if participating in psychological testing was no more complex for a client than taking a blood test" (p. 441). Finn's approach involves talking with the client about assessment results, and engaging in a productive discussion that yields valuable qualitative information (i.e., the client's thoughts, reactions, etc.). These concepts were emphasized by Betts and Groth-Marnat (2014) in their summary of the hallmarks of positive psychological assessment: validating assessment data (artwork, etc.) based on clients' own interpretations, downplaying an over-reliance on test scores by blending all available sources of information about a person, focusing on the quality of the relationship (Dudley, 2004), and working collaboratively with the client (Bornstein, 2009; Fischer, 2000; Snyder, Ritschel, Rand, & Berg, 2006), ensuring that both "outside" and "inside" environmental assets and problems are considered (Snyder et al., 2006), and including hopes and strengths in reports. In summary, the *integrative* approach to assessment is the recommended approach in the research and validation of our instruments and the position upon which this chapter is based.

Much work remains to be done to further establish the rigor and utility of art therapy assessments (Betts, 2006), even those that have been used for the past decade or more. The subsequent section provides instruction on traditional constructive (formerly, projective) assessment development, validation, and application of assessments and scoring systems and their impact on clinical judgment and decision making. As examples that are recognized in the art therapy profession, the Bird's Nest Drawing (BND; Kaiser, 1996), the Diagnostic Drawing Series (DDS; Cohen & Mills, 2016; Cohen, Hammer, & Singer, 1988), the Face Stimulus Assessment (FSA; Betts, 2003), the Human Figure Drawing (HFD; Deaver, 2009; Harris, 1963), and the Person Picking an Apple from a Tree (PPAT; Gantt, 1990) are referenced (and described in Box 7.1) to provide the reader with practical understanding as to how the traditional psychological assessment research approaches to validity and reliability apply to art therapy assessment research.

---

### Box 7.1 Overview of Some Recognized Art Therapy Assessments Referenced in this Chapter

**Art Therapy-Projective Imagery Assessment (AT-PIA).** The AT-PIA (Deaver & Bernier, 2014; Raymond et al., 2010) is a comprehensive direct-observation clinical interview that includes a series of six discrete constructive drawing tasks collected under standardized conditions. The AT-PIA was developed to provide a systematic method of assessment that is compatible with psychological and psychiatric evaluation processes. The AT-PIA is to be administered and interpreted by art therapists or art therapy students (under the supervision of a registered art therapist) who are trained to assess mental status, personality dynamics, and diagnostic indicators expressed through artwork, verbal associations, and behavior. It is designed for use with children, adolescents, and adults to identify developmental level, areas of clinical concern, strengths, defenses, diagnostic information, and potential for engaging with art materials and processes. The six drawing tasks are: projective scribble drawing, favorite weather drawing, human figure drawing, kinetic family drawing, reason for being here drawing, and free choice drawing. Clinicians must be trained in AT-PIA administration, and adhere to specific instructions as provided in the AT-PIA manual (Raymond et al., 2010).

**Bird's Nest Drawing (BND).** The BND is a process-based, constructive assessment that was developed by art therapist Donna Kaiser (1996) to assess attachment security. Clients should be provided with a set of ten Crayola® fine-line markers and an 8" x 12" piece of white paper and directed to "draw a picture of a bird's nest." Clients should be given 15 minutes to complete the drawing and, after that, asked to write a story about the drawing in at least 3–5 sentences (Yoon, Betts, & Holttum, submitted). Further details are provided in the separate section on the BND in Chapter 8, Section III.

**Diagnostic Drawing Series (DDS).** The DDS (Cohen & Mills, 2016; Cohen, Hammer, & Singer, 1988) is a three-picture series in which the respondent produces a range of psychological and graphic responses. A process-based, constructive assessment, each picture reflects an individual's response to a specific directive and structure. The drawings are the free picture, the tree picture, and the feelings picture. The materials must include a 12-color pack of Alphacolor or Blick chalk pastels and white (60 or 70 lb.) drawing paper (18" x 24"). A 1993 paper describes the early development of the DDS and its validity and reliability (Mills, Cohen, & Meneses, 1993), and a bibliography is available at www.diagnosticdrawingseries.com.

**Expressive Therapies Continuum (ETC) assessment.** The ETC (Hinz, 2009; Kagin & Lusebrink, 1978; Lusebrink, 2010) is a comprehensive assessment. It has been theoretically tied to neurobiology, because it assesses kinesthetic and sensory, perceptual and affective, cognitive and symbolic content. The ETC elucidates people's behavior as they are presented with arousing stimuli and work with color and a range of fluid to resistive media. Process-based assessments such as the ETC provide information about functioning during a state of emotional arousal (Finn, 2012). Hinz (2009) recommended three to five sessions for conducting the ETC assessment protocol, with each session serving as its own data point. If this is not possible, clinicians can alternately conduct the protocol in one to two sessions. As per Graves-Alcorn and Green (2014), the choice of materials or projects should rest with the client. A range of fluid to resistive media needs to be available but not so many choices that it becomes overwhelming. Materials are not standardized.

**Face Stimulus Assessment (FSA).** Betts (2003) developed a performance-based drawing assessment as an outcome of her work using the face as a stimulus with clients with communication disorders. The client is provided with a standard packet of eight Crayola® markers, and a packet of eight Crayola® multicultural markers. Three stimulus pictures (copyrighted templates) are then provided, one at a time (#1, complete face stimulus; #2, face and neck outline; #3, blank white paper). The directive for each consecutive picture is held constant: "Use the markers and this piece of paper." The FSA has demonstrated some utility as an assessment of cognitive/neuropsychological and developmental level: In a study of 193 children in South Korea, Kim, Kim, and Seo (2014) validated the FSA as distinguishing children with ADHD from normal children. G. Kim (personal communication, February 28, 2016) examined 206 adults over the age of 65 to determine the FSA's ability to differentiate older adults with and without dementia. Older adults with dementia showed significantly lower performances on the clock drawing test (CDT) and the FSA than did those without dementia. These findings suggest that the FSA can be used to complement mainstream measurements used to diagnose dementia.

**Human Figure Drawing (HFD).** The HFD (Deaver, 2009; Golomb, 1974; Harris, 1963; Koppitz, 1968; Naglieri, 1988) has demonstrated value as a constructive assessment of cognitive/neuropsychological and developmental level. For instance, Deaver (2009) investigated the HFDs of 316 fourth graders (mean age = 9.69 years) and 151 second graders (mean age = 7.56 years). Fourth graders scored significantly higher than second graders on the *developmental level* scale, demonstrating congruence with Lowenfeld and Brittain's (1987) stages of children's normative artistic development. Furthermore, ethnic group identity was not a significant variable, which is consistent with Naglieri's (1988) findings and lends some support to the generalizibility of developmental stages in artwork across ethnic groups. Participants in Deaver's (2009) study adhered to a standardized administration procedure for the HFDs: they were provided with a pencil and eraser, a set of eight markers, a box of 12 oil pastels, and gray 9" x 12" 80 lb. paper. As per Koppitz (1968), participants were instructed: "use any of the drawing supplies to draw a person from head to toe. Try to draw a whole person, not a cartoon or stick figure. You will have up to 15 minutes to complete this drawing.

**Person Picking an Apple from a Tree (PPAT).** The PPAT (Gantt, 1990) has shown some utility as a constructive assessment of cognitive/neuropsychological (Bat Or, Ishai, & Levi, 2015) and developmental (Stafstrom, Havlena, & Krezinski, 2012; White, Wallace, & Huffman, 2004) levels. For PPAT administration, white drawing paper (12" x 18") and a set of 12 Sanford® "Mr. Sketch"® watercolor markers should be used. The directive is, "Draw a person picking an apple from a tree." There is no established time limit on completing the drawing. PPAT drawings are scored with the Formal Elements of Art Therapy Scale (FEATS; Gantt & Tabone, 1998) rating system. Note that the FEATS is a *rating system*, not an *assessment* – the PPAT is the assessment.

Next, quantitative levels of measurement are described, so as to provide background on the ways in which formal elements of artwork are quantitatively scored – essential to understanding development of sound methodology for the pursuit of assessment research.

## Quantitative Levels of Measurement

Some art therapy assessments include accompanying rating systems to enable the researcher to score artwork using defined measurement scales. Four different scale types or "levels of measurement" are commonly used, as developed by psychologist Stanley Smith Stevens (1946). These are nominal, ordinal, interval, and ratio scales, classifications that provide different ways for a researcher to measure variables of interest. Table 7.1 provides examples of how these scales are used in art therapy rating systems.

A rating system in art therapy is understood as a standardized procedure that the rater uses to generate scores for formal elements of artwork. A well-known example is the rating manual known as the Formal Elements Art Therapy Scale (FEATS; Gantt & Tabone, 1998). The FEATS enables art therapists to quantify formal elements in artwork by assigning a score to 14 variables of interest. For example, to measure the amount of space a PPAT drawing fills on a piece of paper (as is shown in Table 7.2), the art therapist would refer to FEATS scale #4, which is a type of ratio scale. For this scale, *space*, the art therapist would estimate the total amount of paper covered by the image, and assign a score from 0–5. The PPAT drawing example shown in Figure 7.1 would be scored a 3, as approximately 50 percent of the paper's space is used. Here, the FEATS *space* scale is used to enable the art therapist to make a judgment about the artwork variable "space" based on the instructions provided (operationalized) in the manual. Training in the proper use of such scoring systems is important so as to reduce the subjectivity inherent in the rating process.

### *Nominal (Categorical) Scales*

When a rater is presented with options based upon categories in which order does not matter, such a scale is known as nominal (categorical or, as is discussed in Chapter 3, "discrete"). Such a scale is the most basic of the four types. In art therapy, the Diagnostic Drawing Series (DDS; Cohen, Hammer, & Singer, 1988) is scored in conjunction with the Drawing Analysis Form II (DAF2; Cohen & Mills, 2016), which includes a combination of 21 nominal scales, one ordinal scale (*color*) and one ratio scale (*space usage*). As an example of a DDS nominal scale, consider *idiosyncratic color*, for which the rater is required to indicate whether or not each of the three DDS drawings has "idiosyncratic

Table 7.1 Art therapy rating systems and levels of measurement

| Level of Measurement | Description | Art Therapy Rating Scale Example | Art Therapy Assessment |
|---|---|---|---|
| Nominal (categorical, or "discrete") | For mutually exclusive, but not ordered, categories. | DDS Drawing Analysis Form<br>*Idiosyncratic Color*<br>□ yes  □ no | DDS |
| Ordinal (continuous) | The order matters but not the difference between values, which simply express an order. | DDS Drawing Analysis Form<br>*Color*<br>□ Mono  □ 2–3 colors  □ 4+ colors  □ Blank | DDS |
| Interval (Likert) (continuous) | The difference between two values is meaningful because the difference between sets of neighboring values is the same. | FEATS manual<br>*Color Fit (Likert-type)*<br>No markings on page  **0 – 1 – 2 – 3 – 4 – 5**  *All colors appropriate* | PPAT |
| Ratio (continuous) | Shares the same qualities as an interval variable, but also has a "true zero." | FEATS Manual<br>*Space*<br>*0% (no space) used*  **0 – 1 – 2 – 3 – 4 – 5**  *100% of space used* | PPAT |

176   Assessment Research

*Table 7.2* Characteristics of levels of measurement used in rating artwork content and formal elements variables

| Characteristics | Nominal and Ordinal | Interval and Ratio |
| --- | --- | --- |
| Rating time | Shorter | Longer |
| Inter-rater reliability | Higher (due to more consistency in responses) | Lower (more variability in scores due to more specificity in scales) |
| Amount of data gleaned | Less (e.g., presence or absence of Idiosyncratic Color) | More (five interval Color Fit scale plus true zero) |
| Comparison of data in terms of direction or magnitude | Not possible | Possible |

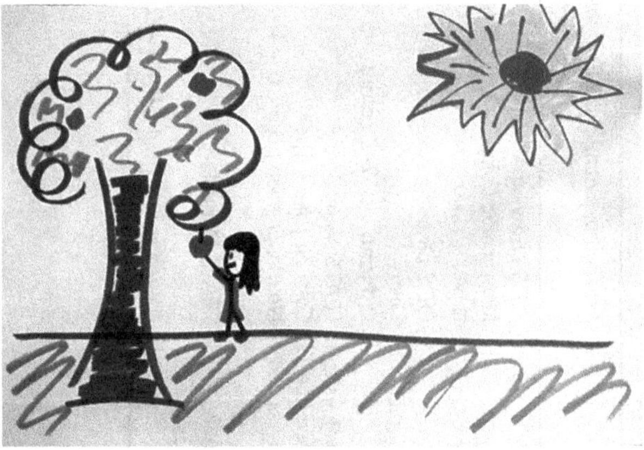

*Figure 7.1* PPAT example with FEATS scale #4, *space*

color" by checking either the "no" box or the "yes" box – the rater is forced to choose only one of these. Nominal scales are also used in the DDS to indicate presence or absence of people, animals, objects, symbols, and other content that may be relevant. They allow the rater to indicate categories of content such as "Tree" by selecting one of the following choices: *unrecognizable, chaotic, falling apart,* or *none*. Whereas these tree designations represent distinct tree types or categories, they do not have meaning in relation to one another. In other words, they do not have numerical values that can be placed in a meaningful order. An "unrecognizable" tree is not better or worse than a "chaotic" tree. It is neither worth more nor worth less. These are merely categories for the purpose of tracking content.

The FEATS manual includes a content tally sheet comprised of nominal/categorical scales, used to track data from PPAT drawings that may have meaning when compared to a group of drawings from a similar patient group (Gantt & Tabone, 1998). The content categories enable the art therapy researcher to capture specific details about PPAT drawings that are not accounted for in the 14 main FEATS scales. For instance, Gantt and Tabone noticed a trend in some of the drawings – that only these particular PPATs included people drawn completely in one color, typically yellow. In order to capture such data (i.e., use of a single color to draw the person), one would check the relevant box in the "Color used for person" category.

## Ordinal Scales

When the order of items in a scale matters, but not the difference between values, these are known as ordinal variables (also referred to as one of the "continuous" types of scales in Chapter 3). The DDS includes at least one ordinal scale – *color*. it contains the following categories: *mono (one color)*, *2–3 colors*, *4+ colors*, and *blank*. The rater selects one of these choices when rating a DDS drawing. The order of these scales is meaningful because the scales increase in numerical value incrementally. However, the difference between the neighboring values is not the same, so the scale is designated as ordinal (not interval, described next).

Table 7.2 shows the characteristics of levels of measurement used in rating artwork and their weaknesses and strengths. For *rating time*, the amount of time it takes to rate a drawing, nominal and ordinal scales are better because they typically include fewer and more simplified variables for rating.

Nominal and ordinal scales also perform well in terms of *inter-rater reliability*, as shown in Table 7.2. Inter-rater reliability is the frequency with which two or more raters consistently assign the same scores to test results. To determine inter-rater reliability, it is recommended that three individuals who are trained in using the given rating procedure (such as the FEATS) score the samples (such as a set of PPAT drawings). The raters' sets of scores are then compared, and a determination is made as to how closely their scores match.

Nominal and ordinal scales tend to yield higher inter-rater reliability results because of the increased likelihood of consistency in responses. In other words, such scales tend to be simple enough that raters are more likely to indicate similar answers. Consider this example: on the DDS drawing analysis form, a rater must indicate whether *idiosyncratic color* is present or not present. Idiosyncratic color is defined as "any color used to depict a representational image which is unnatural for that image depicted" (Cohen & Mills, 2016, p. 12). To rate this variable, the rater must simply check the "yes" box or the "no" box. Now contrast this with the FEATS approach to rating this variable. In the FEATS, idiosyncratic color is rated on scale #2, *color fit*, to assess "whether the colors used in the PPAT are appropriate to the objects depicted" (Gantt & Tabone, 1998, p. 31). Given that the 14 FEATS scales are Likert/interval-type, we know that the difference between values on any scale is meaningful because the difference between sets of neighboring values is relatively similar. So, rather than rating color fit as simply present or not present, we are enabled to make a more refined decision about the amount of color fit. We actually have six choices – between a rating of zero through 5 – on that scale.

In terms of the *amount of data* that can be gleaned from nominal, ordinal, interval or ratio scales, the nominal and ordinal yield less data than interval or ratio. Similarly, comparison of data in terms of *direction or magnitude* is not possible with nominal and ordinal data. These concepts are explained in the subsequent sections on interval scales and ratio scales.

### *Interval Scales*

When the difference between a continuum of neighboring values is the same, and therefore meaningful, such variables are known as interval (also referred to as one of the "continuous" types of scales in Chapter 3). For instance, the difference between a temperature of 50 and 60 degrees is the same as between 40 and 50 degrees. As was previously described, the 14 FEATS scales are designated as equal-*appearing* interval (or Likert) scales because the intervals between the numbers on the FEATS scales aren't necessarily equivalent all along the scale. A four on a FEATS scale cannot be assumed to be exactly twice as much as a two. Consider scale #1, *prominence of color*. The scale descriptions are qualitative, and require subjective interpretation on the part of the rater. A score of 1 is intended for PPAT drawings for which "color is used only to outline the forms or objects in the picture, or to make lines; none of the forms are colored in" (Gantt & Tabone, 1998, Prominence of Color). A drawing is scored 2 when "color is used for outlining most of the forms or objects, but only one form or object is filled in (such as a tree trunk or a person's body)." Although the scale appears to be interval as it provides a range of values from 0 through 5, because subjective interpretation plays a role, the numerical differences are imprecise (hence, "equal-*appearing*").

### *Ratio Scales*

A ratio variable has the same properties as an interval variable, but in addition it uses a true, or absolute, zero. Of the four scale types, the ratio is the most complex. An example of ratio scales used in art therapy research is described in Chapter 3 as a "continuous" scale, in relation to the variable of behavior – specifically, as applied to counting the *frequency of observed behaviors*.

In art therapy assessment research, the absolute zero typically indicates the absence of that variable. To help conceptualize the ratio scale, first consider measures such as weight and height – these are ratio variables because they are interval scales (numerical values with equal intervals between each unit of measurement) with an absolute zero. A pole can be 10 inches tall, or 20, or 1, and "zero inches" means the pole doesn't exist. Similarly, consider the example of money – it is also measured on a ratio scale because zero dollars means no money. It can be determined that having 100 dollars is twice as much as 50 dollars, for instance.

When applied in art therapy assessment research, at first glance, some of the FEATS scales may appear to have properties of a ratio scale because they do include the zero. In some cases, the zero does mean that none of that variable exists. On many scales, a rating of zero is qualified by Gantt and Tabone (1998) to mean, "this variable cannot be rated; or, the person did not do the drawing." Not doing the drawing, leaving the page untouched and blank, would constitute a true zero. However, the subjective process involved in scoring drawings using the FEATS rating system, combined with the fact that the difference between sets of neighboring values on many of the scales varies, renders the scales to be interval/Likert-*type*. As described in relation to Table 7.2, the FEATS *space* scale most closely resembles a ratio scale. In Chapter 3, the variable "space" was also described as a continuous ratio scale used with Human Figure Drawings (Deaver, 2009), through the use of a grid on transparent plastic placed over the drawing, to objectively measure the amount of space used in increments of 25, 50, 75, or 100 percent.

A main strength of the ratio scale is that it enables more advanced statistical analyses. Both interval and ratio scales yield a greater *amount of data* and comparison of data in terms of *direction or magnitude* as compared to nominal and ordinal scales. However, it is the true zero and equal intervals between each consecutive rating that make the ratio scale the most precise level of measurement available (Aiken, 1997). The ratio scale enables use of descriptive statistics, such as frequency distribution and median and percentiles, as well as mean and standard deviation, and inferential computations such as standard error of the mean and coefficient of variation. The trade-off, though, is that it takes longer to rate using a ratio scale and the greater number of choices on interval and ratio scales causes more variation in scoring that impact inter-rater reliability. Consider the FEATS scale, color fit – the rater has six options (zero through 5) on which to rate appropriateness of the colors used in a PPAT drawing, which takes longer than it would were it a two-point scale (such as the nominal scale, idiosyncratic color, from the DDS, with "no" or "yes" as the only options). On the other hand, it can be desirable to gain a more nuanced sense of a variable such as is offered with the FEATS scales. A "yes" or "no" doesn't capture the range of possibilities that can exist along a continuum.

The ability of an art therapy assessment to be clinically useful depends on how the data derived from it is interpreted. If a formal elements rating system is used to gather quantitative (numerical) data, how accurate is that system? If qualitative data are derived, such as through a recording of client comments about the artwork and the process, how effectively has the clinician recorded this content, and how well does she summarize it? If a behavioral observation checklist is used during the assessment session, is the assessor tracking the most salient behaviors? In the summary and report writing phase, how well is the assessor integrating all data points in order to come up with a valid and fair assessment of the client? It is important to consider these questions when approaching art therapy assessment in research and clinical work.

## Establishing Rigor in Art Therapy Assessment Research

This section addresses the need for methodological rigor in establishing the usefulness of an assessment. Rigor is important in assessment research when a researcher's primary aim is to *further establish* an existing instrument (by contributing to its validity and reliability; see Chapter 8), and also during test selection, when a researcher's purpose is to design a study of a client population and a well-established pretest and posttest instrument is required. In either case, this section provides information to help you make informed decisions about both assessment research and test selection. The art therapy assessments summarized in Box 7.1 are cited to illustrate the types of validity and reliability that are needed in order to justify the use of assessments in clinical practice. For information about rigor in the collection of qualitative assessment data, refer to the concepts of credibility, transferability, dependability, and conformability described in Chapter 4.

### *Validity*

Validity is an attribute of the dependent variable (described in Chapter 3). An instrument can be deemed as valid when it measures what it is supposed to measure. An assessment is valid only for a specific use, because validity is relative to the assessment's purpose and subject characteristics. For example, to establish the validity of a test to measure the dependent variable "artistic skill," we might correlate the scores on the test we are using with scores on other tests that purport to measure artistic ability and have been shown to demonstrate a minimal level of psychometric validity. If a high correlation across the tests can be determined, then we have established the validity of our test, and can feel confident using it in our study. Finally, note that an instrument's validity should be determined based on the extent or amount of validity – an assessment can't simply be valid or invalid.

Let's consider an example of validity for the researcher whose aim is to study a population that requires use of a pretest and posttest assessment. The researcher wants to investigate the effect of participation in an adult art therapy group (the independent variable) on level of depression (the dependent variable). To measure the levels of depression, she wants to use an established assessment before and after the intervention. The researcher consults the literature for validation studies and also reviews various instruments known to measure depression. In this way, she determines that the Beck Depression Inventory, second edition (BDI-II; Beck, Steer, & Brown, 1996) is a well-established instrument for her purposes. The BDI studies inform her as to how often in the past it has successfully measured depression with adults, so she can proceed in using it with confidence. This is the traditional approach to validity.

Another area for validity research is the process-focused (PF) model, wherein the "intra- and interpersonal factors that lead to differential performance (and differential prediction) in different groups" (Bornstein, 2011, p. 532) is studied. Whereas the traditional approach to validity focuses on quantifying a relationship between test score and criterion, the PF model manipulates variables in an experimental format to determine *moderating* variables – those factors that impact outcomes in vivo. For example, how a person reacts to the assessment situation in terms of how the testing environment affects his or her performance, and what psychological processes are triggered.

Thus, to determine an assessment's validity, researchers should attempt to collect an array of evidence. Three main types of evidential (research-based) validity examine a test's ability to provide useful, accurate, and unbiased data (Bornstein, 2011): content validity, criterion validity, and construct validity (see Figure 7.2). Importantly, not all methods of validation are relevant for all methods of assessment. Further, in contrast to evidential validity, consequential (impact-based) validity represents the degree to which an assessment successfully yields useful, accurate, and unbiased data in vivo (ibid.).

### Content Validity

Content validity is the extent to which an instrument measures all aspects of a particular social concept. Here, we are concerned with how well the assessment results reflect a client's presenting symptoms or a targeted variable. Content validation is a multimethod, primarily qualitative, process applicable to all aspects of an instrument (Haynes, Richard, & Kubany, 1995). As a qualitative measure of validity, it is normally not quantified

## 182 Assessment Research

**Construct Validity**
*The ability of an instrument to perform well in clinical practice.*

**Convergent Validity**
*The extent to which constructs that should be related to one another are in fact related.*

**Discriminant Validity**
*Serves to confirm that constructs that should not be related to one another are in fact not related.*

**Content Validity**
*Extent to which instrument measures all aspects of a particular social concept.*

**Criterion Validity**

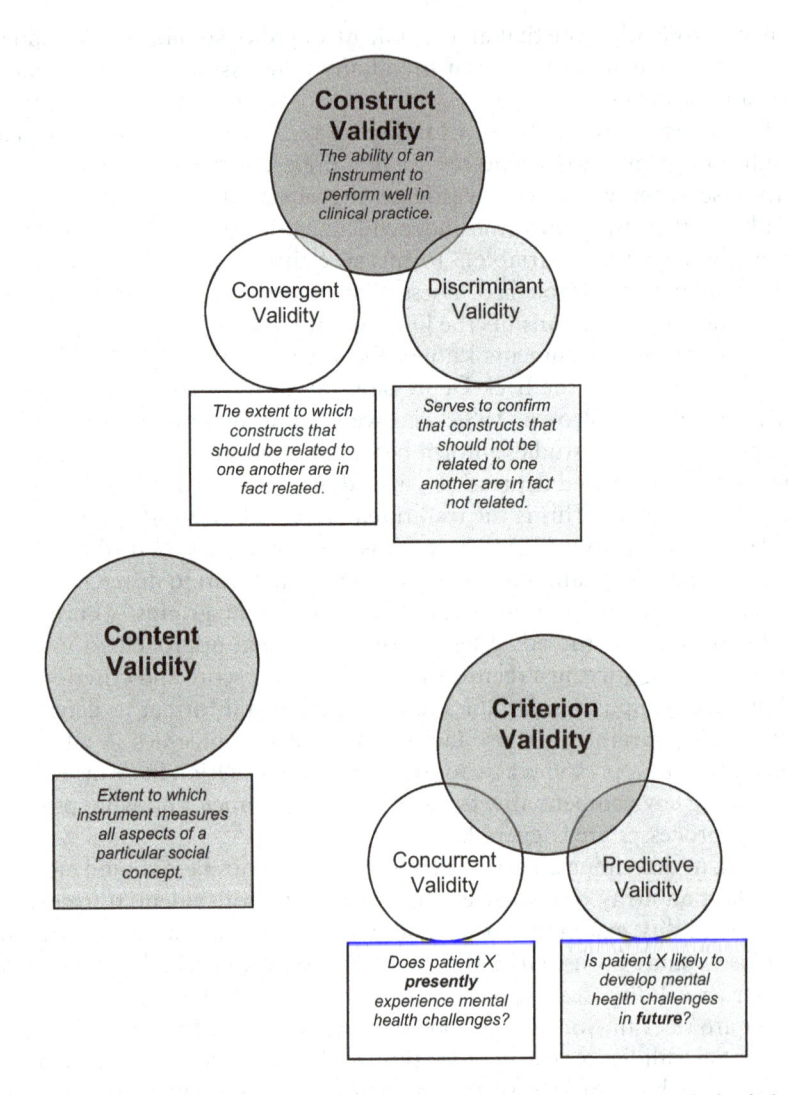

**Concurrent Validity**
*Does patient X **presently** experience mental health challenges?*

**Predictive Validity**
*Is patient X likely to develop mental health challenges in **future**?*

*Figure 7.2* Three main types of evidential validity in assessment research (and their sub-types)
Source: Based on Haynes et al.'s (1995) assertion that "construct validity subsumes all categories of validity" (p. 239), in that each type supplies evidence about an assessment's construct validity.

with statistics. For example, subject matter experts can be consulted to help establish a test's content validity. Content validity should not be confused with face validity (Groth-Marnat & Wright, 2016). Whereas content validity refers to a test's relevance from the perspective of *experts*, face validity is based upon judgments made by a test's *users*.

During the early phases of a test's development, content validation serves to diminish potential error variance and to increase the likelihood of attaining supportive construct validity indices in additional studies (Haynes et al., 1995). In this way, content validity is related to construct validity: Content validity is the degree to which an instrument is representative of the targeted construct. Whereas content validity has traditionally been important in the early phases of a test's development, recently it has been deemed as more closely matching empirically based, rigorous approaches to construct validity. Furthermore, psychological assessment researchers have promoted the establishment of content validity more rigorously from multiple perspectives to include the support of criterion and construct validity in a study's findings (Groth-Marnat & Wright, 2016; Kazdin, 1995). Art therapy assessment research should follow suit by employing a triangulation approach to establishing content validity. Achieving this would require analysis of formal elements scores in addition to behavioral observation data and participant verbalization data. Kortesluoma, Punamaki, and Nikkonen (2008) suggested that verbal discussion might enhance a drawing's content validity. In addition, the clinician should take a sufficient sample of a client's responses on a test and examine each response of interest under varying stimulus conditions as well as different but connected responses (Bruscia, 1988). This would encompass approaches such as systematic observation and qualitative interviewing. Also relevant would be examination of practitioners' interpersonal style and skills used in clinical inference, such as cognitive flexibility, intuition, and empathy, as put forth by psychologist Leonard Handler and colleagues (see Handler & Riethmiller, 1998; Scribner & Handler, 1987). Examples of art therapy assessments that have built this triangulation approach into the protocol (which can be adopted for purposes of validity research) are the AT-PIA (Deaver & Bernier, 2014; Raymond et al., 2010) and the ETC assessment (Hinz, 2009; Van Meter, in press).

A system for establishing content validity for the AT-PIA is already built in to its protocol. This is one of its hallmark features as a comprehensive assessment. Client verbalizations and behavioral observations are a required component – the "Template for AT-PIA Report" (Raymond et al., 2010, p. 9) stipulates that interpretations about the client's psychological dynamics be supported with content derived from the artwork, verbalizations, and behavior. For example, "Poor body image was noted both in behavior (posture when drawing, attire, verbal associations about self) and in the artwork (small distorted human figures)" (p. 8). The artwork is considered based upon its formal elements as well as latent metaphoric and symbolic content.

Another strength of the AT-PIA is its required completion of six drawings in a standardized sequence because collecting a series of drawings on a variety of topics can enhance the assessment's content validity. Deaver and Bernier (2014) described the case example of "Susie Smith," a seven-year-old female living with her mother at a shelter for victims of domestic violence. Based on the AT-PIA's comprehensive system, Susie's imagery and verbal associations pointed to "primitive, oral-level preoccupations" (p. 141) and, taken together, provided preliminary support for establishing the AT-PIA's content validity as a measure of adjustment disorder with anxiety in traumatized children (among other symptoms identified in this complex case). Additional research with clients who have presenting problems and diagnoses similar to Susie's would further validate the AT-PIA.

Another well-known assessment, the Diagnostic Drawing Series (DDS; Cohen & Mills, 2016; Cohen, Hammer, & Singer, 1988) could establish content validity if researchers were to study formal elements scores, verbalizations, and behaviors simultaneously. A study by Fowler and Ardon (2002) that investigated the drawings of those with dissociative disorders could be replicated and built upon to help establish content validity for the DDS, if researchers were to obtain data on client verbalizations and behaviors. The DDS protocol includes a method for gathering client verbalizations using the DDS Drawing Inquiry Form (DIF; Cohen & Mills, 2016), comprising a series of semi-structured interview questions. Although Fowler and Ardon (2002) did not report on DIF data in their study, a future team could do so, thereby augmenting the research. In terms of behavioral observations, the DDS protocol (Cohen & Mills, 2016) includes a section on how to write an evaluation using the DDS, which suggests that the evaluation include behavior: "Mr. X was deeply involved/compliant/hostile," etc. Ideally, participant verbalizations and behaviors would also be examined in conjunction with the drawing variables derived from patient DDSs constituting a step toward content validation for the DDS with the population under investigation.

*Criterion Validity*

The criterion validity of an assessment is a measure of agreement between the results derived from a test and results for the same population, measuring the same construct (variable) obtained either by direct measurement or a well-established instrument that shares the same theoretical orientation (Groth-Marnat & Wright, 2016). These results are compared, and criterion validity is measured by the correlation coefficient between the two assessment methods. Depending on the nature of the resulting data, the criterion validity measures are organized into concurrent validity and predictive validity measures. Both types of criterion-related validity are measured using the correlation coefficient, a number that quantifies relationships between variables, such as the Pearson product-moment correlation coefficient, Pearson's *r*. These concepts are further elucidated below.

An example of establishing criterion validity is found in Deaver's (2009) Human Figure Drawing (HFD) study based upon her approach to strengthening her instrumentation. She established the criterion validity of five modified FEATS/HFD scales by determining relationships (correlations) between: (a) the two sets of scores (the second graders' set and the fourth graders' set) on the five scales used (*color fit, prominence of color, space, developmental level,* and *details of objects and environment*); and (b) scores on ten test HFDs (an existing group of children's HFD drawings not included in the study) rated with the FEATS/HFD. Additionally, she suggested that calculating correlations between scores derived from ten PPAT drawings using the original FEATS (Gantt & Tabone, 1998) and scores on the ten test FEATS/HFDs would be a next step to take to increase concurrent validity of the assessment rating instrument. Correlations of 0.80 and above would establish acceptable criterion validity of the FEATS/HFD scales (Deaver, 2009), because the results would enable comparison of these newly established scales that measure the same five variables to the data derived from the same five variables using the well-established instrument, the FEATS. Establishing criterion and construct validation for the FEATS/HFD would further augment this.

*Concurrent Validity*

Concurrent validity is a type of criterion validity that is determined by gathering data from two different instruments at the same time and comparing the results (Groth-Marnat & Wright, 2016). The goal is to decide to what extent the results of a relatively new or unsubstantiated test relate to results derived from a well-established measurement for the same construct. If the results of the newer test are shown to correspond with the results from the well-established measure, then this helps to establish concurrent validity for the newer test. Consider a study by Lack (1997) that evaluated the concurrent validity of the Person-in-the-Rain (PITR) projective drawing as a measure of children's coping capacity. Scores obtained from the PITR rating system were correlated with demographic variables, nine Rorschach variables, the presence or absence of three psychiatric symptoms, and Wechsler Intelligence Scale for Children-Revised (WISC-R; Wechsler, 1974) scores. In addition, the presence of clinically relevant stressful life events was also compared across participant groups. Results suggested that Lack's PITR rating system measures intelligence. Rorschach variables and psychiatric symptoms supported (offered the most consistent evidence of) concurrent validity for the PITR as a measure of coping capacity, coping style, appraised stress, and depression. So, in this example, a measure of agreement was determined by comparing the PITR data to more "objective," valid results for the same study participants derived from the Rorschach data.

As another example, Groth-Marnat and Roberts (1998) examined the concurrent validity of House-Tree-Person (HTP; Buck & Warren, 1992) drawings and Human Figure Drawings (HFDs) as measures of self-esteem. Forty undergraduate psychology students completed measures of psychological adjustment – the Tennessee Self-Concept Scale (TSCS; Fitts & Warren, 1996) and the Coopersmith Self-Esteem Inventory (SEI; Coopersmith, 2002) – as well as the HTP and HFD drawings. The quantitative composite ratings for psychological health derived from the two drawing instruments did not correspond to the self-esteem measure outcomes. Based on their findings, the researchers suggested that the HTP and the HFD should not be used as measures of psychological health (specifically, self-esteem) for normative groups such as undergraduate students. Instead, they proposed that clinical populations would yield more meaningful discriminations between indicators of psychological health. Further, their nonsignificant findings might have been due to the comparatively subtle differences in self-esteem that they attempted to assess. As such, their conclusions are instructive for art therapy assessment researchers – Groth-Marnat and Roberts (1998) recommended that future studies include clinical and normative groups with a broad range in self-esteem scores or more "impressionistic, global ratings" (p. 221) as opposed to the quantitative total scores that they used. This is precisely the approach undertaken by art therapy researchers such as Gantt and Tabone and their FEATS manual (1998), which is based upon global ratings.

*Predictive Validity*

Predictive validity is an important sub-type of criterion validity. It involves assessing clients on a particular construct (e.g., depression), and then comparing the results with those obtained from the same sample at a future point in time. Mental health professionals would be most interested in predictive validity when needing to determine course of treatment or assess potential for risk of a client engaging in self-harm. Another application of predictive validity includes advising a prospective employer about whether to hire a job candidate based on his or her likelihood of developing an emotional disorder (Groth-Marnat & Wright, 2016). In terms of statistical procedures, predictive validity coefficients tend to diminish each time a client takes a test, as is also true of test-retest reliability.

Given that predictive validity is most appropriate for assessments used to select job candidates and that it is more complex, time consuming, and more expensive to determine than is concurrent validity, it is not surprising that there are no studies of predictive validity of assessments developed by art therapists to date. However, psychologists have been able to establish predictive validity of drawing-based measures such as HFDs. For example, Matto, Naglieri, and Clausen (2005) examined the incremental predictive validity of the Draw-A-Person: Screening Procedure for Emotional Disturbance (DAP:SPED) relative to strengths-based emotional and behavioral functioning criterion measures. They studied 109 youth, aged 9 to 14 years, in general education classes or receiving special education services. The DAP:SPED was found to be a valuable youth-report instrument as an efficient and nonthreatening means to identify children and adolescents who may be in need of "more specialized attention" (p. 41).

In a study on predictive validity to determine whether children's academic achievements could be predicted from independent judgments of their HFDs, ter Laak et al. (2005) examined drawings of 115 students, aged seven to nine years, attending regular or special education schools. The results of multiple regression analysis indicated that social and emotional development and drawing skill did not predict academic achievement. It was concluded that the DAP can be considered "good enough" because of its sensitivity to developmental levels based on children's age and school type, but with only moderate predictive validity (p. 89). This result points to the limited ability of the global approach to measure social and emotional development and cognition in human figure drawings. Thus, predictive validity has been useful in psychology for forecasting job suitability and academic achievement, and for identifying children in need of clinical attention. Art therapists could test predictive validity for identifying individuals who might benefit from art therapy services or who might be at risk for self-harm.

*Construct Validity*

Construct validity refers to the ability of an instrument to perform well in clinical practice. "The most critical psychometric issue involves construct validity and the establishment of linkages between psychophysiological measures and specific psychological processes" (Tornarken, 1995, p. 387). How useful is a given assessment from the perspective of the art therapist using it, in terms of how it may help to identify what's going on with a client and how she or he can best be helped? Construct validity is the most valuable indicator of an instrument's validity. An assessment with good construct validity helps the clinician make important decisions about treatment planning.

To illustrate construct validity in art therapy, consider the case of a researcher whose primary aim is to help *establish* an assessment. In the Deaver (2009) HFD study, two groups that were close together in age – second and fourth graders – were studied to determine if five modified FEATS scales could distinguish the HFDs of the groups. Results established construct validity for the modified scales, such as Scale IV, *developmental level* – fourth graders scored significantly higher on the scale, reflecting congruence with Lowenfeld's stages of artistic development (Lowenfeld

& Brittain, 1987). Thus, we can say that, based on this preliminary research, the Deaver (2009) FEATS/HFD scale for *developmental level* shows promise for testing that construct.

To cite an example from the occupational therapy literature, construct validity for the Sensory Processing Scale (SPS; Schoen, Miller, & Sullivan, 2014) was supported by its differentiation between children with sensory modulation challenges and typically developing control children. Sensory over-responsivity (SOR), sensory under-responsivity (SUR), and sensory craving (SC, also termed sensory seeking) behaviors were compared between the two groups. The clinical group demonstrated more evidence of these behaviors and group differences on all sensory domain scores were significant with large effect sizes, thus providing support for the test's construct validity. The SPS has the potential to aid in differential diagnosis of sensory modulation issues.

Two sub-types of construct validity are convergent validity and discriminant validity. If an assessment can be found to demonstrate both types of validity, then it is said to have robust construct validity. *Convergent validity* determines the extent to which constructs that should be related to one another are in fact related. *Discriminant validity* (also known as divergent validity) serves to confirm that constructs that should not be related to one another are in fact not related. Construct validity is important because of the complex nature of the human psyche. Constructs don't exist independently and they often overlap with one another, so the researcher is challenged to separate them out, to the extent possible, to ensure that the assessment used measures exactly what it is supposed to measure. Well, as close to exact as possible! It's important to gather enough solid data to be able to demonstrate rigor in results and support claims made about an assessment's validity.

An example: A researcher wants to establish construct validity of the FEATS (Gantt & Tabone, 1998) *developmental level* scale. This construct is very difficult to measure in psychological assessment research on adults as its complexity has confounded researchers given the multifaceted constructs it attempts to measure, such as premorbid social competence, moral reasoning, and ego development, to name just a few (Luthar, Burack, Cicchetti, & Weisz, 1997). However, in art therapy assessment research, developmental level is considered primarily in the context of *artistic* developmental level. Nonetheless, other factors impact artistic developmental level, primarily the individual's innate artistic skill and artistic experience (the person's previous exposure to art and art training). Figure 7.3 illustrates the overlapping nature of some of the constructs and variables that comprise developmental level.

Consider a researcher who wants to validate the *developmental level* scale of the FEATS. At the outset, she is aware that at least two other constructs and variables moderate and overlap *developmental level*. What

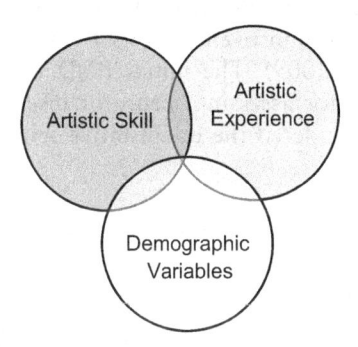

*Figure 7.3* Constructs and variables that comprise developmental level

she needs to do is single out *developmental level*. She would apply *convergent validity* to determine whether and how the two main constructs are actually related to *developmental level*. She would also determine how the demographic variables might be related and how they moderate the assessment outcomes. This can be achieved by including a demographic survey to gather salient demographic information that can then be used in the data analysis process. To check for *discriminant validity*, the researcher would be cautious in how she handled and reported her data in terms of ensuring to the extent possible that the non-overlapping (or more accurately, semi-overlapping) constructs of artistic skill and artistic experience do not overlap too much. It is this kind of complication that makes research of human subjects challenging.

Two additional types of validity with important implications for practice and research are incremental validity and conceptual validity. *Incremental validity* is used to determine whether a new assessment will successfully identify a client's presenting problems and provide accurate diagnostic information better than would an established test. In other words, can the new test increase predictive ability better than the established test against which it is compared? It's increasingly important to demonstrate that a test provides incremental validity more than do other tests, due to the demands of the healthcare system. The idea is to make the assessment process more efficient, so a test deemed to have poor incremental validity would be redundant.

For example, if the Bird's Nest Drawing (in conjunction with a psychological interview) gives a clinician more useful information about a client's attachment security than do other measures, then it would be seen as having incremental validity and the applicability of other measures used may be deemed less relevant. Importantly, *incremental validity* also relates to an assessment's validity based upon modifications made to it over time, typically informed by clinical use or research. For example, the BND has undergone successive refinements in the way the data is collected and analyzed, in order to improve its ability to measure attachment security (Kaiser & Deaver, 2009). The initial BND rating checklist was later replaced by a scale for assessing secure or insecure attachment (Kaiser, 2016), which has rendered the quantitative scoring process more accurate.

### Conceptual Validity

Conceptual validity is considered in the context of generating accurate conclusions about a client. Do the results of the assessment make sense clinically in the context of the client's history and presenting problem? If the assessment results point to depression, is that finding consistent with observed behaviors and/or the reason for referral and the person's family history? As another example, a client referred to treatment for a violent act of rage, who upon intake presents as having lack of empathy and remorse, with a family history of abuse, is administered the BND. If it has high conceptual validity in this case, the BND results should point to disorganized attachment. Conceptual validity can appear to be similar to construct validity, but they differ in an important way – construct validity is based upon previously developed constructs, whereas conceptual validity yields constructs as its outcome. With conceptual validity, the resulting constructs relate to the individual rather than to the test itself, and in this way, it serves as a means of integrating data from the assessment into the report.

In order for an assessment to be relevant, both validity and reliability must be taken into account. A reliable test with poor validity is not useful – results may be consistent but erroneous. Conversely, a valid but unreliable assessment can be of some use, so from this perspective, validity can be deemed more important than reliability. To be of true value, though, a test must be both reasonably valid and reliable.

### Reliability

An assessment's *reliability* depends upon its ability to maintain consistency, accuracy, predictability, and stability. Of interest is the extent to which a client's assessment results remain consistent if the person takes the same test more than once. In psychological assessment research, there are four main methods to determine reliability: test-retest ("time to time"), alternate-form ("form to form"), internal consistency (determined by split-half reliability and coefficient alpha – "item to item"), and inter-rater (or inter-scorer – "scorer to scorer") (Groth-Marnat & Wright, 2016, pp. 13–14).

To grasp the concept of reliability, think about it in this way: Its purpose is to estimate the degree of test variance caused by error. In other words, when individuals are administered a test, the behavior exhibited within a single administration of the test, or across several administrations, will vary. So, we can always expect some fluctuation, or range of error, in such results. Since error is always a factor, it's a matter of reducing the degree of measurement error, to the greatest extent possible (Groth-Marnat & Wright, 2016). *Measurement error* refers to the approximation of the range within which a person's score varies. Moreover, test scores are only an estimate of the constructs we attempt to measure, because it is not possible to assess psychological constructs directly or with 100 percent accuracy!

So, the *degree of error* reminds us to expect that our measures cannot be totally reliable. A number of factors influence an individual's performance on a test. Contributing factors to degree of error include lack of precision in the testing method and fluctuation in the test-taker's performance. Lack of precision in the testing method can be caused by the test itself (no test is perfect), differences in the testing situation (such as interruptions, a different assessor, change in room temperature) or the test administrator (change in demeanor, manner of administering the test, etc.). Good test construction helps to reduce an assessment's inherent imprecision. The test-taker's performance can vary based upon such factors as the individual's energy level, motivation, and anxiety level. The assessor cannot control these factors. Higher reliabilities should be anticipated for an intelligence test than for an assessment of a personality variable such as depression because personality states and traits are more dependent on influential factors such as mood. The assessor must be aware of what variable is being measured, and the potential degree of error.

Due to the above factors, the task of accurate measurement is difficult. Although considered high, 0.80 is the aim for a measure of reliability. If this is attained, the difference between scores, whether time to time, form to form, or item to item, is more likely to result from a true difference than from chance fluctuation. In order to determine how much variation to expect in test scores, a reliability estimate is used, known as the *reliability coefficient*. This coefficient is another expression of the correlation coefficient. Like the validity coefficient, a reliability coefficient expresses a relationship between scores. However, whereas the validity coefficient looks at scores derived from the same people on two different tests, the reliability coefficient explains the difference between people's scores on the same assessment at two different intervals or on two parts of the same assessment. Reliability coefficients differ from other uses of the correlation coefficient, as they cannot have negative values – they must range from 0.00 to 1.00.

An example of the application of reliability coefficients in art therapy assessment research is included in Kim, Kim, and Seo (2014). The authors found the Face Stimulus Assessment (FSA; Betts, 2003) to be both valid and reliable in distinguishing children with ADHD from normal children. They determined reliability in two ways – internal consistency and intra- and inter-rater consistency. *Internal consistency* (reliability) is the extent to which all of the items of a test measure the same latent variable (i.e., those not directly observed but statistically *inferred* based on other variables that are directly measured). The statistical operation Cronbach's alpha is calculated from the pairwise correlations identified between items. Its internal consistency ranges between negative infinity and one. Coefficient alpha is negative whenever there is greater within-subject variability than between-subject variability. Kim et al. (2014) determined internal consistency by computation of the reliability coefficient of assessment items for each FSA drawing. This yielded Cronbach's alpha scores of = 0.778, 0.835, and 0.831 for FSA drawings #1, #2, and #3, respectively. These results were similar to the range of Cronbach's alphas of 0.773–0.910 for the FSA assessment items suggested by Kim (2010). So, Kim et al.'s (2014) research found the FSA to be reliable in measuring the difference between FSA drawing scores (different items on the same test), from "item to item," based on a true difference (rather than from chance fluctuation). In other words, the data was able to successfully demonstrate that FSA drawing items that were assumed to measure the same general construct (symptoms of ADHD) did in fact produce similar scores. To provide a similar example from a word-based test, if a person were to indicate his or her agreement with the concepts "I like to swim" and "I've enjoyed swimming in the past," and disagreement with "I hate swimming," the test would be deemed to have good internal consistency.

Another application of reliability coefficients is found in the Groth-Marnat and Roberts (1998) HTP and HFD study that was described above in relation to concurrent validity. They demonstrated *internal consistency* (reliability) for all 40 of the HFDs and HTPs using Cronbach's alpha, which resulted in reliabilities of 0.69 (HFD1), 0.50 (HFD2), and 0.76 (HTP). Furthermore, the Cronbach's alpha increased to 0.77 when the total number of items encompassing HFD1 and HFD2 was combined into a single 20-item scale. Despite the establishment of internal consistency, however, the quantitative, composite ratings of psychological health for the HTP and HFD did not relate to the formal measures of self-esteem.

Green, Chen, Helms, and Henze (2011) explored reliability reporting practices in psychological assessment research, and identified interesting implications for internal consistency reporting. They conducted a stratified random review of the literature and found that researchers misrepresented reliability "as a property of *scales* as opposed to a property of the samples' *responses* from which their data were derived" (p. 666). They further elucidated:

> If researchers understand that reliability is calculated by using a sample's pattern of responses, then it should become apparent that internal consistency is a property of the sample rather than the scale.

Thus, researchers can accurately interpret their reliability coefficients not as characteristics of measures but as data about test scores that potentially have real-life implications for the people behind the data.
(p. 667)

This team further examined previous data in order to determine the real-life repercussions of researchers' ongoing misappropriation of reliability data. Since the reliability coefficients of research on depression were found to vary across gender and racial or ethnic subgroups, for example, they recommended that preliminary analyses of data be done by researchers to determine whether their data fit the assumptions of their reliability analyses. Doing so has implications for test selection and interpretation of results, which subsequently affect treatment recommendations. Future art therapy assessment researchers and statisticians should consider Green et al.'s recommendations when examining study data – to recognize the people whom we are studying by adopting better practices in internal consistency interpretation, analysis, and reporting.

The *standard error of measurement* is an index that helps us describe, statistically, the extent to which test results change in different situations. Standard error of measurement provides an established range of possible scores that give us context for understanding how much variation, or error, is considered typical for a given test item. A commonly used reference to standard error is poll results reporting a margin of error + or – 3 points. As another example, if a subject takes the same test on multiple occasions, and if all factors are held constant (no memory of questions carrying over, no new learning of the test material), the standard deviation between the subject's test scores is signified as the standard error of measurement. To illustrate, Mouradian, DeGrace and Thompson (2013) examined 40 parents to determine whether an art-based occupation group using scrapbooking in the neonatal intensive care unit (NICU) would reduce their stress, operationalized as anxiety, and found it to be effective. They conducted two repeat administrations of the State-Trait Anxiety Inventory (STAI; Spielberger, 1983), and compared the results to generate estimates and confidence intervals on how the scores changed. The investigators obtained the reliable change index (RCI) by dividing each participant's change in state scores during the intervention by the standardized difference. Since a criterion for the RCI of 1.96 establishes an α for significance of approximately 0.05, a change in state scores was considered meaningful if its RCI exceeded 1.96. They found that, although the RCI is not truly a measure of clinical significance, it provides a rigorous assessment of "whether the observed change in state or trait score is beyond a range that could be attributed to measurement variability" (p. 694). The decline in parents' mean state anxiety (12.7 points, SD = 11.8; $p < 0.0001$) was clinically significant, and the decline in mean trait anxiety (2.6 points, SD = 5.2; $p$ = 0.0036) was statistically significant but not clinically meaningful.

*Test-retest reliability* is measured by comparing two (or more) sets of a client's scores derived from an assessment taken at different time intervals that are carefully determined. If the scores are close, then the assessment is deemed to have test-retest reliability. This is typically achieved through statistical computation of a reliability coefficient between the sets of scores. The amount of time that passes between the assessment administration intervals impacts the coefficient results. Furthermore, test-retest reliability coefficients vary across samples and are therefore not solely the properties of a test.

The *alternate-form reliability* of an assessment aims to correct a problem that can occur with test-retest reliability – the "practice effect." Alternate-form reliability is only applicable with tests that are word-based, not art-based, because it involves changing the wording of questions while preserving the integrity (or "equivalency") of their meaning. To test for this type of reliability, two diverse but parallel forms of a test are administered to the same group of individuals during the same time frame. Simply changing the sequence of the questions in the second version of the assessment is another way to measure alternate form reliability. Alternate form reliability is determined by calculating the correlation coefficient between the test results, and comparing the first version's scores to the second version's scores. Some researchers combine the test-retest and equivalent-forms methods by administering two different forms of an assessment with a coordinated time lapse between the two administrations.

*Inter-rater reliability*, as previously described, is a measure of how often two or more (usually two to three) raters consistently assign the same numbers (scores) to an assessment, such as FEATS scores for PPAT drawings. The goal is to determine how closely raters' scores match. Researchers can then select the appropriate statistical procedure to calculate inter-rater reliability. To achieve optimal results, art therapy researchers are encouraged to consult with a statistician to determine the most appropriate procedure for computing inter-rater reliability. A number of art therapy assessment studies have previously been found to use inadequate methods of rating pictures, and erroneous approaches to determining inter-rater reliability (Betts, 2006). A common problem was the use of the correlation coefficient; as noted by Hacking (1999), Pearson's $r$ does not measure agreement. Rather, it is used to determine the quality of a linear relationship between two variables. Also, given that the correlation coefficient is sensitive to the type of participants studied, using $r$ to assess agreement constitutes a flawed approach. The chi-square statistical procedure is also incorrect in determining inter-rater reliability, as it is yet another test of association. A study by Kay (1979) was cited for incorrectly judging agreement using chi-square. Johnson (2004) used intraclass correlations (coefficient alpha and percent agreement) to compute inter-rater reliability, Gussak (2009) employed the kappa κ statistic, and Bat Or, Ishai, and Levi (2015) used Cronbach's alpha, to cite a few examples of the ways in which art therapy researchers have computed inter-rater reliability.

## Summary

Factors involved in ensuring methodological rigor in establishing the usefulness of an assessment were described earlier in this chapter. We emphasized the importance of understanding rigor in assessment research when attempting to *further establish* an existing instrument (by contributing to its validity and reliability). A resource section at the end of Chapter 8 provides a step-by-step guide for students and researchers who seek to design and conduct an assessment research study. Those interested in pursuing art therapy assessment research are encouraged to investigate those assessments that have already been established, and to follow the recommendations put forth in this chapter. These include triangulation of qualitative and quantitative data, as well as the impact of media dimension variables and the process of art-making, particularly based upon the work of Hinz (2009), Kagin and Lusebrink (1978), and Lusebrink (2010).

## References

Aiken, L. R. (1997). *Psychological testing and assessment* (9th ed.). Boston, MA: Allyn & Bacon.

American Art Therapy Association (AATA). (2013). *Ethical principles for art therapists*. Alexandria, VA: Author.

Bat Or, M., Ishai, R., & Levi, N. (2015). The symbolic content in adults' PPAT as related to attachment styles and achievement motivation. *The Arts in Psychotherapy, 43*, 49–60. Retrieved from https://doi.org/10.1016/j.aip.2014.12.005

Beck, A. T., Steer, R. A., & Brown, G. K. (1996). *Manual for the Beck Depression Inventory-II*. San Antonio, TX: Psychological Corporation.

Beck, A. T., Ward, C. H., Mendelson, M., Mock, J., & Erbaugh, J. (1961). An inventory for measuring depression. *Archives of General Psychiatry, 4*, 561–571. Retrieved from https://doi.org/10.1001/archpsyc.1961.01710120031004

Betts, D. J. (2003). Developing a projective drawing test: Experiences with the face stimulus assessment (FSA). *Art Therapy: Journal of the American Art Therapy Association, 20*(2), 77–82. Retrieved from https://doi.org/10.1080/07421656.2003.10129393

Betts, D. J. (2006). Art therapy assessments and rating instruments: Do they measure up? *The Arts in Psychotherapy, 33*(5), 371–472. Retrieved from https://doi.org/10.1016/j.aip.2006.08.001

Betts, D. J. (2012). Positive art therapy assessment: Looking towards positive psychology for new directions in the art therapy evaluation process. In A. Gilroy, R. Tipple, & C. Brown (Eds.), *Assessment in art therapy* (pp. 203–218). New York, NY: Routledge.

Betts, D. J. (2013). A review of the principles for culturally appropriate art therapy assessment tools. *Art Therapy: Journal of the American Art Therapy Association, 30*(3), 98–106. Retrieved from https://doi.org/10.1080/07421656.2013.819280

Betts, D. J. (2017). *Assessment*. Retrieved from https://donnabettsphd.wordpress.com/assessment/

Betts, D. J. & Groth-Marnat, G. (2014). The intersection of art therapy and psychological assessment: Unified approaches to the use of drawings and artistic processes. In L. Handler & A. Thomas (Eds.), *Figure drawings in assessment and psychotherapy: Research and application* (pp. 268–285). New York, NY: Routledge.

Bornstein, R. F. (2007). Toward a process-based framework for classifying personality tests: Comment on Meyer and Kurtz (2006). *Journal of Personality Assessment, 89*(2), 202–207. Retrieved from https://doi.org/10.1080/00223890701518776

Bornstein, R. F. (2009). Heisenberg, Kandinsky, and the heteromethod convergence problem: Lessons from within and beyond psychology. *Journal of Personality Assessment, 91*(1), 1–8. Retrieved from https://doi.org/10.1080/00223890802483235

Bornstein, R. F. (2011). Toward a process-focused model of test score validity: Improving psychological assessment in science and practice. *Psychological Assessment, 23*(2), 532–544. Retrieved from https://doi.org/10.1037/a0022402

Bruscia, K. E. (1988). Standards for clinical assessment in the arts therapies. *The Arts in Psychotherapy, 15*, 5–10. Retrieved from https://doi.org//10.1016/0197-4556(88)90047-0

Buck, J. N. & Warren, W. L. (1992). *The House-Tree-Person projective drawing technique: Manual and interpretive guide* (rev. ed.). Los Angeles, CA: Western Psychological Services.

Butcher, J. N., Graham, J. R., Ben-Porath, Y. S., Tellegen, A., Dahlstrom, W. G., & Kaemmer, B. (2001). *Minnesota Multiphasic Personality Inventory–2: Manual for administration, scoring and interpretation* (rev. ed.). Minneapolis, MN: University of Minnesota Press.

CAAHEP (Commission on Accreditation of Allied Health Education Programs). (2016). *Standards and guidelines for the accreditation of educational programs in art therapy*. Clearwater, FL: Author.

Cohen, B. M., Hammer, J. S., & Singer, S. (1988). The Diagnostic Drawing Series: A systematic approach to art therapy evaluation and research. *The Arts in Psychotherapy, 15*(1), 11–21. Retrieved from https://doi.org/10.1016/0197-4556(88)90048-2

Cohen, B. M. & Mills, A. (2016). *The Diagnostic Drawing Series (DDS) handbook*. Alexandria, VA: Self-published e-packet.

Coopersmith, S. (2002). *Coopersmith Self-Esteem Inventories: Manual*. Palo Alto, CA: Mindgarden.

Deaver, S. (2002). What constitutes art therapy research? *Art Therapy: Journal of the American Art Therapy Association, 19*(1), 23–27. Retrieved from https://doi.org/10.1080/07421656.2002.10129721

Deaver, S. (2009). A normative study of children's drawings: Preliminary research findings. *Art Therapy: Journal of the American Art Therapy Association, 26*(1), 4–11. Retrieved from https://doi.org/10.1080/07421656.2009.10129309

Deaver, S. P. & Bernier, M. (2014). The art therapy projective-imagery assessment. In L. Handler & A. Thomas (Eds.), *Figure drawings in assessment and psychotherapy: Research and application* (pp. 131–147). New York, NY: Routledge.

Dudley, J. (2004). Art psychotherapy and the use of psychiatric diagnosis. *Inscape, 9*(1), 14–25.

Elliott, R., Fischer, C. T., & Rennie, D. L. (1999). Evolving guidelines for publication of qualitative research studies in psychology and related fields. *British Journal of Clinical Psychology, 38* , 215–229. Retrieved from https://doi.org/10.1348/014466599162782

Exner, J. (2003). *The Rorschach: A comprehensive system* (4th ed.). New York, NY: Wiley.

Finn, S. E. (2007). *In our clients' shoes: Theory and techniques of therapeutic assessment.* New York, NY: Routledge.

Finn, S. E. (2011). Journeys through the valley of death: Multimethod psychological assessment and personality transformation in long-term psychotherapy. *Journal of Personality Assessment, 93*, 123–141. Retrieved from https://doi.org/10.1080/00223891.2010.542533

Finn, S. E. (2012). Implications of recent research in neurobiology for psychological assessment. *Journal of Personality Assessment, 94*(5), 440–449. Retrieved from https://doi.org/10.1080/00223891.2012.700665

Fischer, C. T. (2000). Collaborative, individualized assessment. *Journal of Personality Assessment, 74*, 2–14. Retrieved from https://doi.org/10.1207/S15327752JPA740102

Fischer, C. T. (2001). Collaborative exploration as an approach to personality assessment. In K. J. Schneider, J. F. T. Bugenthal, & J. F. Pierson (Eds.), *The handbook of humanistic psychology: Leading edges in theory, research and practice.* Thousand Oaks, CA: Sage.

Fitts, W. H. & Warren, W. L. (1996). *Tennessee Self-Concept Scale* (2nd ed.). Torrance, CA: Western Psychological Services.

Fowler, J. P. & Ardon, A. M. (2002). Diagnostic Drawing Series and dissociative disorders: A Dutch study. *The Arts in Psychotherapy, 29*, 221–230. Retrieved from https://doi.org/10.1016/S0197-4556(02)00171-5

Gantt, L. (1990). A validity study of the Formal Elements Art Therapy Scale (FEATS) for diagnostic information in patients' drawings (doctoral dissertation, University of Pittsburgh, Pittsburgh, PA).

Gantt, L. & Tabone, C. (1998). *The Formal Elements Art Therapy Scale: The rating manual.* Morgantown, WV: Gargoyle Press.

George, C. & West, M. (2012). *The Adult Attachment Projective Picture System: Attachment theory and assessment in adults.* New York, NY: Guilford Press.

Golomb, C. (1974). *Young children's sculpture and drawing.* Cambridge, MA: Harvard University Press.

Graves-Alcorn, S. & Green, E. (2014). The expressive arts therapy continuum: History and theory. In E. Green & A. Drewes (Eds.), *Integrating expressive arts and play therapy with children and adolescents* (pp. 1–16). Hoboken, NJ: Wiley.

Green, C. E., Chen, C. E., Helms, J. E., & Henze, K. T. (2011). Recent reliability reporting practices in *Psychological Assessment*: Recognizing the people behind the data. *Psychological Assessment, 23*(3), 656–669. Retrieved from https://doi.org/10.1037/a0023089

Groth-Marnat, G. & Roberts, L. (1998). Human Figure Drawings and House Tree Person Drawings as indicators of self-esteem: A quantitative approach. *Journal of Clinical Psychology, 54*(2), 219–222.

Groth-Marnat, G. & Wright, A. J. (2016). *Handbook of psychological assessment* (6th ed.). New York, NY: Wiley.

Gussak, D. (2009). The effects of art therapy on male and female inmates: Advancing the research base. *The Arts in Psychotherapy, 36,* 5–12. Retrieved from https://doi.org/10.1016/j.aip.2008.10.002

Hacking, S. (1999). The psychopathology of everyday art: A quantitative study (doctoral dissertation, University of Keele, Sheffield, UK). Retrieved from www.wfmt.info/Musictherapyworld/modules/archive/stuff/papers/Hacking.pdf

Handler, L. & Riethmiller, R. (1998). Teaching and learning the administration and interpretation of graphic techniques. In L. Handler, M. J. Hilsenroth, L. Handler, & M. J. Hilsenroth (Eds.), *Teaching and learning personality assessment* (pp. 267–294). Mahwah, NJ: Lawrence Erlbaum.

Harris, D. B. (1963). *Children's drawings as measures of intellectual maturity.* New York, NY: Harcourt, Brace.

Haynes, S. N., Richard, D. C. S., & Kubany, E. S. (1995). Content validity in psychological assessment: A functional approach to concepts and methods. *Psychological Assessment, 7*(3), 238–247. Retrieved from https://doi.org/10.1037/1040-3590.7.3.238

Hinz, L. D. (2009). *Expressive Therapies Continuum: A framework for using art in therapy.* New York, NY: Routledge.

Johnson, K. M. (2004). The use of the Diagnostic Drawing Series in the diagnosis of bipolar disorder (doctoral dissertation, Seattle Pacific University, Seattle, WA).

Kagin, S. L. & Lusebrink, V. B. (1978). The Expressive Therapies Continuum. *The Arts in Psychotherapy, 5,* 171–180. Retrieved from https://doi.org/10.1016/0090-9092(78)90031-5

Kaiser, D. H. (1996). Indications of attachment security in a drawing task. *The Arts in Psychotherapy, 23*(4), pp. 333–340. Retrieved from https://doi.org/10.1016/0197-4556(96)00003-2

Kaiser, D. H. (2016). Assessing attachment with the Bird's Nest Drawing. In D. E. Gussak & M. L. Rosal (Eds.), *The Wiley-Blackwell handbook of art therapy* (pp. 641–657). Hoboken, NJ: Wiley-Blackwell.

Kaiser, D. H. & Deaver, S. (2009). Assessing attachment with the Bird's Nest Drawing: A review of the research. *Art Therapy: Journal of the American Art Therapy Association, 26*(1), 26–33. Retrieved from https://doi.org/10.1080/07421656.2009.10129312

Kay, S. R. (1979). Significance of torque in retarded mental development and psychosis: Relationship to antecedent and current pathology. *American Psychologist, 34*(4), 357–362. Retrieved from https://doi.org/10.1037/0003-066X. 34.4.357

Kazdin, A. E. (1995). Preparing and evaluating research reports. *Psychological Assessment, 7*(3), 228–237. Retrieved from https://doi.org/10.1037/1040-3590. 7.3.228

Kim, S. R. (2010). A study on development of FSA evaluation standard and its validation (doctoral dissertation, Yeungnam University, Daegu, South Korea).

Kim, J., Kim, G., & Sco, S. (2014). Validation of the FSA as a screening tool for children with ADHD. *The Arts in Psychotherapy, 41*, 413–423. Retrieved from https://doi.org/10.1016/j.aip.2014.04.006

Koppitz, E. M. (1968). *Psychological evaluation of children's human figure drawings*. New York, NY: Grune and Stratton.

Kortesluoma, R., Punamaki, R., & Nikkonen, M. (2008). Hospitalized children drawing their pain: The contents and cognitive and emotional characteristics of pain drawings. *Journal of Child Health Care, 12*(4), 284–300. Retrieved from https://doi.org/10.1177/1367493508096204

Laak, J. der, de Goede, M., Aleva, A., & van Rijswijk, P. (2005). The Draw-A-Person Test: An indicator of children's cognitive and socioemotional adaptation? *The Journal of Genetic Psychology, 166*(1), 77–93. Retrieved from https://doi.org/10.3200/GNTP.166.1.77-93

Lack, H. S. (1997). The Person-in-the-Rain projective drawing as a measure of children's coping capacity: A concurrent validity study using Rorschach, psychiatric, and life history variables (doctoral dissertation, California School of Professional Psychology, Alameda, CA).

Lowenfeld, V. & Brittain, W. L. (1987). *Creative and mental growth* (8th ed.). New York, NY: Macmillan.

Lusebrink, V. B. (2010). Assessment and therapeutic application of the Expressive Therapies Continuum: Implications for brain structures and functions. *Art Therapy: Journal of the American Art Therapy Association, 27*(4), 168–177. Retrieved from https://doi.org/10.1080/07421656.2010.10129380

Luthar, S. S., Burack, J. A., Cicchetti, D., & Weisz, J. R. (Eds.). (1997). *Developmental psychopathology: Perspectives on adjustment, risk, and disorder*. New York, NY: Cambridge University Press.

Matto, H. C., Naglieri, J. A., & Clausen, C. (2005). Validity of the Draw A Person: Screening Procedure for Emotional Disturbance (DAP: SPED) in strengths-based assessment. *Research on Social Work Practice, 15*(1), 41–46. Retrieved from https://doi.org/10.1177/1049731504269553

Mihura, J. L., Meyer, G. J., Dumitrascu, N., & Bombel, G. (2012). The validity of individual Rorschach variables: Systematic reviews and meta-analyses of the Comprehensive System. *Psychological Bulletin, 139*(3), 548–605. Retrieved from https://doi.org/10.1037/a0029406

Mills, A., Cohen, B. M., & Meneses, J. Z. (1993). Reliability and validity tests of the Diagnostic Drawing Series. *The Arts in Psychotherapy, 20*(1), 83–88.

Mouradian, L. E., DeGrace, B. W., & Thompson, D. M. (2013). Art-based occupation group reduces parent anxiety in the neonatal intensive care unit: A mixed-methods study. *American Journal of Occupational Therapy, 67*(6), 692–700. Retrieved from https://doi.org/10.5014/ajot.2013.007682

Naglieri, J. (1988). *DAP, Draw a Person: A quantitative scoring system manual.* New York, NY: Psychological Corporation.

National Institute of Mental Health (NIMH). (2016). *NIMH strategic plan for research, strategic objective 3.2: Develop ways to tailor existing and new interventions to optimize outcomes.* Retrieved from www.nimh.nih.gov/about/strategic-planning-reports/strategic-research-priorities/srp-objective-3/priorities-for-strategy-32.shtml

Raymond, L., Bernier, M., Rauch, T., Stovall, K., Deaver, S., & Sanderson, T. (2010). Art therapy projective imagery assessment (training manual, Graduate Art Therapy and Counseling Program, Eastern Virginia Medical School, Norfolk, VA).

Rosal, M. (1992). Illustrations of art therapy research. In H. Wadeson (Ed.), *A guide to conducting art therapy research.* Mundelein, IL: American Art Therapy Association.

Schoen, S. A., Miller, L. J., & Sullivan, J. C. (2014). Measurement in sensory modulation: The Sensory Processing Scale Assessment. *American Journal of Occupational Therapy, 68,* 522–530. Retrieved from https://doi.org/10.5014/ajot.2014.012377

Schore, A. N. (2011). *The science of the art of psychotherapy.* New York, NY: Norton.

Scribner, C. & Handler, L. (1987). The interpreter's personality in Draw-a-Person interpretation: A study of interpersonal style. *Journal of Personality Assessment, 51*, 112–122. Retrieved from https://doi.org/10.1207/s15327752jpa5101_10

Snyder, C. R., Ritschel, I. A., Rand, K. L., & Berg, C. J. (2006). Balancing psychological assessments: Including strengths and hope in client reports. *Journal of Clinical Psychology, 62*(1), 33–46. Retrieved from https://doi.org/10.1002/jclp.20198

Spielberger, C. D. (1983). *Manual for the State-Trait Anxiety Inventory (Form V).* Palo Alto, CA: Consulting Psychologists Press.

Stafstrom, C., Havlena, J., & Krezinski, A. (2012). Art therapy focus groups for children and adolescents with epilepsy. *Epilepsy & Behavior, 24*(2), 227–233.

Stevens, S. S. (1946). On the theory of scales of measurement. *Science, 103*(2684), 677–680. Retrieved from https://doi.org/10.1126/science.103.2684.677

Tornarken, A. J. (1995). A psychometric perspective on psychophysiological measures. *Psychological Assessment, 7*(3), 387–395. Retrieved from https://doi.org/10.1037/1040-3590.7.3.387

Van Meter, M. L. (in press). *The Expressive Therapies Continuum and parallels in neuroscience.* New York, NY: Routledge.

Wechsler, D. (1974). Wechsler intelligence scale for children–revised. New York, NY: Psychological Corporation.

White, C. R., Wallace, J., & Huffman, L. C. (2004). Use of drawings to identify thought impairment among students with emotional and behavioral disorders: An exploratory study. *Art Therapy: Journal of the American Art Therapy Association, 21*(4), 210–218.

Yoon, J. Y. & Betts, D. J., & Holttum, S. (submitted). Bird's Nest Drawing stories in the assessment of attachment security.

Chapter 8

# Designing and Executing an Art Therapy Research Study

Research course objectives in graduate art therapy programs typically include research concepts as applied to the profession and contextualize these in the broader sphere of mental health. Students also need experientially based learning opportunities toward completion of the requirements for their degree, such as a research proposal and/or a capstone project or thesis. Experiential learning is facilitated through identification of a topic that interests the student and engagement in related hands-on activities such as reviewing literature and planning out the steps to conduct a study using a particular design. This also permits the teaching of related important concepts such as ethical implications and institutional review board (IRB) requirements for research with human subjects.

As described in Chapter 1, it behooves art therapy educators who teach research to be familiar with the criteria for "Thesis or Culminating Project" set forth in the CAAHEP (2016) Standards and Guidelines. The required knowledge, skills, and behaviors that students must develop for competency in this content area include the ability to "organize research on the literature in the field as the basis for an extensive thesis or culminating project" (*knowledge*); "create an in-depth study of one aspect of art therapy or an integration of knowledge and clinical skill in art therapy" and "complete a thesis or culminating project based on established research methods (e.g., quantitative, qualitative, mixed methods, arts-based), innovative methods of inquiry, clinical practice, or a synthesis of clinically based personal and professional growth (e.g., service learning, designing a program, designing a "tool kit" for art therapists) (*skills*); and "participate in opportunities and support for sharing thesis or culminating project outcomes in a public forum (e.g., thesis presentations, written article for publication, submission of grant application)" (*affective/behavior*) (p. 22). Additional desired learning outcomes for graduate art therapy research can include augmentation of students' understanding of the purpose, benefits, and challenges of conducting art therapy research; knowledge of foundational approaches, theories, techniques, and evaluation methods of art therapy and the mental health professions; proficiency as art therapy researchers, with consideration of the inter-relationships among theory, practice, and science; self-evaluation and critical-thinking skills through art making and written critique of research; and knowledge of methods of data collection and analysis, interpretation, and reporting results.

In this chapter, specific guidelines for writing a research proposal are delineated. We describe the development of the first three chapters of the research report: the introduction, the literature review, and the methods (procedures). Techniques for optimal teaching and learning of each unit are suggested, with references to the book's supplemental materials. Factors unique to art therapy research are described – those related to enhancing study quality, and special considerations pertaining to controls for the extraneous variables of artistic skill and background, cultural appropriateness of art-based instruments and interventions, and variability in the artwork of children. Materials to supplement this chapter include a sample table of contents/headings template for the proposal and worksheets to guide students/researchers in the development of proposals; research idea, research question, review of the literature, research designs (quantitative, qualitative, mixed methods, program development, case study, heuristic, arts-based), sampling plan, ethics, and rigor and integrity (see Appendices).

A flow chart (Figure 8.1) is provided to illustrate a schema for conceptualizing the research process, from development of the research problem, through the proposal phases, to study completion. Research for art therapists should be embraced in the way we approach the creative process. When embarking on a research pursuit, envision the potential for creative flow through all stages of the project, as is shown in Figure 8.1. The outlined arrows indicate the ideal flow through the stages, and the black arrows indicate the reality of research as a circular – not linear – cycle, emphasizing that the process should be approached accordingly. As described by Alon (2009), research involves "meandering" (p. 3). Each stage informs the other as we meander through the stages and learning to embrace this as a creative process encourages students to engage more fully in research pursuits. Additionally, as the results of a study begin to emerge, we are reminded that new or unexpected discoveries that may diverge from the original research idea, problem, question, or hypothesis can be more fully embraced, rather than perceived as a failure.

The traditional model for the research report includes five chapters: (I) the Introduction, (II) the Literature Review, (III) the Methods/Procedures, (IV) the Results, and (V) the Discussion. The present chapter provides specific guidelines for writing the research report in two main sections: "The Research Proposal" and "Completing the Research Report." In "Section I: The Research Proposal," specifics about the development of a sound art

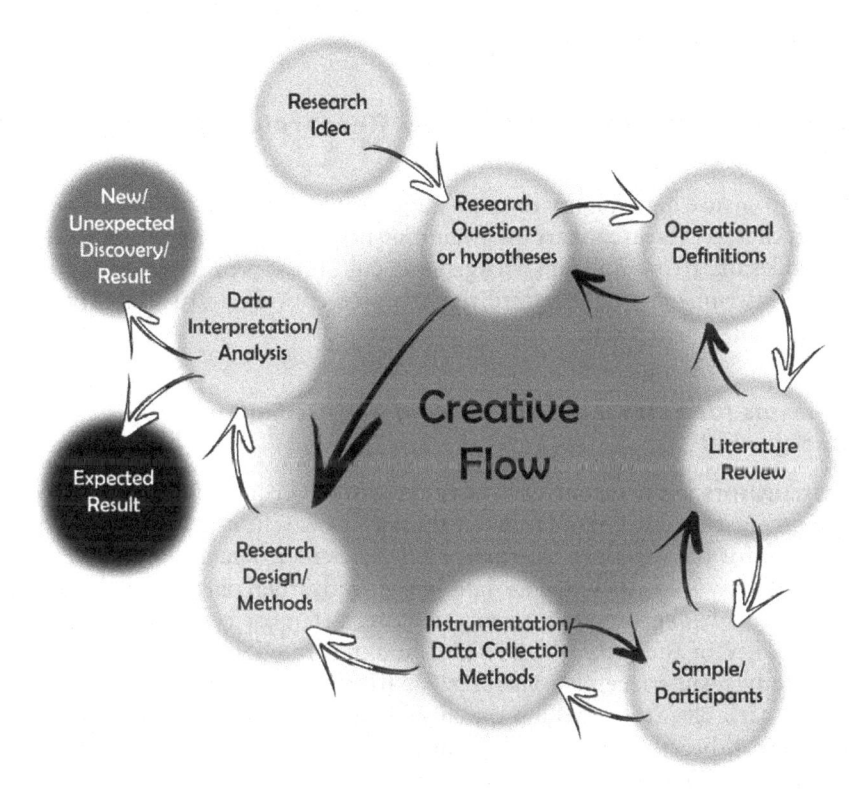

*Figure 8.1* The art therapy research process: flow chart
Source: Adapted from Fraenkel, Wallen, and Hyun (2015).

therapy research proposal are provided. The first three chapters that serve as the research proposal are detailed, based on the traditional model for the research report that comprises the research proposal: the Introduction, the Literature Review, and the Methods (or Procedures). Material to supplement this section includes worksheets to guide students/researchers in the development of proposals, for components such as: research idea and problem – curiosity and inquiry; research question; literature review; research design; sampling; ethical considerations; rigor and integrity; and data interpretation/analysis.

"Section II: Completing the Research Report" focuses on writing up Chapter IV (Results) and Chapter V (Discussion), based on the traditional research report model. Finally, as an aid to educators, students, and practitioner-researchers, this chapter culminates with "Section III: How to Conduct an Art Therapy Research Study (and Judge its Quality)," which offers a practical step-by-step guide on this process.

First, three topics unique to art therapy research and study quality are briefly discussed.

## Factors Unique to Art Therapy Research Impacting Study Quality

To help ensure high quality through all phases of research, factors unique to art therapy research warrant attention such as controls for extraneous variables of artistic skill and background, cultural appropriateness of art-based instruments and standardized art interventions, and variability in the artwork of children.

### Controls for Extraneous Variables of Artistic Skill and Background

Investigators need to control for variables that affect study outcomes to the greatest extent possible. In art therapy research, it is imperative to account for the variables of *artistic skill* and *artistic background/experience*. If artwork is included as data in the study, then participants' skill/talent and background/experience making art most certainly impacts the quality of the artwork that is to be interpreted and factored in to the study results (see also Chapter 7). To control for these two extraneous variables (those which the investigator has limited or no ability to control directly), data can be collected through asking questions on a demographic questionnaire (see the "Demographic Questionnaire for Art Therapy Research" form in Appendix A) or, such controls can be directly built into the study. For instance, participants can be invited to draw a still life or another means of determining artistic skill in real time.

### Cultural Appropriateness of Art-Based Instruments and Interventions

The researcher should be aware of the ways in which artwork is interpreted in different clinical settings and according to cultural variations, and how this informs the approach to interpretation in the context of research. Betts (2013) addressed in depth the considerations necessary for successful adaptations of art therapy assessments in multicultural and cross-cultural contexts. Very few drawing-based assessments developed in the United States by psychologists and art therapists were originally tailored for use with a range of culturally diverse groups, so there is a need for increased awareness of the implications of using such instruments with diverse populations with respect to cultural sensitivity and relevance.

In terms of artwork interpretation from a culturally relevant and ethical perspective, it's also important to consider the ways in which art therapists are able to "harness the potential of visual communication" (Curtis, 2011, p. 9). Meaning-making in art therapy is "cyclical, relational, and personal" (p. 6), which brings to the foreground the viewer's relationship to the image. Citing the work of Arnheim (1966) and Acosta (2001), Curtis (2011) recommended that "observers come to know themselves and the image (its separate elements, the gestalt, and their relation to each other), rather than thinking about the image as just a sum of its parts" (p. 5). To this end, use of Betts' Art Therapy Inquiry Form (2016; Appendix B) is recommended.

Also relevant to artwork interpretation is individual variation in observation and inference skills and other intrapersonal factors on the part of researchers. As psychologists Handler and Riethmiller (1998, paraphrasing Emanuel Hammer) stated: "In the hands of some, figure drawings are like disconnected telephones" (p. 270). Accordingly, they recommended validating the person interpreting the artwork, to assess his or her skill. Scribner and Handler's (1987) work revealed that interpreters with affiliative interpersonal orientations were significantly more accurate in their interpretations of artwork, as compared to those who were found to be disaffiliative. Another study found that traits needed to attain success in artwork interpretation include cognitive flexibility, intuition, and empathy (Burley & Handler, 1997). Each of these sources points to the need for consideration of a relational approach to the art therapy session and the artwork produced by the client or research participant. This is especially true for investigations of mechanisms of change – examining how and why clients experience change during art therapy treatment, and which variables are most salient to this process.

### Variability in the Artwork of Children

Through clinical experience, art therapists come to appreciate that children vary greatly in their approach to artwork depending upon a range of factors such as cultural background, socioeconomic status, age, gender, and so forth. We know that the artwork of children can show indicators of various developmental stages and that development does not occur in a predictable manner for all children. These issues have been explored in the scholarly literature. Deaver (2009) underscored the need for establishment of normative data on children's artistic development and the importance of factoring for cultural differences. Citing the work of Hess-Behrens (1973), Deaver (2009) emphasized that Piaget's (Piaget & Inhelder, 1971) stages of cognitive development do not apply to children universally. A few studies have since been undertaken by art therapists, including Levick's (2009) and Alter-Muri and Vazzano's (2014). An investigation of 700 children from 13 African countries, Asia, Europe, North America, and Central America was pursued by Alter-Muri and Vazzano (2014). They examined gender typicality in artwork and scrutinized Lowenfeld and Brittain's (1987) theory of artistic development. Alter-Muri and Vazzano's (2014) study offers a different perspective on understanding normative development in children's artwork in its finding of disparity between Lowenfeld and Brittain's (1987) ages and stages of artistic development, with important implications for clinical practice and research, especially regarding the importance of factoring individual and cultural differences when interpreting artwork.

It's important to keep in mind the factors unique to art therapy research when designing a study. Doing so helps to ensure high quality through the stages of the research, as one takes the first step toward deriving a plan and creating the research proposal.

## Section I: The Research Proposal

Development of a research proposal helps graduate art therapy students become acclimated to concepts important to the research process. Whether they go on to develop their proposals to conduct an actual study or not, proposal development is considered a fundamental part of the art therapy master's degree curriculum. This section offers practical guidelines for introducing students to research toward development of the first three chapters that comprise the research proposal: the Introduction, the Literature Review, and the Methods/Procedures. Each of these is outlined in Box 8.1, and further elucidated in "Section III: How to Conduct an Art Therapy Research Study (and Judge its Quality)."

### Box 8.1 The Research Proposal: Overview

- The following sections are typically included in a dissertation or research report and are intended to serve as a guide.
- The *Publication Manual of the American Psychological Association* (APA, 2010) style for formatting should be followed.
- Some of the suggested categories are not necessary or appropriate for all studies, and the order of items within chapters may vary somewhat.
- Note that, for the proposal, use of future tense ("I propose to investigate…" and "I will employ an experimental design…," etc.) is applied. Following completion of the study, the proposal language is converted to past tense ("In this study, I investigated…" and "I employed an experimental…").

## Chapter I: Introduction (Problem to be investigated)

- *Background of the problem*: Describe trends in the art therapy profession related to the problem, unresolved topics, and/or related social concerns.
- *Statement of the problem*: State the identified problem that is to be investigated and describe the justification of the need or rationale for the proposed study and its importance.
- *Purpose of the study*: Emphasize the area of concern, explain relationships among variables or comparisons to be considered, describe expected outcomes (including conceptual or substantive assumptions), and describe scope and delimitations (to narrow your focus).
- *Research questions and/or hypotheses*: Describe questions to be answered or objectives to be investigated, and/or state hypotheses (directional or non-directional).
- *Definition of terms*: Provide operational definitions for key variables and terms of study.
- *Brief overview of study*: Outline of the remainder of the proposal or paper.

## Chapter II: Literature Review

- Provide overview and organization of the chapter.
- Summarize and integrate existing studies with focus on who has done work, what has been found, where and when studies were completed, and methods used, including design, data collection, and interpretation/ statistical analyses implemented (literature review of methods can alternately be used in chapter on methods/procedures).
- Establish need for the study and likelihood of obtaining meaningful and/or significant results.
- Draw from various theoretical perspectives to establish and support your research question and/or hypotheses.

## Chapter III: Methods (or Procedures)

- Describe research design and, if quantitative or MMR, study variables (independent and dependent).
- Describe the sample (selection of participants and their relevant characteristics).
- Describe the instruments used (tests, questionnaires, observational data, scales, data interpretation, and/or scoring procedures and information about the validity and reliability of each).

- Describe procedures followed (detailing how the study will actually be carried out).
- Discuss the study's internal and external validity.
- Describe the data analysis methods to be used (and justification for these).

Sources: Adapted from Isaac and Michael (1995, pp. 239–241) and Fraenkel, Wallen, and Hyun (2015, p. 624).

## Embarking on Research and Developing the Proposal

In preparation for embarking on a research pursuit, students' natural wonder and curiosity can be tapped through experiential and art-based activities. Suggestions are offered in this book's supplemental materials – the unit outlines, and worksheets and experientials for this section, which are also referenced below. Betts and Potash (2018) developed a unique and effective research simulation experiential that brings research to life by actively engaging students in generating qualitative and quantitative data while teaching research concepts. Educators are invited to try out this approach and modify any part of the protocol to best suit their preferences. The data generated by the students yields material that is used throughout a one-semester course to illustrate research concepts in a dynamic and lively manner that promotes deep engagement.

### Research Simulation Experiential

Students and their research methods instructor meet at a local art gallery, where students are invited to participate by agreeing to partake in the mock study, through an informed consent process. The instructor leads the students into a gallery space, where they complete a mood scale (pre-test), and then engage in the mock experiment, which involves a series of activities. They are asked to view the exhibit, and to select one artwork that is the most meaningful to them (see Figure 8.2). Then, they are asked to respond to a series of questionnaires that generate qualitative and quantitative data.

The data collection materials are included in Appendix A and are explained forthwith:

1. The *Art Exhibit Visit* form is designed to gather information about the artwork's title, artist, year, materials, and dimensions.
2. The *Art Characteristics* questionnaire includes nine categories, including *Number of Elements, Arrangement of Elements*, and

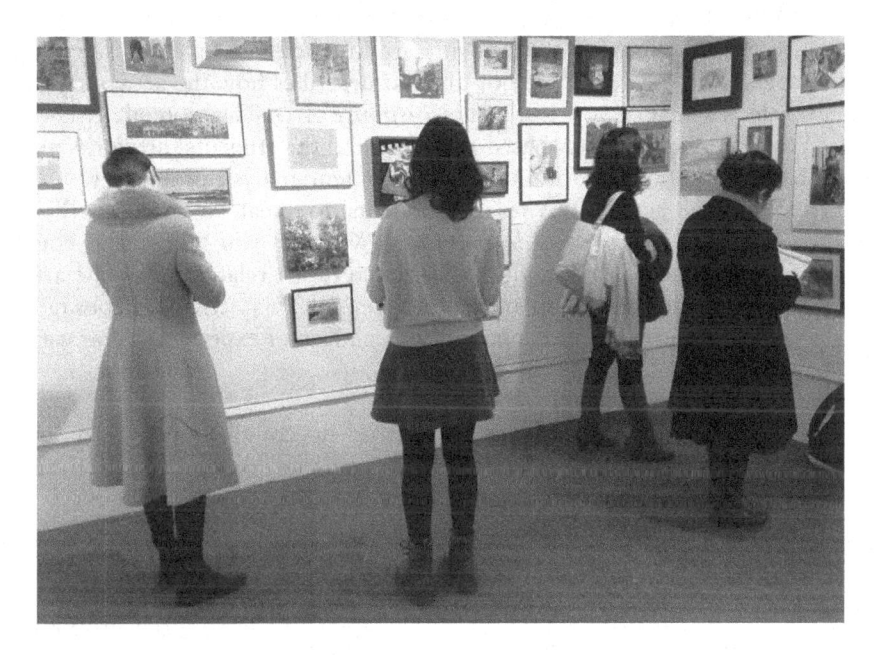

*Figure 8.2* Research simulation experiential: students in an art gallery

*Clarity of Presentation*, and respondents are invited to circle structural descriptions that best match their selected artwork (in a dichotomous or categorical format). For example, the category *Number of Elements* is described as either "simple" (least number necessary, focus) or "complex" (many forms, intricate, distracts). Input from this form yields nominal and ordinal data that are used in the course later to elucidate categorical data analysis procedures.

3. The *Relational Aesthetics Questionnaire* invites students to explore their choice in a meaningful way based on a relational aesthetics framework, defined as: "A set of artistic practices which take as their theoretical and practical point of departure the whole of human relations and their social context, rather than an independent and private space" (Bourriaud 1998, p. 113). Specifically, this task asks participants to consider the degree to which each of ten statements was a factor in selecting their artwork (on a five-point Likert scale), beginning with the statement, "I was interested in the colors used in this art." The responses yield numerical data which are later used to illustrate concepts of quantitative analysis and, to generate qualitative data, participants are invited to write (in long-hand) in the space provided a description of why the artwork was meaningful.

4. A blank page is provided for the *Response Art* activity, to generate art-based data, and the students are instructed to "please use color pencils to create a sketch or art that describes how the artwork you selected makes you feel" (the *Response Art*). This content is later used in teaching arts-based research, and the students' artworks are referenced in class for a unit about content analysis of imagery.
5. The final activity invites respondents to create a *title* for their Response Art, write a *description* ("What do you see?"), and construct *meaning* ("How does this sketch or art relate to how the artwork from the exhibit makes me feel?"). This activity encourages reflective learning and enhances articulation of experiences that usually remain tacit.

Following completion of these tasks, students complete the post-mood scale, and answer basic demographic questions (age, gender, undergraduate degree major, race, and ethnicity).

### Chapter I: Introduction (Problem to be Investigated)

As is delineated in Box 8.1, the first chapter of the research proposal typically includes the following sections: background of the problem, statement of the problem, purpose of/rationale for the study, research questions and/or hypotheses, definition of terms, and brief overview of study. Students are taught about these components through the experiential and supplemental course materials, described forthwith.

The Research Idea – Curiosity and Inquiry (Worksheet 1)

To engage and excite students it is of central importance in the first few weeks of the research course to elicit their buy-in to the research endeavor. Research in art therapy is framed as enhancing understanding of how people's experiences affect their lives, enabling increased awareness of how art therapy helps, and yielding more precise knowledge that can impact quality of practice (Kapitan, 2018). Students are invited to come up with ideas that are of interest to them toward development of the research problem, so they are called upon to consider various sources of inspiration. These ideas can come from internship experiences, art therapist role models, theories and approaches learned in other courses, and so forth.

As they generate ideas using Worksheet 1 (see Appendix C), students are encouraged to consider questions that serve as a bridge to Worksheet 2, such as why, what, and how they want to learn about the selected topic. The content in Box 8.2 is offered as an example of research questions relevant to art therapy that can serve to generate ideas for areas of inquiry.

## Box 8.2 Components to inform an art therapy assessment research proposal using the Expressive Therapies Continuum

The use of art media and art processes in art therapy is core to practice and should therefore be a prioritized area of inquiry. As is described in Chapter 7, the Expressive Therapies Continuum provides this central theory for art therapy practice and, as such, some key research questions (suggested by Hinz, 2014) are offered here to assist in generating ideas that would be important to pursue:

1. What types of experiences are evoked by the basic media used in art therapy? How can we best describe basic media properties and their therapeutic effects?
2. How can we best define task structure and task complexity? What are the effects of task structure and task complexity on participant experience in art therapy?
3. Can we gather factor analysis data to demonstrate the three-level structure of the Expressive Therapies Continuum?
4. Can we investigate the basic principles involved in art therapy assessment based on the model of the Expressive Therapies Continuum; that is, catalogue the normal range of visual expressions and their pathological variations (similar to studies of other art therapy assessments)?
5. Can we conduct ongoing investigation to define what media and task instructions are most effective in addressing symptoms/challenges associated with different disorders/difficulties?
6. Can we explore the creative transition area of the Expressive Therapies Continuum?

The ETC assessment could also be researched through the Research Domain Criteria (RDoC) framework (NIMH, n.d.). As explained in Chapter 1 of this book, the RDoC is a research framework for new ways of studying mental disorders. It integrates many levels of information (from genomics to self-report) toward improved understanding of the range of human behavior from normal to abnormal. There are five RDoC categories: (1) negative valence systems, (2) positive valence systems, (3) cognitive systems, (4) systems for social processes, and (5) arousal/regulatory systems.

Sources: Hinz (2009), Kagin and Lusebrink (1978), and Lusebrink (2010).

## The Research Question (Worksheet 2)

This unit (see Appendix D) is organized around the theme "How can I expand my curiosity?" with the aim of teaching concepts to aid in development of good research questions. Students are encouraged to refine their research ideas and questions through specific activities. This content also relates to the content from Box 8.1 on research questions (hypotheses are covered later, in Worksheet 4) and definition of terms.

Students are next guided to restate their research idea as a researchable question, using Worksheet 2. They are invited to brainstorm and consider what they already know about their chosen subject. Then they are asked to generate a list of questions. To support this process, class time is dedicated to teaching characteristics of good research questions, such as that they must be feasible, ethical, clear, and meaningful (Fraenkel, Wallen, & Hyun, 2015). In teaching the art of question development, new vocabularies for talking about research are explored (Gillis, 2014). One way to approach this is by encouraging students to ask odd-angled questions (Lesnick, 2009). Students are invited to brainstorm characteristics of good questions, which include such elements as questions that can't be answered with yes or no, that are unexpected, that draw connections, that cannot remain general, that allow for multiple answers, and that examine a problem from multiple angles (Gillis, 2014). This approach relies on the idea that, when embarking on exploration of the unfamiliar, we almost always start with what is familiar or obvious. From this, additional questions can be developed sequentially, with each building upon the previous question. Such questions can initially be posed in a basic form, such as "I'm curious about," "I'd like to know more about," "I wonder about," etc. This process is intended to enable students to delve deeper into question development, until a feasible research question emerges.

Step 4 on Worksheet 2 invites students to then divide their list of questions into two categories: (1) questions that can be answered through a series of activities involving the gathering of new data, such as through direct observation, artifact description, analysis, interpretation, or interviews (primary or "field" research); and (2) questions that can be answered by reading and reflecting on what answers others have provided about the topic of interest, such as through a search of the literature (secondary or "desk" research). The associated exercise is to review their list of questions, choose one from the first category (primary research), and write down some ways in which they might answer this question.

Definition of terms is also covered in Worksheet 2. Students are instructed on how to compose definitions of key terms for their proposed study. This includes explanation of constitutive (dictionary) versus operational definitions (assign meaning to a variable or concept by clarifying the operations or activities needed to measure it [quantitative] or observe it [qualitative]).

*Chapter II: Literature Review (Worksheet 3)*

*The Literature Review (Worksheet 3)*

The literature review serves several purposes. Primarily, it enables students to become familiar with the previous work of others on their topic of interest. Students need to know what has already been accomplished, how it was accomplished, the quality of the published scholarship about the work, and the extent to which each source is relevant to their research question. Students should read widely and then conduct a selective evaluation to decide what to include in their literature review, known as the selective literature review.

Worksheet 3 (see Appendix E) is used in conjunction with a hands-on activity in the classroom. Each student is equipped with computer access to the university library database and the class is instructed on optimal search techniques. Instructors and peers provide each student with individualized support during this session in formulating search terms pertinent to the research problem. Based on their research idea, students are invited to consult "experts" (the literature) or, put another way, to inquire, "Who do I need to invite to my research party?"

*Chapter III: Methods (or Procedures)*

In the methods chapter, the goal is to delineate and describe the ways in which students propose to carry out their research. By way of introduction to the different methodologies associated with research paradigms, an overview is provided, prior to more in-depth exploration of each spanning several instructional classroom hours or sessions. One approach to the methodology overview is illustrated through the *Still Life Experiential* (Betts & Potash, 2018). Students are invited to sketch a still life (Figure 8.3) and the images are displayed as a group once they are completed (Figure 8.4). Instructors facilitate a discussion on the range of perspectives represented in the drawings, and how this experience relates to the selection of methodology as informed by one's worldview. Students tend to home in on the metaphors of this experiential as mirroring the process of selecting a research design. For instance, they can determine that looking at a still life from different angles offers different perspectives, which then points to the subjective nature of research, trustworthiness of data, inductive versus deductive reasoning, etc.

Four worksheets are used to supplement teaching various research designs: 4. Quantitative and Experimental; 5. Qualitative; 6. Program Development and Case Study; and 7. Heuristic and Arts-Based (see Appendices F, G, H, and I). Following is an orientation to each of these and recommendations for their use. It is suggested that instructors teach students all the methodologies, but that particular attention be given to

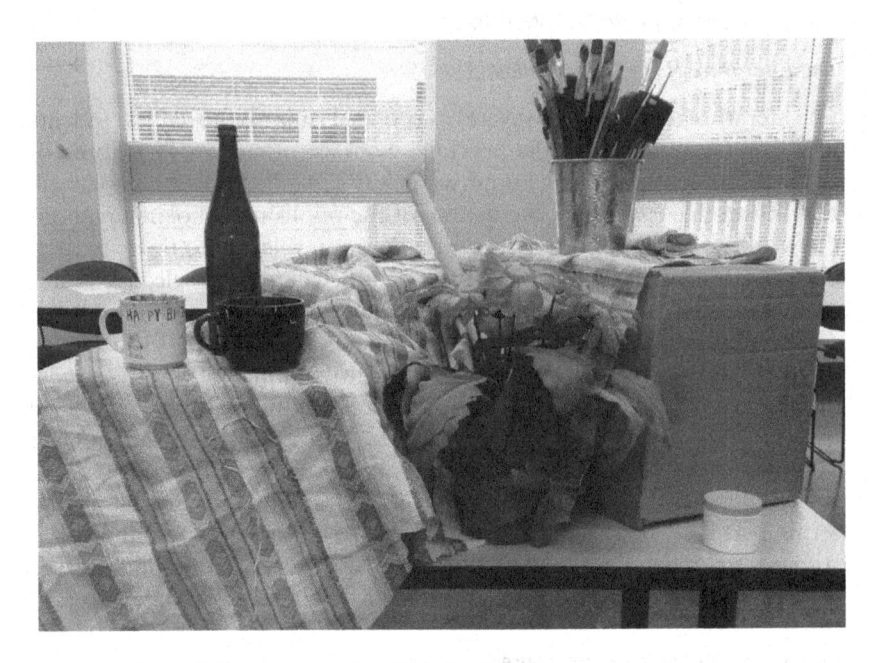

*Figure 8.3* The still life experiential: still life display

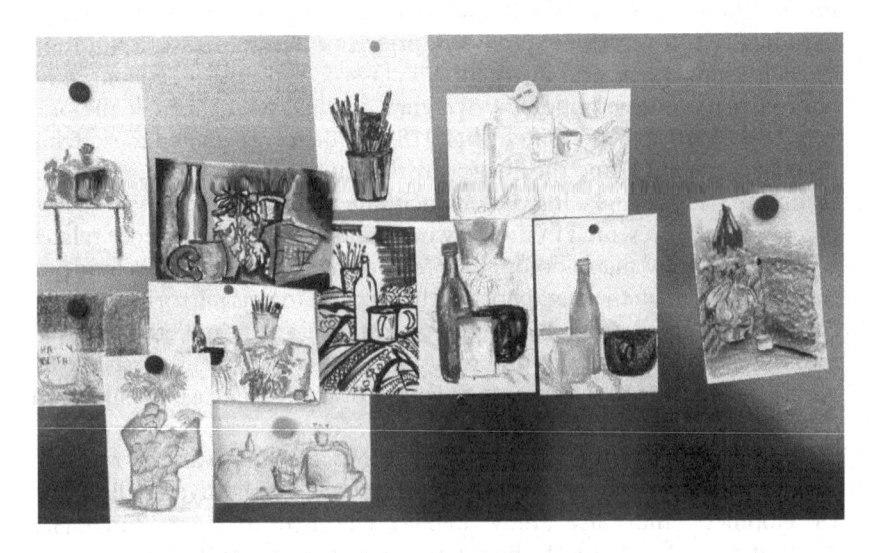

*Figure 8.4* The still life experiential: students' still life drawings

methods most conducive to art therapy research. As such, an instructor may choose to adapt the four worksheets related to the methodologies (Worksheets 4–7) according to the preferred research approach on a particular graduate art therapy program.

Research Design – Quantitative and Experimental (Worksheet 4)

Worksheet 4 (Appendix F) guides students in quantitative, experimental, (and non-experimental) research designs, as a supplement to Chapter 3 of this book. With Worksheet 4, students are asked to generate a hypothesis (directional or non-directional) related to their idea that can be answered using quantitative experimental and non-experimental means, in an attempt to explain cause and effect or to establish relationships that are not causal, such as in survey and assessment research. They are asked to consider their hypothesis/assumption as suggesting a relationship between at least two variables. In designating the functions of their dependent and independent variables, students determine extraneous variables that might affect their proposed study results. A final purpose of Worksheet 4 is to describe the types of instruments and/or means of data collection (tasks, activities) the students can consider for their study.

Research Design – Qualitative (Worksheet 5)

Worksheet 5 (Appendix G) guides students in tailoring their research idea and research question to form a qualitative framework. It can be used in conjunction with Chapter 4. The qualitative method is described as the use of stories, narratives, images, and lived experience to understand an event, circumstance, or process in-depth, with the aim of answering *how* or *what* in relation to a phenomenon of interest. Students are asked to specify a question related to their idea that can be answered using qualitative methods, and to describe the concepts or topics related to their idea. This worksheet is also used to describe types of data collection that can be proposed for use in the qualitative framework, such as interviews and observations.

Research Design – Program Development and Case Study (Worksheet 6)

Students are guided in tailoring their research question into the format of a program development proposal (i.e., development of an art therapy program) or a case study proposal using Worksheet 6 (Appendix H). These are combined in one worksheet, as program development and case study research aim to use direct observation and involvement to understand a specific person or program (see also Chapter 4). These methods also generally involve immersing oneself in the participants' circumstances. Students are thereby guided in formulating a question related to their idea that can be answered through direct observation and/or involvement with an individual case or agency. They are further invited to consider the types of data collection (interviews, observations) that are most likely to glean the kind of date that will answer their research question.

Research Design – Heuristic and Arts-Based (Worksheet 7)

The contents of Worksheet 7 (Appendix I) provide students with the opportunity to explore their research questions in the context of heuristic and arts-based designs (see also Chapter 5). Students are instructed that this approach to research aims to harness their own life experiences to augment self-awareness or personal development, and generally involves immersing oneself in a topic by being interviewed, engaging in reflective writing, and/or making art. In the worksheet, they develop a question related to their topic and describe the types of qualitative data collection procedures they might use.

At this point in the course timeline, students are provided with individualized guidance on the selection of a method that would be most feasible for their chosen research focus. To remain on track with the course's timeline, students are asked to commit to one particular method that is consistent with their personal values and worldview. This enables them to proceed in developing their proposal and further tailor aspects of their study accordingly, such as regarding the sampling plan, ethical considerations, rigor and integrity, and instrumentation.

Sampling (Worksheet 8)

Worksheet 8 (Appendix J) is structured to support consideration of quantitative sampling procedures (see also Chapter 3), as well as how participants are recruited in qualitative research (see also Chapter 4). To begin, students are asked to consider the demographic characteristics of their proposed sample. For quantitative proposals, students need to identify the intended sampling procedure (simple random, convenience, etc.), and how they plan to obtain their sample. Instruction is provided on external validity, and, if a quantitative study is proposed, students must consider how their results may or may not be generalizable in terms of accessible population and target population. Considerations for ecological validity (the extent to which study procedures match up with the real world) are also included in reference to accessible population and target population.

Ethical Considerations (Worksheet 9)

Worksheet 9 (Appendix K) should be used in conjunction with Chapter 2 of this book. The worksheet invites student comments on possibilities for harm to their proposed participants, and how they would handle such harm. Possible problems are offered for consideration, including any that may be related to confidentiality, deception, conflict of interest, use of images of research participants' art in the final research report, and so forth.

Rigor and Integrity (Worksheet 10)

The ways in which rigor and integrity are achieved in research are explored in the various chapters of this book that address the various research paradigms. Worksheet 10 (Appendix L) is designed to help students explore concepts central to rigor and integrity, as applied to their methodology of choice. Students are asked to identify threats that apply to their proposed study and explain how they would attempt to control for these. Possible threats include subject characteristics, mortality, location, instrumentation, testing, history, maturation, subject attitude, regression, and implementation. Each of these threats, and the means for addressing them, is described in Chapter 3 on quantitative research. For qualitative research, students must describe how they will ensure integrity.

Concepts of validity and reliability are also explored by the student using Worksheet 10. For studies employing quantitative methods, internal validity, external validity, reliability, and objectivity must be considered (see Chapter 3). Students with a qualitative proposal are required to consider credibility, transferability, dependability, and conformability (see Chapter 4).

Finally, Worksheet 10 is a useful guide for students who plan to use instrumentation in their design, such as scales, measures, surveys, and observations. Students are asked to list any existing instruments/means of data collection they have chosen to answer their research questions or hypotheses. Further, they must express what they have learned about the validity and reliability of these instruments/means of data collection; relevant psychometrics are salient to the overall rigor in research. If the students intend to develop their own instruments/means of data collection, they must explain how they propose to ensure the internal consistency, reliability, and validity of the results.

## Section II: Completing the Research Report

### *Proposal Complete – What's Next?*

Once the research proposal is complete, those who go on to conduct their studies will write up their outcomes and findings in the form of Chapters IV (Results) and V (Discussion). This section explains how to write up these sections of a research report for a capstone paper or thesis, including issues unique to writing reports on qualitative, quantitative, and other research paradigms described in this book (see Box 8.3). Finally, the process of preparing the report for publication is briefly described.

*Chapter IV: Results*

In Chapter IV, the results of the collected data and analysis are reported and displayed visually using figures (such as photographs of artwork) and tables. Such graphics are referred to and summarized descriptively in the text of the chapter. Descriptive data is typically presented first, and results are organized to consistently parallel the research questions (or hypotheses), which are restated. For qualitative studies, verbatim quotes are used to exemplify findings, and patterns, themes, and sub-themes are explained. Any new or unexpected results that emerged (see Figure 8.1) can be reported and related to questions that emerged during the later stages of the research process. The chapter closes with a summary statement.

*Chapter V: Discussion*

This chapter entails the discussion in the form of a summary of all salient aspects of the study's findings and includes the researcher's own speculations about the results. Whereas the purpose of Chapter IV is to report and present the study's results, Chapter V is intended for discussion of the implications of the results through meaningful interpretation of the findings, conclusions derived from the results, and implications of these results and their relevance as compared to previous literature on the topic. When discussing how the study confirms or contradicts previous research, the relevant literature presented in Chapter II (Literature Review) is cited. Recommendations for practical applications of the findings to establish how the study advances the knowledge base and informs art therapy practice are described. Limitations of the study and how it could be improved in future research endeavors are also provided. This content informs suggestions for future explorations of the topic, which are offered to assist other researchers and promote cohesive investigations.

---

**Box 8.3 Completing the Research Report: Overview**

The following sections are typically included in a research dissertation or report and are intended to serve as a guide.

Not all suggested categories are necessary or appropriate for all studies, and the order of items within chapters may vary somewhat.

(Follow APA for formatting and begin with: Title page, Table of Contents, List of Figures, List of Tables.)

### Chapter IV: Results

- Description of findings related to each research question and/or hypothesis posed in problem statement.
- Presentation of findings in tables or charts when applicable.
- Use of headings that correspond to each research question and/or hypothesis.
- Factual presentation of information (avoid interpretation and inference as these are addressed in Chapter V).

### Chapter V: Summary, Conclusions, and Recommendations

- Brief summary of everything covered in first three chapters and in findings portion of Chapter IV.
- Discussion of findings tied together with theory and review of literature (connect findings cited in your Chapter II and compare with your findings, and if your results are surprising and unrelated to the literature already cited, you may introduce a few key sources).
- Restatement of questions and/or hypotheses as inferences with some degree of certainty and generalizability (quantitative) or transferability (qualitative).
- Discussion of limitations.
- Recommendations (practical suggestions for implementation of findings, such as implications for clinical practice, or for additional research).

Sources: Isaac and Michael (1995) and Fraenkel, Wallen, and Hyun (2015).

### *Preparing for Publication*

Upon completion of their research papers and typically following graduation, students can be encouraged to pursue publication of their work. Those who wish to undertake writing up their work for submission to a journal should consider authorship. You may choose to publish as the sole author of your work, to publish in collaboration with a colleague, or, if you're a recent graduate, to produce a co-authored manuscript with the program faculty member(s) who worked with you (as advisor or thesis chair, for instance). The *Publication Manual of the American Psychological Association* (APA, 2010) is an essential resource for art therapists seeking to publish, and many other books and online resources are also available. Prospective authors should be aware that writing for publication involves investing considerable personal resources in terms of time and energy, along with a commitment to advancing the knowledge base of one's discipline. In addition, condensing a lengthy work such as a master's thesis to meet the parameters for article publication presents the challenges of summarizing key points, homing in on the main findings, and minimizing less relevant content. Art therapists are encouraged to surmount the difficulties and forge ahead in conducting and publishing research! The results of these efforts will enrich our body of knowledge and enhance the services we provide for all who may benefit from art therapy.

## Section III: How to Conduct an Art Therapy Research Study (and Judge Its Quality)

The present section provides a step-by-step guide for students and researchers in setting up an art therapy research study and includes benchmarks related to study quality to aid in evaluation of a research report. We've chosen to tailor the example to a correlational study of an assessment currently under investigation, the Bird's Nest Drawing (BND; Kaiser, 1996) as a measure of attachment security. The BND is presented to more fully explore key concepts such as operationalization and measurement of theoretical constructs and indicators of study quality. Moreover, much of the content of this section will be useful as a general resource for assembling the main components of a research study, as its contents parallel the suggested format delineated in Box 8.1 and Box 8.3. First, a brief overview of the BND is offered.

Kaiser's (1996) study on indications of attachment security in a drawing task was her foundational work in developing the standardized art therapy directive that later came to be known as the Bird's Nest Drawing (BND) assessment (see also Chapter 7). The Bird's Nest Drawing and story was developed over 20 years ago by Donna Kaiser (1996), based on her interest in a measure of attachment that could serve as a graphic representation of Inner Working Models (IWMs; Bowlby, 1969), which would be easy to administer; access unconscious dimensions of a person's mental models, feelings, and expectations about family and intimate relationships; and circumvent defenses that tend to arise when a person is asked to complete a family drawing. The BND was also deemed attractive for its potential ability to evoke attachment concerns that could be addressed therapeutically. Moreover, the BND is a process-based, constructive assessment, in that it involves drawing a bird's nest and writing a story about it. Since Kaiser's (1996) paper, a collection of small thesis studies has attempted to improve the BND's validity and reliability (Kaiser & Deaver, 2009). Procedures for BND administration have been standardized whereas the methods for assessing the drawing and story remain in development. Numerous iterations of the BND rating system, which began as a sign-based approach examining individual indicators, have since evolved and now the BND includes a scale to determine secure or insecure attachment based on a more global approach. This is further detailed in Kaiser (2016). Fourteen items are rated using an interval scale to determine the extent to which each variable is evident. Kaiser's system also includes themes and looks at the coherence of the story, and efforts are underway to establish the first in-depth system for coding BND stories (Yoon, Betts, & Holttum, submitted).

## Chapter I: Introduction

First, begin with conceptualization of Chapter I, the Introduction (problem to be investigated). The main sections in Chapter I include: background of the problem, statement of the problem, purpose of the study, research questions and/or hypotheses, definition of terms, and a brief overview of the study.

### Background of the Problem

In this opening section you briefly detail industry trends related to a problem and its corresponding unresolved issues. For example, Kaiser (1996) began her paper with a clear rationale related to a trend in art therapy, "Drawing tasks for diagnosis and screening can prove to be valuable instruments for art therapists" (p. 333). From there she developed this argument with specifics such as how image making helps to augment client insight and build rapport between the art therapist and the client.

### Statement of the Problem

Here, you describe the specific area of concern and justify the need for the study. What is the basic difficulty or felt need for the proposed investigation? Based upon the background of the problem she identified, Kaiser (1996) delineated the problem of a need for research on the theoretical construct of attachment in art therapy assessment research. Specifically, she explored whether "an individual's depiction of a bird's nest may tap unconscious psychic representations of early caregiving experiences that contribute to secure or insecure attachment patterns" (p. 334). She provided justification for her study through the literature she cited (see Chapter II, below, on the literature review for more on this).

### Purpose of the Study

This segment should emphasize the area of concern, explain relationships among variables or comparisons to be considered, elucidate expected outcomes including conceptual or substantive assumptions, and describe scope and boundaries (delimitations) to help narrow your focus. Kaiser's (1996) area of concern was to examine how drawing a bird's nest might elicit graphic indicators of secure or insecure attachment style in women. Thus, she set out to investigate the relationship between graphic indicators in a bird's nest drawing and attachment patterns as determined by the Attachment to Mother (ATM) scale of the Inventory of Parent and Peer Attachment (Armsden & Greenberg, 1987), and developed a descriptive and correlational study design to explore her hypotheses.

In terms of expected outcomes, Kaiser (1996) conceptually assumed that an individual's drawing of a bird's nest would "tap unconscious (internalized) ... representations of early caregiving experiences that contribute to secure or insecure attachment patterns" (p. 334). The scope and boundaries (delimitations) of the study included a focus on 41 women of ages 21–38 using the services of a university day care center.

*Research Questions and/or Hypotheses*

In this section, you describe questions to be addressed by your study or objectives to be examined, and/or, if it's a quantitative study, state a hypotheses (directional or non-directional). Kaiser (1996) hypothesized that nine specific characteristics in bird's nest drawings (determined by a checklist devised by Kaiser, the Attachment Rating Scale – ARS) would serve as indicators of attachment security. The first four items related to the "containing function" of the nest, and the other five items related to the use of formal elements including space, line quality, color, and placement and size of the nest (p. 335).

*Definition of Terms*

This section provides an opportunity to define (operationalize) key variables and terms that are to be included in the study. Drawing from our example, relevant terms from Kaiser (1996) that would need to be defined include variables of interest (levels of attachment security) as measured by the Attachment to Mother (ATM) scale, and the nine graphic indicators she identified. To provide an example of an operational definition from the Kaiser study, consider *line quality*: This indicator should be noted when the line quality in a BND "suggests excessive energy and fills most of the paper space" (Kaiser, 2016, p. 651). (Note that this definition came later than the original 1996 study and was based on additional research indicating that many BNDs by insecure individuals have been drawn with excessive energy, filling most of the page space, suggesting anxiety.)

*Brief Overview of the Study*

In this section, which wraps up Chapter I, you provide an outline of the remainder of the proposal or paper. This would summarize next steps, including study procedures and methods of data interpretation and analysis.

## Chapter II: Literature Review

This chapter is your opportunity to compile and convey information relevant to your study based on what has been previously written about your topic. Kaiser (1996) further delineated the rationale for the use of drawing tasks for screening and diagnosis based on the art therapy literature, and the use of attachment theory as a foundation for research on measures of individuals' attachment systems. Citing the groundbreaking work of Bowlby (1969), Ainsworth, Blehar, Waters, and Wall (1978) and others, Kaiser (1996) made a solid case for the relevance of understanding and making use of attachment theory at all stages of mental health treatment, beginning with assessment and evaluation. She further delineated the need for a new approach to assessing the individual's perception of interpersonal conflict and familial and relational dynamics, and the need for tasks that provide "greater emotional distance" (p. 334). To establish her use of the bird's nest as a drawing directive, Kaiser cited the work of Edinger (1972), who described the nest as a protective and maternal symbol, and Naumann (1955), who observed its quality of containment, among others. Additionally, Kaiser (1996) argued that, "the theoretical concept of an unconscious internal working model of secure or insecure attachment" (p. 333) is conducive to symbolic manifestation of this unconscious content through the process of creative expression (making a drawing) that is an integral part of art therapy practice. Once completed, she argued that the drawing can then be used to examine the client's past experiences and how these affect current relationships toward the identification and reworking of insecure attachment patterns.

## Chapter III: Methods or Procedures

In this chapter, describe your research methods or approach, beginning with the research design.

*Research Design*

In this section, provide details on the variables involved in your study, including independent, dependent, and others as applicable (moderating variables, for instance). Optionally, and if statistical analysis of results is planned, you may formulate an operational statement of your research hypotheses. The variables of interest in Kaiser (1996) – i.e., as related to attachment theory – are described below in the context of her subject selection and participant demographics.

## Selection of Subjects

The selection or sampling of participants is important, to ensure that the correct variables are being measured in keeping with the purpose of the assessment under investigation. Three main factors should guide the researcher in determining selection of participants appropriate to the study goals (Weiner, 1995). In normative studies, the participants should share similarities with the types of people to whom the results are intended to be generalized (to the extent possible). In comparison studies, the groups under investigation should resemble each other in particular ways. Finally, in both normative and comparison studies, participants should be grouped "independently of the measures that are being used to assess them" (p. 330). Weiner warned that, without such independence, study variables may be contaminated in ways that adversely impact any positive findings. You want to consider inclusion and exclusion criteria as well; that is, the characteristics that your prospective subjects must possess to be included in the study, and the characteristics that would render prospective subjects excluded from the study.

When researching the BND, Kaiser (1996) set out to establish an instrument that could help "provide a framework for the therapist and client to explore past experiences as they impact current attachment patterns" (p. 333). Since the population for which the BND is intended to be used includes a range of people of all ages in individual, couples, family and group art therapy, as a means of assessment as well as to introduce attachment concepts, a range of populations would need to be investigated to augment the BND's validity and reliability. Kaiser began this endeavor with a descriptive and correlational study of mothers, as an obvious population of study when it comes to attachment.

The subjects in Kaiser's (1996) study were 41 women, aged 21–38, from a university day care center. Because research has shown that secure attachment organization is found in approximately 60% of the population, the remaining 40% would be thought to be insecurely attached, defined as either insecure-avoidant or insecure-ambivalent (Campos, Barrett, Lamb, Goldsmith, & Sternberg, 1983). Therefore, Kaiser created two groups of study – one group designated as high (secure) attachment, and the other as low (insecure) attachment, making it a "comparison" study. She considered it likely that there would be an adequate number of subjects in each attachment category to achieve correlation.

*Instrumentation*

In the instrumentation section of Chapter III, the methods that you use in your study to test your hypotheses (or examine your research questions) are described. These methods are specified as scales, tests, observations, measures, and/or questionnaires. The instrumentation you choose for your study is an opportunity for you to build in controls for extraneous variables. This can be accomplished by asking questions with a demographic questionnaire, or by asking participants to complete a still-life drawing. In a study on the concurrent validity of Human Figure Drawings and House-Tree-Person drawings as measures of self-esteem, Groth-Marnat and Roberts (1998) measured the effect of artistic ability by asking participants to rate their own drawing ability on a five-point scale ranging from "excellent" to "poor" (p. 220).

Kaiser's (1996) instrumentation is described in her article under the heading, "Assessment Procedures" (p. 335). Also included is a description of her research procedures (e.g., what instructions were provided to subjects or how materials were distributed), as well as methods used for data collection and recording and data processing and analysis. These elements are also important to include in the methods chapter. Methodological assumptions and study limitations (weaknesses) can be described here as well, and the ways in which they impacted the study results should be addressed in Chapter V (Discussion). A summary can be written to wrap up the chapter and lead in to the next.

## Chapter IV: Results

The purpose of Chapter IV is to present study results. Typically, this is accomplished through presentation of findings in the form of charts or tables, which are accompanied by descriptive text. Importantly, in this chapter results should simply be presented, not discussed. The results section of Kaiser's (1996) paper (beginning on p. 335) includes tables to display statistical results, and specific results are described. Discussion of your findings should be addressed solely in Chapter V. In Chapter IV, you should focus on reporting findings by providing evidence for your hypotheses and/or research questions. Organize the chapter by designating relevant headings that correspond with each hypothesis or question. Remember to keep factual information separate from discussion of any evaluation or interpretation of potential implications. Conclude with a summary of the chapter that leads into Chapter V, the discussion.

## Chapter V: Discussion

This chapter is your opportunity to provide a summary, conclusions, and recommendations based on your study's findings. You can begin with a summary of main points covered in the first three chapters and the highlights of your results. The hypotheses can be restated definitively and implications for generalizability should be mentioned. Recommendations should be included as suggestions for additional research and for implementation of findings. For example, Kaiser (1996) concluded that, "The results of this study are consistent with the view that less securely attached women may be unconsciously expressing felt lack of support from significant others when they leave out parent and/or baby birds" (p. 337). Kaiser further suggested that the study be repeated to determine whether gender or age impact the way in which the BND is drawn with adult men, adolescents, and elementary school-age children. For instance, she wondered whether a population of men who are in treatment for addiction "would express different aspects of relational patterns in their drawings" (p. 340).

## Summary

In this chapter, guidelines for writing a research proposal and report based on the traditional five-chapter model were provided in two sections: I. The Research Proposal, and II. Completing the Research Report. Techniques for optimal teaching and learning of each unit were offered, with references to the book's supplemental materials. Factors unique to art therapy research were described – those related to enhancing study quality, and special considerations pertaining to controls for the extraneous variables of artistic skill and background, cultural appropriateness of art-based instruments and interventions, and variability in the artwork of children. A practical step-by-step guide was offered in Section III, How to Conduct an Art Therapy Research Study (and Judge its Quality).

## References

Acosta, I. (2001). Rediscovering the dynamic properties inherent in art. *American Journal of Art Therapy, 39*(3), 93–97.

Ainsworth, M. D., Blehar, M. C., Waters, E., & Wall, S. (1978). *Patterns of attachment: A psychological study of the strange situation.* Hillsdale, NJ: Lawrence Erlbaum.

Alon, U. (2009). How to choose a good scientific problem. *Molecular Cell, 35*, 1–3. Retrieved from https://doi.org/10.1016/j.molcel.2009.09.013

Alter-Muri, S. B. & Vazzano, S. (2014). Gender typicality in children's art development: A cross-cultural study. *The Arts in Psychotherapy, 41,* 155–162. Retrieved from https://doi.org/10.1016/j.aip.2014.01.003

American Psychological Association (APA). (2010). *Publication manual of the American Psychological Association* (6th ed.). Washington, DC: Author.

Armsden, G. & Greenberg, M. (1987). The inventory of parent and peer attachment: Individual differences and their relationship to psychological well-being in adolescence. *Journal of Youth and Adolescence, 16*(5), 427–453. Retrieved from https://doi.org/10.1007/BF02202939

Arnheim, R. (1966). *Toward a psychology of art*. Berkeley, CA: University of California Press.

Betts, D. J. (2013). A review of the principles for culturally appropriate art therapy assessment tools. *Art Therapy: Journal of the American Art Therapy Association, 30*(3), 98–106. Retrieved from https://doi.org/10.1080/07421656.2013.819280

Betts, D. J. & Potash, J. (2018). Research simulation experiential: Bringing research to life! (personal collection of D. Betts and J. Potash, the George Washington University, Washington, DC).

Bourriaud, N. (1998). *Relational aesthetics*. Dijon: Les Preses du réel.

Bowlby, J. (1969). *Attachment and loss: Vol. I. Attachment*. New York, NY: Basic Books.

Burley, T. & Handler, L. (1997). Personality factors in the accurate interpretation of projective tests. In E. F. Hammer (Ed.), *Advances in projective drawing interpretation* (pp. 359–377). Springfield, IL: Charles C Thomas.

CAAHEP (Commission on Accreditation of Allied Health Education Programs). (2016). *Standards and guidelines for the accreditation of educational programs in art therapy*. Clearwater, FL: Author.

Campos, J. J., Barrett, K. C., Lamb, M. E., Goldsmith, H. H., & Sternberg, C. (1983). Socioemotional development. In M. M. Haith & J. J. Campos (Eds.), *Handbook of child psychology: Vol. 2. Infancy and Psychobiology* (pp. 783–915). New York, NY: Wiley.

Curtis, E. K. (2011). Understanding client imagery in art therapy. *Journal of Clinical Art Therapy, 1*(1), 9–15. Retrieved from http://digitalcommons.lmu.edu/jcat/vol1/iss1/6

Deaver, S. (2009). A normative study of children's drawings: Preliminary research findings. *Art Therapy: Journal of the American Art Therapy Association, 26*(1), 4–11. Retrieved from https://doi.org/10.1080/07421656.2009.10129309

Edinger, E. F. (1972). *Ego and archetype*. Harrisonburg, VA: R. R. Donnelly & Sons.

Fraenkel, J. R., Wallen, N. E., & Hyun, H. (2015). *How to design and evaluate research in education* (9th ed.). New York, NY: McGraw-Hill.

Gillis, B. (2014). *The art of the question* (personal collection of B. Gillis, the George Washington University, Washington, DC).

Groth-Marnat, G. & Roberts, L. (1998). Human Figure Drawings and House Tree Person Drawings as indicators of self-esteem: A quantitative approach. *Journal of Clinical Psychology, 54*(2), 219–222.

Handler, L. & Riethmiller, R. (1998). Teaching and learning the administration and interpretation of graphic techniques. In L. Handler, M. J. Hilsenroth, L. Handler, & M. J. Hilsenroth (Eds.), *Teaching and learning personality assessment* (pp. 267–294). Mahwah, NJ: Lawrence Erlbaum.

Hess-Behrens, N. (1973). *The development of the concept of space as observed in children's drawings: Cross-nation/cross-cultural study*. National Center for Educational Research and Development Publication No. R02-06110. Washington, DC: US Department of Health, Education, and Welfare.

Hinz, L. D. (2009). *Expressive Therapies Continuum: A framework for using art in therapy*. New York, NY: Routledge.

Hinz, L. D. (2014). Art therapy research guided by the framework of the Expressive Therapies Continuum (unpublished paper).

Kagin, S. L. & Lusebrink, V. B. (1978). The Expressive Therapies Continuum. *The Arts in Psychotherapy: An International Journal, 5*, 171–180.

Kaiser, D. H. (1996). Indications of attachment security in a drawing task. *The Arts in Psychotherapy, 23*(4), pp. 333–340. Retrieved from https://doi.org/10.1016/0197-4556(96)00003-2

Kaiser, D. H. (2016). Assessing attachment with the Bird's Nest Drawing. In D. E. Gussak & M. L. Rosal (Eds.), *The Wiley-Blackwell handbook of art therapy* (pp. 641–657). Hoboken, NJ: Wiley-Blackwell.

Kaiser, D. H. & Deaver, S. (2009). Assessing attachment with the Bird's Nest Drawing: A review of the research. *Art Therapy: Journal of the American Art Therapy Association, 26*(1), 26–33. Retrieved from https://doi.org/10.1080/07421656.2009.10129312

Kapitan, L. (2018). *Introduction to art therapy research* (2nd ed.). New York, NY: Routledge.

Lesnick, A. (2009). Odd questions, strange texts and other people. In T. Vilardi & M. Chang (Eds.), *Writing-based teaching: Essential practices and enduring questions* (pp. 71–94), Albany, NY: State University of New York Press.

Levick, M. F. (2009). *Levick Emotional and Cognitive Art Therapy Assessment: A normative study*. Bloomington, IN: AuthorHouse.

Lowenfeld, V. & Brittain, W. L. (1987). *Creative and mental growth* (8th ed.). New York, NY: Macmillan.

Lusebrink, V. B. (2010). Assessment and therapeutic application of the Expressive Therapies Continuum: Implications for brain structures and functions. *Art Therapy: Journal of the American Art Therapy Association, 27*(4), 168–177. Retrieved from https://doi.org/10.1080/07421656.2010.10129380

Naumann, E. (1955). *The great mother*. Princeton, NJ: Princeton University Press.

Piaget, J. & Inhelder, B. (1971). *Mental imagery in the child*. New York, NY: Basic Books.

Scribner, C. & Handler, L. (1987). The interpreter's personality in Draw-a-Person interpretation: A study of interpersonal style. *Journal of Personality Assessment, 51*, 112–122. Retrieved from https://doi.org/10.1207/s15327752jpa5101_10

Weiner, I. B. (1995). Methodological considerations in Rorschach research. *Psychological Assessment, 7*(3), 330–337. Retrieved from https://doi.org/10.1037/1040-3590.7.3.330

Yoon, J. Y., Betts, D. J., & Holttum, S. (submitted). Bird's Nest Drawing stories in the assessment of attachment security.

# Appendix A

# Research Simulation Experiential Materials Packet

The following materials are provided as a supplement to the book and may optionally be used and adapted by instructors to teach art therapy students about the research approaches described in this book: a "mock" Informed Consent form; a Baseline Survey (Brief Mood Introspection Scale); Art Exhibit Visit Surveys; a Post Survey (Brief Mood Introspection Scale); and a Demographic Questionnaire for Art Therapy Research. These activities were designed by graduate art therapy educators Donna Betts and Jordan Potash (2018) as a way to bring research to life and engage students in hands-on experientials that relate to their own experiences and that incorporate art-based activities.

## Informed Consent

*(Alternatively, instructors may use the "waiver of documentation of consent" approach and provide an information sheet about the study.)*

**Principal investigators:** Name(s) of instructor(s)
**Sponsor:** Name of university

*Please note, as this experiential workshop is a learning exercise meant to simulate a research experience, this activity does not constitute legitimate research. The data and results generated will only be used within our classroom. Therefore, ethical approval was not obtained.*

**Introduction:** You are invited to participate in a study conducted by (name of instructor) of (name of university) Graduate Art Therapy Program. You are being asked if you want to take part in this study. Please read this form and ask any questions that will help you decide if you want to participate in the study. You must be at least 18 years old to take part in this study.

**Participation and withdrawal:** Taking part is completely voluntary. Even if you decide you want to participate, you can quit at any time without penalty. The status of your employment and/or your academic standing will not, in any way, be affected should you choose not to participate or if you decide to withdraw from the study at any time.

**Purpose:** The purpose of this study is to understand how engaging with an art exhibit may affect wellbeing.

**Procedures:** As part of this study, you will be asked to spend some time in an art exhibit and a discussion group. During that time you will complete questionnaires, create art, engage in reflective writing and participate in discussion. The whole process is expected to last approximately 30–60 minutes.

**Confidentiality:** Your confidentiality will be maintained at all times. In follow-up reports and publications, your identifying information will be obscured or omitted.

**Risks:** There is minimal risk involved in participating in this study. It is possible that you could experience some discomfort depending on the nature of some of the art in the exhibit. Please speak to the facilitators if you experience distress. There is also a possibility that your confidentiality could be compromised. To minimize this risk, you will be assigned a participant identification number.

**Potential benefits:** We hope that you will experience satisfaction from being a part of this study. Your experience will help us develop innovative art exhibit practices that will inform guidelines for how to better help art exhibit attendees have a meaningful experience.

**Documentation and photography:** The art you create will be collected and photographed. In addition, your participation may be documented by photographing you at the exhibit. If there is a photograph of your face, it will be obscured or cropped to ensure your anonymity.

**Compensation:** You will not be compensated for participating in this study.

**Questions and concerns:** If you have any questions about this workshop and the evaluation procedures, or if you want to know more about your rights as a research participant, please contact (name of instructor and contact information).

Documentation of consent
By signing below, I:
- affirm that I am at least 18 years old;
- agree to participate in this project and allow my information to be used for the stated purposes; and
- give my permission to allow photographs of my process and art to be used for educational presentations and scholarly publications.

Print name          Today's date

Signature

Participant identification number: \_\_\_ \_\_\_ \_\_\_ \_\_\_
(last 4 digits of phone number)

## Baseline Survey

### *Brief Mood Introspection Scale*

**Instructions:** Circle the response on the scale below that indicates how well each adjective or phrase describes your present mood.

|  | **Definitely do not feel** |  | **Do not feel** |  | **Slightly feel** |  | **Definitely feel** |
|---|---|---|---|---|---|---|---|
| **Lively** | 1 | 2 | 3 | 4 | 5 | 6 | 7 |
| **Happy** | 1 | 2 | 3 | 4 | 5 | 6 | 7 |
| **Sad** | 1 | 2 | 3 | 4 | 5 | 6 | 7 |
| **Tired** | 1 | 2 | 3 | 4 | 5 | 6 | 7 |
| **Caring** | 1 | 2 | 3 | 4 | 5 | 6 | 7 |
| **Content** | 1 | 2 | 3 | 4 | 5 | 6 | 7 |
| **Gloomy** | 1 | 2 | 3 | 4 | 5 | 6 | 7 |
| **Jittery** | 1 | 2 | 3 | 4 | 5 | 6 | 7 |
| **Drowsy** | 1 | 2 | 3 | 4 | 5 | 6 | 7 |
| **Grouchy** | 1 | 2 | 3 | 4 | 5 | 6 | 7 |
| **Peppy** | 1 | 2 | 3 | 4 | 5 | 6 | 7 |
| **Nervous** | 1 | 2 | 3 | 4 | 5 | 6 | 7 |
| **Calm** | 1 | 2 | 3 | 4 | 5 | 6 | 7 |
| **Loving** | 1 | 2 | 3 | 4 | 5 | 6 | 7 |
| **Fed up** | 1 | 2 | 3 | 4 | 5 | 6 | 7 |
| **Active** | 1 | 2 | 3 | 4 | 5 | 6 | 7 |

Overall, my mood is (circle one number):

| Very unpleasant |  |  |  |  |  |  |  |  |  |  |  |  |  |  |  |  |  |  |  | Pleasant |
|---|---|---|---|---|---|---|---|---|---|---|---|---|---|---|---|---|---|---|---|---|
| −10 | −9 | −8 | −7 | −6 | −5 | −4 | −3 | −2 | −1 | 0 | 1 | 2 | 3 | 4 | 5 | 6 | 7 | 8 | 9 | 10 |

Source: Mayer and Gaschke (1988). The authors give permission for its general research use.

Participant identification number: ___ ___ ___ ___
(last 4 digits of phone number)

## Art Exhibit Visit Surveys

**Instructions:** Enter the exhibit and take a few minutes to walk around and view the display. Select one artwork that is the most meaningful to you right now. Record the information about this artwork below.

| | |
|---|---|
| **Title** | |
| **Artist** | |
| **Year** | |
| **Art materials** | |
| **Size** (actual dimensions if known or approximate: small, medium, large, ...) | |

On the following pages, please tell us more about this artwork.

## Art Characteristics

For each of the following characteristics (indicated in the bold text in the left-hand column), please circle the description that best matches your selected artwork.

| | | | |
|---|---|---|---|
| **Number of elements** | simple (least number necessary, focus) | | complex (many forms, intricate, distracts) |
| **Arrangement of elements** | sequential (arranged, patterned) | | randomness (disorganized or haphazard) |
| **Clarity of presentation** | boldness (clarity and directness) | | diffusion (gradation, soft-focused) |
| **Manipulation of images** | distortion (beyond natural state) | exaggeration (amplify, overstate) | no manipulation (appears naturally) |
| **Interrelationship of images** | juxtaposition (adjacent images) | symmetry | asymmetric |
| **Special effects** | movement (implied movement) | dimensionality (implied depth) | stillness or none |
| **Form** | recognizable images | | abstract |
| **Style or attitude** (see definition in right-hand column) | **Naturalism** | (appears as it would in the natural world) ||
| | **Elementalism** | (simple, general, iconographic, elegance, restraint) ||
| | **Expressionism** | (manipulated, dynamic, uninhibited implied movement) ||
| | **Surrealism** | (unexpected, irrational) ||
| | **Decorativism** | (complex, may appear similar to surrealism but not disturbing) ||
| | **Formalism** | (unity, purposeful organization, logical defensive) ||
| | **Impressionism** | (tentative, unsure) ||

| **Dominant colors** (circle all that apply) | red | orange | yellow | green | blue | violet |
|---|---|---|---|---|---|---|
| | black | brown | beige | pink | white | gray |

## Relational Aesthetics Questionnaire

For each of the following statements, please place a check (✓) to indicate to which degree the statement was a factor in selecting your artwork.

|  | Does not describe my reason for choosing ... |  |  | Describes my reason for choosing ... |  |
|---|---|---|---|---|---|
|  | 1 | 2 | 3 | 4 | 5 |
| I was interested in the colors used in this art. |  |  |  |  |  |
| I was interested in the subject matter and content of the art. |  |  |  |  |  |
| I was interested in the style that the artist used to create the art. |  |  |  |  |  |
| I wanted to know more about this art. |  |  |  |  |  |
| I wanted to know more about the artist. |  |  |  |  |  |
| The artist seems to be expressing important feelings. |  |  |  |  |  |
| The art reminds me of an experience I had. |  |  |  |  |  |
| The art reminds me of an experience someone I know had. |  |  |  |  |  |
| The artist seemed to be passionate about creating this art. |  |  |  |  |  |
| The art moves me. |  |  |  |  |  |

In the space below, please describe why this artwork is meaningful to you:

## *Response Art*

In the space below, please use color pencils to create a sketch or art that describes how the artwork you selected makes you feel:

## 238 Appendices

For the art you created, please answer the following:

| | |
|---|---|
| **Title** | |
| **Description** (What do you see?) | |
| **Meaning** (How does this sketch or art relate to how the artwork from the exhibit makes you feel?) | |

Thank you for your participation. Please return this form to one of the facilitators.

Participant identification number: ___ ___ ___ ___
(last 4 digits of phone number)

## Post Survey

### *Brief Mood Introspection Scale*

**Instructions:** Circle the response on the scale below that indicates how well each adjective or phrase describes your present mood.

|  | Definitely do not feel |  | Do not feel |  | Slightly feel |  | Definitely feel |
|---|---|---|---|---|---|---|---|
| Lively | 1 | 2 | 3 | 4 | 5 | 6 | 7 |
| Happy | 1 | 2 | 3 | 4 | 5 | 6 | 7 |
| Sad | 1 | 2 | 3 | 4 | 5 | 6 | 7 |
| Tired | 1 | 2 | 3 | 4 | 5 | 6 | 7 |
| Caring | 1 | 2 | 3 | 4 | 5 | 6 | 7 |
| Content | 1 | 2 | 3 | 4 | 5 | 6 | 7 |
| Gloomy | 1 | 2 | 3 | 4 | 5 | 6 | 7 |
| Jittery | 1 | 2 | 3 | 4 | 5 | 6 | 7 |
| Drowsy | 1 | 2 | 3 | 4 | 5 | 6 | 7 |
| Grouchy | 1 | 2 | 3 | 4 | 5 | 6 | 7 |
| Peppy | 1 | 2 | 3 | 4 | 5 | 6 | 7 |
| Nervous | 1 | 2 | 3 | 4 | 5 | 6 | 7 |
| Calm | 1 | 2 | 3 | 4 | 5 | 6 | 7 |
| Loving | 1 | 2 | 3 | 4 | 5 | 6 | 7 |
| Fed up | 1 | 2 | 3 | 4 | 5 | 6 | 7 |
| Active | 1 | 2 | 3 | 4 | 5 | 6 | 7 |

Overall, my mood is (circle one number):

| Very unpleasant |  |  |  |  |  |  |  |  |  |  |  |  |  |  |  |  |  |  |  | Pleasant |
|---|---|---|---|---|---|---|---|---|---|---|---|---|---|---|---|---|---|---|---|---|
| -10 | -9 | -8 | -7 | -6 | -5 | -4 | -3 | -2 | -1 | 0 | 1 | 2 | 3 | 4 | 5 | 6 | 7 | 8 | 9 | 10 |

(Please complete the demographic form on the reverse side.)

Source: Mayer and Gaschke (1988). The authors give permission for its general research use.

Participant identification number: ___ ___ ___ ___
(last 4 digits of phone number)

## Demographic Questionnaire for Art Therapy Research

Please complete this questionnaire as honestly as possible.

1. What is your current age: _____

2. What is your gender:
   □ Male   □ Female   □ Other (please specify): _____

3. What is your ethnic background (please check only one):
   □ White, not of Hispanic origin   □ Hispanic
   □ Black                           □ Mixed: _____
   □ Asian or Pacific Islander       □ Other (please specify): _____

4. What is your marital status?
   □ Single, never married   □ Divorced
   □ Married                 □ Widowed
   □ Separated               □ Other (please specify): _____

5. What is the highest level of education you have completed?
   □ Grade 9, 10 or 11                    □ Associate's degree
   □ High school diploma or equivalent    □ Bachelor's degree
   □ Some college credit, less than 1 year □ Master's degree
   □ 1 or more years of college, no degree □ Professional or doctoral degree

6. What was your Bachelor's degree major? _____

7. What is your religious affiliation (please check only one):
   □ Protestant        □ Muslim
   □ Catholic          □ Other: _____
   □ LDS/Mormon        □ No religious affiliation
   □ Jewish

8. In what educational institution(s) have you had formal art training (check all that apply):
   □ Elementary school   □ Junior high school   □ Senior high school
   □ College   □ Other (e.g., post-college art classes): _____

9. When was the last time you made art (prior to today)? *Please check only one* and indicate what materials you used (e.g., drawing, painting, photography, computer graphic art):

| Please check only one: |  | Art materials used |
|---|---|---|
|  | Yesterday |  |
|  | Last week |  |
|  | In the past month |  |
|  | In the past six months |  |
|  | In the past year |  |
|  | One year ago or more |  |

10. How often do you make art (please check only one):
    □ At least once a week   □ About once per month   □ Once a year
    □ Once every few years   □ Never

11. Do you consider yourself to be an "artist"? (please check only one):
    □ Yes        □ Sometimes        □ No

**Thank you for your participation. Please return this form to one of the facilitators.**

## References

Betts, D. J. & Potash, J. (2018). Research simulation experiential: Bringing research to life! (personal collection of D. Betts and J. Potash, the George Washington University, Washington, DC).

Mayer, J. D. & Gaschke, Y. N. (1988). The experience and meta-experience of mood. *Journal of Personality and Social Psychology, 55*, 102–111. Retrieved from https://doi.org/10.1037/0022-3514.55.1.102

# Appendix B

# Art Therapy Inquiry Form

In order to work effectively with art productions in psychotherapy, clinicians must first learn to identify, describe, and interact with all aspects of a picture (Cohen & Cox, 1995). This includes both qualitative (subjective) and quantitative (objective) aspects. Qualitative aspects can include the artist/client's thoughts/feelings/reactions to his/her work, as well as the therapist's thoughts/feelings/reactions.

In examining an artwork using both qualitative and quantitative approaches, *triangulation* is achieved. Triangulation is an important concept in research – it is a powerful technique that facilitates validation of data through cross-verification from more than two sources (Bogdan & Biklen, 2006). In particular, it refers to the application and combination of several research methodologies in the study of the same phenomenon. In our work with clients, triangulation of methods enables us to make a more well-rounded assessment of our clients' functioning (Betts, 2012).

This *Art Therapy Inquiry Form* is based upon methodologies developed by Feldman (1994) and Anderson (1997). The form is for use by art therapists to *evaluate their own subjective response to client artwork*, to help hone skills in comprehension of an artwork's message, i.e., the "gestalt" of the image. In using this form, the art therapist is invited to identify, describe, and interact with various aspects of an artwork using a qualitative line of questioning. Completing this form will enable the art therapist to:

- Increase his or her visual literacy skills.
- Understand a client via his or her artwork.
- Use art as a bridge to strengthen the therapeutic alliance.
- Determine appropriate treatment goals and design effective treatment plans.

This form is for use by art therapists to facilitate in-depth engagement with an art product. It can be used both as a device to increase the therapists' understanding of and empathy for the client and a research tool. It can also be a valuable supplement to the formal assessment of artworks, adding a qualitative, yet systematic, approach to gaining meaning based on the art therapist's reactions to a client's artwork.

1. How does this work of art make you feel?

2. What does it make you think of?

3. What mood is presented?

4. How are we meant to feel in the presence of this piece, and why? What's the evidence?

5. Would you like to have it for your own? Why or why not?

6. Do you think the work is good in and of itself? Why or why not? What criteria do you base that on? *(Answers can be about technique, skill level, expressive power, beauty, and other qualities to be found in the work.)*

7. What cultural significance does the artwork have? How is it important in society?

8. Do you have any further observations of the artwork that you feel are important in better understanding the artist who made it?

Source: Donna Betts, PhD, ATR-BC.
Note: This form is based on Anderson's (1997) CritCard method, a systematic approach for examining artworks; Anderson based his method on that of Feldman (1994).

## References

Anderson, T. (1997, September). A model for art criticism: Talking with kids about art. *SchoolArts*, 21–24.

Betts, D. J. (2012). Positive art therapy assessment: Looking towards positive psychology for new directions in the art therapy evaluation process. In A. Gilroy, R. Tipple, & C. Brown (Eds.), *Assessment in art therapy* (pp. 203–218). New York, NY: Routledge.

Bogdan, R. C. & Biklen, S. K. (2006). *Qualitative research in education: An introduction to theory and methods*. Boston, MA: Allyn & Bacon.

Cohen, B. M. & Cox, C. T. (1995). *Telling without talking: Art as a window into the world of multiple personality*. New York: W.W. Norton.

Feldman, E. B. (1994). *Practical art criticism*. Upper Saddle River, NJ: Prentice Hall.

# Appendix C

# Art Therapy Research: A Practical Guide

## Worksheet 1: Research Idea – Curiosity and Inquiry

*Donna J. Betts & Jordan S. Potash*

---

1. Pick a topic about art therapy that interests you, one you are curious about, or one that you want to know more about, and describe it briefly here:

2. Why is the topic of interest to you?

3. Why do you want to learn about this topic?

4. What do you want to learn about this topic?

5. Come up with a longer list of questions related to your topic using the words *when, why, what,* and *how*.

Source: Adapted from Gaillet, L. L. & Eble, M. F. (2016). *Primary research and writing: People, places, and spaces.* New York, NY: Routledge.

# Appendix D

# Art Therapy Research: A Practical Guide

## Worksheet 2: Research Question

*Donna J. Betts & Jordan S. Potash*

1. Restate your research idea (from Worksheet 1) here:

2. Without searching for any information on your subject, first brainstorm and write down what you already know about your subject.

3. Generate a list of questions related to your topic.

4. Divide your list into two categories:
   a. Questions that can be answered through a series of activities such as observation; artifact description, analysis, and interpretation; or interviews (primary research).
   b. Questions that can be answered by reading and reflecting on what answers others have provided about your questions (secondary research).

5. Look back at your list, pick one of the questions from the first category (primary research) and write down some ways in which you might answer this question.

6. Identify the key words in your idea or question that need clarification:
   a. _____
   b. _____
   c. _____
   d. _____
   e. _____

7. Write down your operational definitions of these terms:

Sources: Adapted from Fraenkel, J. R., Wallen, N. E., & Hyun, H. (2015). *How to design and evaluate research in education* (9th ed., Problem Sheet 6). New York, NY: McGraw-Hill, and Gaillet, L. L. & Eble, M. F. (2016). *Primary research and writing: People, places, and spaces.* New York, NY: Routledge.

# Appendix E

# Art Therapy Research: A Practical Guide

## Worksheet 3: Literature Review

*Donna J. Betts & Jordan S. Potash*

1. Write down your research idea and question(s):

2. To learn more about your topic, create a list of "experts" you would need to consult (or, put another way, who do you need to invite to your "research party?"). For example, if you are interested in how art therapy benefits children with communication disorders, you might consult a speech-hearing pathologist, an art therapist who works in a school, etc.

3. Based on your answers for Question 2, next consider the areas that you need to focus on in order to search for literature that relates to your idea/question(s). Come up with a list of search terms that you can use in the online library database system:

4. Write down the results of your literature search:

Source: Adapted from Fraenkel, J. R., Wallen, N. E., & Hyun, H. (2015). *How to design and evaluate research in education* (9th ed., Problem Sheet 5). New York, NY: McGraw-Hill.

# Appendix F

# Art Therapy Research: A Practical Guide

Worksheet 4: Research Design – Q
and Experimental (for use with Cha

*Donna J. Betts & Jordan S. Potash*

---

Quantitative and experimental research both aim to use numbers and objective data to determine a relationship between two events. These approaches generally answer *why* a phenomenon occurs.

1. Write down your research idea and question(s):

2. Formulate a hypothesis related to your idea that can be answered using quantitative or experimental means:

3. Your hypothesis/assumption suggests a relationship between at least two variables; write them down here:
   _____ and _____

4. More specifically, one of these variables is dependent and the other is independent. Add them here:
   a. Dependent _____ _____
   b. Independent _____

consider which extraneous variables might affect your results and write them down:
   a.
   b.
   c.
   d.

6. Determine which types of instrument and/or means of data collection (tasks, activities) you can use:

Source: Adapted from Fraenkel, J. R., Wallen, N. E., & Hyun, H. (2015). *How to design and evaluate research in education* (9th ed., Problem Sheet 13). New York, NY: McGraw-Hill.

# Appendix G

# Art Therapy Research: A Practical Guide

Worksheet 5: Research Design – Qualitative (for use with Chapter 4)

*Donna J. Betts & Jordan S. Potash*

---

Qualitative research aims to use stories, narratives, images, and lived experience to understand an event in depth. It generally aims to answer *how* or *what* in relation to a phenomenon.

1. Write down your research idea:

2. Come up with a question related to your idea that can be answered using qualitative methods:

3. Determine which types of data collection (interviews, observations) you can use:

Source: Adapted from Fraenkel, J. R., Wallen, N. E., & Hyun, H. (2015). *How to design and evaluate research in education* (9th ed.). New York, NY: McGraw-Hill.

Appendix H

# Art Therapy Research: A Practical Guide

## Worksheet 6: Research Design – Program Development and Case Study

Donna J. Betts & Jordan S. Potash

Program development and case study research aims to use direct observation and involvement to understand a specific person or event. It generally involves immersing oneself in the circumstances of the participants.

1. Write down your research idea:

2. Come up with a question related to your idea that can be answered through direct observation and/or involvement with an individual case or agency:

3. Determine which types of data collection (interviews, observations) you can use:

Source: Adapted from Fraenkel, J. R., Wallen, N. E., & Hyun, H. (2015). *How to design and evaluate research in education* (9th ed.). New York, NY: McGraw-Hill.

Appendix I

# Art Therapy Research: A Practical Guide

Worksheet 7: Research Design – Heuristic and Arts-Based (for use with Chapter 5)

*Donna J. Betts & Jordan S. Potash*

---

Heuristic research aims to use personal experience in order for researchers to learn more about themselves or increase their own development through a self-study. It generally involves immersing oneself in a topic by being interviewed, engaging in reflective writing, and/or making art.

1. Write down your research idea:

2. Come up with a question related to your idea that can be answered by allowing yourself to be interviewed, creating your own art, and/or engaging in your own reflective writing:

3. Determine which types of data collection (interviews, observations) you can use:

Source: Adapted from Fraenkel, J. R., Wallen, N. E., & Hyun, H. (2015). *How to design and evaluate research in education* (9th ed.). New York, NY: McGraw-Hill.

Appendix J

# Art Therapy Research: A Practical Guide

## Worksheet 8: Sampling and Participant Selection (for use with Chapters 3 and 4)

*Donna J. Betts & Jordan S. Potash*

---

1. Sampling pertains to specific procedures for recruiting individuals to participate in a research study. The goal of sampling is to obtain a group of research participants – or "subjects" – who represent the larger population of people to whom the results of the study are to be generalized. Consider the characteristics of the individuals you'd like to include in your study, briefly describe them here, and indicate how many participants you would select:

2. Describe the more specific demographic features of your intended participants:
   a. Age range:
   b. Gender distribution:
   c. Ethnic distribution:
   d. Location:
   e. Other participant characteristics that are important for your study:

3. Consider the sampling method you would use and circle it:
   a. Random sampling
   b. Stratified random sampling
   c. Cluster random sampling
   d. Purposive sampling
   e. Convenience sampling

4. Describe how you will access your participants:

5. Describe how you will generalize your study's findings (external validity):
   a. To what accessible population will you be able to generalize?

   b. To what target population will you be able to generalize?

Source: Adapted from Fraenkel, J. R., Wallen, N. E., & Hyun, H. (2015). *How to design and evaluate research in education* (9th ed., Problem Sheet 6). New York, NY: McGraw-Hill.

Appendix K

# Art Therapy Research: A Practical Guide

## Worksheet 9: Ethical Considerations (for use with Chapter 2)

*Donna J. Betts & Jordan S. Potash*

1. Write down your research question:

2. Consider what possibilities for harm to the participants may exist in your study and briefly describe them:

3. Describe how you would manage this harm if it were to transpire:

4. Consider whether your study puts your participants at risk for a breach of confidentiality and, if so, describe how:

5. Describe what you would do to manage any potential breach of confidentiality:

6. Consider whether your study puts your participants at risk for deception and, if so, describe how:

7. Describe what you would do to manage any instance of deception:

8. Consider whether your study includes the possibility for the occurrence of conflict of interest:

9. Describe what you would do to manage any conflict of interest:

10. Describe any additional ethical considerations that may pertain to your study:

Source: Adapted from Fraenkel, J. R., Wallen, N. E., & Hyun, H. (2015). *How to design and evaluate research in education* (9th ed., Problem Sheet 4). New York, NY: McGraw-Hill.

Appendix L

# Art Therapy Research: A Practical Guide

## Worksheet 10: Rigor and Integrity (for use with Chapters 3 and 4)

Donna J. Betts & Jordan S. Potash

1. Quantitative and qualitative research employ different approaches for ensuring rigor and integrity. Consider the various approaches listed below, and describe the ways in which you would address these for your study:

   a. Quantitative studies
      - Internal validity (*see next page*)
      - External validity (reactivity, order effects, interaction effects):
      - Reliability:
      - Objectivity:

   b. Qualitative studies
      - Credibility:
      - Transferability:
      - Dependability:
      - Conformability:

2. Instrumentation: as you complete the questions in this section, consider the ways in which the integrity of the instruments (scales, measures, texts, surveys, etc.) you plan to use might impact the rigor of your study:
   a. List any existing (created by others as cited in the literature, for instance) instruments/means of data collection you plan to use and describe what you have learned about the validity and reliability of each:

b. List any instruments/means of data collection that you plan to develop yourself (e.g., a questionnaire, interview questions):

c. Describe how you will attempt to ensure reliability and validity of your study's results gathered through use of these instruments/means of data collection using the following:
   - Internal consistency:
   - Reliability over time (stability):
   - Validity:

3. In quantitative studies, external validity is increased when extraneous and confounding variables are controlled. A number of threats to internal validity (as described in Chapter 3) are listed below. Consider these and indicate which ones may pose a threat to the rigor and integrity of your study. Then describe your reasons for selecting these threats and what you would do to control them:

   a. Selection bias:

   b. History:

   c. Instrumentation:

   d. Experimenter bias

   e. Maturation:

   f. Attrition (mortality):

   g. Statistical regression:

   h. Other:

Source: Adapted from Fraenkel, J. R., Wallen, N. E., & Hyun, H. (2015). *How to design and evaluate research in education* (9th ed., Problem Sheets 8 and 9). New York, NY: McGraw-Hill.

# Glossary

**Action research:** A qualitative research method that stems from social sciences and organizational-based research, where the need for change is not just identified, but implemented and then evaluated.

**Aesthetics – verisimilitude:** One of five components or tensions from Eisner's model of determining credibility in arts-based research emphasizing the need for researchers to be careful to focus on the art while maintaining a focus on the subject of inquiry.

**Alternate-form reliability (form to form):** Aims to correct a problem that can occur with test-retest reliability – the "practice effect" – only applicable with tests that are word-based, not art-based, because it involves changing the wording of questions while preserving the integrity (or *equivalency*) of their meaning.

**American Art Therapy Association:** A 501(c)(3) not-for-profit, non-partisan, professional, and educational organization dedicated to the growth and development of the art therapy profession. Founded in 1969, the AATA is one of the world's leading art therapy membership organizations.

**Analysis of variance:** A statistical test to determine differences in group means, usually when comparing three or more groups.

**Analytical integration:** In arts-based research, an approach to data synthesis that incorporates arts processes, and products to explicate data.

**Art for scholarship's sake:** A term used in arts-based research to distinguish the application of artistic skills to convey research findings in emotionally invested and evocative ways.

**Art Therapy-Projective Imagery Assessment (AT-PIA):** A comprehensive direct-observation clinical art therapy interview that includes a series of six discrete constructive drawing tasks collected under standardized conditions. It provides a systematic method of assessment that is compatible with psychological and psychiatric evaluation processes.

**Arts-based research (ABR):** An approach to research that transforms insights into meaningful actions through harnessing artistic prowess within systematic inquiry to generate theory and inform practice. ABR can build on the work of the art therapist to facilitate the therapists' own search for meaning and expression through the creation of arts products and engaged reflection. The emphasis on *arts* rather than *art* indicates the importance of researchers using a range of creative media (visual, music, performance, movement, poetry, creative writing) depending on researcher capabilities and situational demands. Similar terms used in the literature are *arts-informed research*, *artistic inquiry*, and *a/r/tography*.

**Assessment research:** Research conducted on an assessment when a researcher's primary aim is to *further establish* an existing instrument (by contributing to its validity and reliability).

**Auto-ethnography:** In arts-based research, a self-inquiry method that approximates heuristic inquiry, but intentionally places the subject in a social-cultural context to comment on how these systemic forces impact the researcher's lived experiences.

**Axiology:** Is concerned with researcher values as they manifest in the research process and acknowledges the biases present.

**Belmont Report:** This document published by the US government in 1979 delineates three moral principles underlying research with human participants: respect for persons, beneficence, and justice.

**Beneficence:** This research principle embodies researchers' obligation to safeguard research participants' well-being.

**Better questions – better answers:** One of five components or tensions from Eisner's model of determining credibility in arts-based research emphasizing the need for researchers to invest in the art-making process but retain focus on the study's aims as a test of success because direct answers are needed to explain how research translates into practice.

**Bird's Nest Drawing (BND):** A process-based, constructive art therapy assessment that assesses attachment security through a drawing task (*draw a picture of a bird's nest*) and a corresponding story (narrative) about the drawing.

**Bricolage:** In keeping with the emergent and flexible nature of qualitative research, it involves the piecing together of different methodological strategies using a combination of different historical, philosophical, social, and theoretical lenses intentionally to develop complementary types of data, while recognizing that this gives rise to contradictory ideas and contested arguments that can help create a research approach that addresses both the goals of investigator and the study objectives.

**CAAHEP (Commission on Accreditation of Allied Health Education Programs):** A programmatic postsecondary accrediting agency recognized by the Council for Higher Education Accreditation

(CHEA) that carries out its accrediting activities in cooperation with 25 review Committees on Accreditation. CAAHEP currently accredits more than 2200 entry-level education programs in 32 health science professions.

**Case study:** A qualitative research method that enables in-depth examinations of particular clients, encounters, or contexts, enabling proliferation of data. Case study methods differ depending on the study purpose, discipline, research strategy, and study context. Six different contexts in which a case study method would be appropriate are exploratory, descriptive, instrumental, interpretive, explanatory, and evaluative.

**Central tendency, measures of:** These provide information about the middle of a group of numbers. These measures are mean, median, and mode.

**Collaborative assessment:** A client-centered approach to psychological assessment developed by Connie Fischer, it incorporates traditional psychological assessment with various standardized instruments but with an emphasis on individual narratives and anecdotal evidence to enhance the therapeutic relationship and inform clinical practice.

**Communicative integration:** An approach to data synthesis that incorporates arts processes and products to share findings.

**Conceptual integration:** An approach to data synthesis that incorporates arts processes and products as integral to all stages of the research.

**Conceptual validity:** Considered in the context of generating accurate conclusions about a client, such as in determining whether the results of the assessment make sense clinically in the context of the client's history and presenting problem.

**Concurrent validity:** A type of criterion validity that is determined by gathering data from two different instruments at the same time and comparing the results to determine the extent to which the results of a relatively new or unsubstantiated test relate to results derived from a well-established measurement for the same construct. If the results of the newer test are shown to correspond with the results from the well-established measure, then this helps to establish concurrent validity for the newer test.

**Consequential (impact-based) validity:** In contrast to *evidential* validity, *consequential* validity represents the degree to which an assessment successfully yields useful, accurate, and unbiased data in vivo.

**Construct validity:** The ability of an instrument to perform well in clinical practice. It is the most valuable indicator of an instrument's validity as it helps the clinician make important decisions about treatment planning. Two sub-types of construct validity are *convergent* validity and *discriminant* validity. If an assessment can be found to have both types of validity, then it is said to have robust construct validity.

Constructivism: A research paradigm that is also described as *interpretivism*, because researchers who embrace this paradigm develop interpretations of how their participants make meaning of their experiences. It focuses more on understanding the *why* through taking a relativist position that respects multiple, attainable, and equally valid realities.

Content analysis: A type of qualitative analysis that originated from a need to evaluate mass communication data to develop and apply quantifiable codes derived from written sources of data. The process involves seeing the meaning units, categories, and themes as measurable by how many times they appear in the data set, while also looking for the latent meanings and interconnected patterns and is therefore typically used with online content or a large number of written responses. Unlike thematic analysis, in content analysis, manifested categories (what is written) and latent contents (underlying meaning of what is written) are separated to acknowledge both the quantifiable and qualifying data sources.

Content validity: The extent to which an instrument measures all aspects of a particular social concept or how well assessment results reflect a client's presenting symptoms or a targeted construct. Content validation is a multimethod, primarily qualitative, process applicable to all aspects of an instrument.

Convenience sampling: A type of purposive sampling (nonprobability) that involves selection of participants based primarily on the fact that they are immediately accessible and available.

Convergent parallel research design: Mixed methods research in which quantitative and qualitative data are collected and analyzed separately and then merged.

Convergent validity: A sub-type of *construct* validity that determines the extent to which the constructs that should be related to one another are in fact related.

Creative dialogue: A data collection procedure used in arts-based research that involves engaging in discussion with the art.

Creativity: An ethics principle by which art therapists are obligated to honor and protect art processes and products in practice and in research studies.

Credibility (in arts-based research): Applies to evaluation of quality in the interpretation of arts-based research findings and the level of confidence that the study was conducted in a manner that ensures both rigor and creativity through adherence to criteria for evaluating arts-based research such as through Leavy's approach or Eisner's model.

Credibility (in qualitative research): Applies to evaluation of quality in the interpretation of qualitative findings and the level of confidence that the study was conducted in a rigorous manner through *triangulating* different data sources, methods, investigators, and/or theoretical perspectives; member checking with participants; providing a rich, thick description that is detailed and clearly portrays the study setting; clarifying any bias; presenting negative or counter information that portrays the reality of the findings; spending prolonged time in the field to learn the culture and establish relationships; using a peer debriefer; and using an external auditor.

**Criterion validity:** A measure of agreement between the results derived from a test and results for the same population, measuring the same construct (variable) obtained either by direct measurement or a well-established instrument that shares the same theoretical orientation. These results are compared, and criterion validity is measured by the correlation coefficient between the two assessment methods. Depending on the nature of the resulting data, the criterion validity measures are organized into *concurrent* validity and *predictive* validity measures.

**Critical sampling:** A type of purposive sampling (nonprobability) that involves selection of participants based on unusual or exceptional circumstances that is useful when resources are limited.

**Cronbach's alpha:** A coefficient of reliability that yields the expected correlation of two tests that measure the same construct.

**Data source integration:** An approach to data synthesis that incorporates arts processes and products as data.

**Deductive lens:** An interpretive lens used in the process of qualitative data analysis that focuses on a particular assumption, which is determined through a process of analysis.

**Deductive reasoning:** Thinking from the general to the specific, as in the traditional scientific method, moving from theory to hypothesis testing.

**Degree of error:** A statistical term relating to *margin of error* referring to the extent to which results differ from the actual population value attributable to factors such as lack of precision in a testing method or fluctuation in a test-taker's performance. It serves as a reminder to expect that measures cannot be totally reliable because no test or testing situation is perfect.

**Delphi study:** A consensus survey method that uses a structured multistep process to gather and converge the opinions of a panel of experts to enhance effective decision making in the healthcare realm.

**Diagnostic Drawing Series (DDS):** A process-based, constructive art therapy assessment for which three drawings are produced that reflect an individual's response to a specific directive and structure resulting in a range of graphic and psychological responses.

***Diagnostic and Statistical Manual of Mental Disorders* (DSM):** Published by the American Psychiatric Association (APA), most recently in

2013 (fifth edition), this is the most widely used tool available in the US to categorize mental illnesses and inform diagnosis and treatment planning.

**Discourse analysis:** A qualitative analysis method that evolved from the fields of linguistics, literature, and semiotics, which emphasizes how particular words are used to convey actions, feelings, and thoughts within a certain context. Words are regarded as symbolizing *situated meanings* – assemblies of features that constitute a given time period, relationship, and social/political context.

**Discriminant validity:** A sub-type of *construct* validity (also known as *divergent* validity) serving to confirm that any constructs that should not be related to one another are in fact not related.

**Discussion:** A written section of the traditional research proposal and final report contained in Chapter V that entails the discussion in the form of a summary of all salient aspects of the study's findings and includes the researcher's own speculations about the results.

**Distribution:** The way in which a set of individual scores or values is spread, typically illustrated through frequency tables or graphs.

**Distribution, normal:** A bell shaped distribution of scores or numbers theorized to represent a "normal" or "typical" population, applicable to both descriptive and inferential statistics.

**Economy of means:** In arts-based research, relating to the skills with which an artistic product is created so as to be able to effectively communicate intended meaning and evoke or inspire an audience. The concept of skill is further understood through *hybrid forms* of art and *art for scholarship's sake*.

**Epistemology:** Has to do with ways of knowing and what qualifies as acceptable knowledge. It also is concerned with the researcher-participant relationship.

**Ethics, principle:** Art therapists are *obligated* to abide by the principles embodied in their professional association's ethics documents and, if credentialed, by the entity or board that credentialed them.

**Ethics, virtue:** These *aspirational* ethical values pertain to art therapists' use of their virtuous personality traits in practice and research.

**Ethnography:** A qualitative research method stemming from anthropology that involves documenting or portraying the everyday experiences of individuals to develop an understanding of a particular cultural, social, or political dynamic. Critical ethnography examines social justice issues such as disparities and marginalized groups. *Autoethnography* uses autobiographical narratives of the art therapist's own experiences, thus the researcher is also the participant. A self-narrative is examined through its connection with a social context, which involves systematic analysis based on deep self-reflection and self-observation detailing an often life-changing or altering circumstance.

**Evocative power:** A distinguishing feature of arts-based research related to basing one's art on one's lived experiences, emotions, memories, dreams, and impulses, intended to ensure that the art is emotionally invested for the creator and that it is also provocative to the viewer, thereby encouraging *conspiratorial conversations*; on-going discussions about prevailing worldviews.

**Experimental research:** Research in which the researcher manipulates independent variables, and exerts control over other variables, to observe the effect of the independent variable upon one or more dependent variables.

**Explanatory sequential research design:** Mixed methods research in which quantitative data are collected first, followed by qualitative data intended to amplify or explain the quantitative results.

**Explication:** In arts-based research, a means of emphasizing art making by the researcher in all stages of research to present a new perspective of a phenomenon, raise more questions than answers, and use findings to make changes in the world.

**Exploratory sequential research design:** Mixed methods research designed to develop instruments, measures, or interventions. It involves at least three phases of data collection: qualitative, quantitative, and qualitative.

**Ex-post facto:** "After the fact" studies that examine two or more groups that differ only on a previously existing variable, to discover the cause of the difference. Also called causal-comparative research.

**Expressive Therapies Continuum (ETC) assessment:** A non-standardized comprehensive art therapy assessment that is theoretically tied to neurobiology based on its ability to assess kinesthetic, sensory, perceptual, affective, cognitive, and symbolic content in art products. The ETC elucidates people's behavior as they are presented with arousing stimuli and work with color and a range of resistive to fluid art materials.

**Face Stimulus Assessment (FSA):** A performance-based art therapy assessment that measures cognitive/neuropsychological and developmental level through the use of three standardized stimulus pictures and markers.

**Face validity:** Validity derived from judgments about a test by its *users*, as opposed to *content* validity, which refers to a test's relevance from the perspective of *experts*.

**Factorial designs:** Experimental designs that examine not only the relationship between variables but also their interaction.

**Fidelity:** This ethical principle embodies researchers' scientific integrity and their truthfulness with research participants.

# Glossary 269

**Field notes:** A qualitative data-gathering method that involves note-taking while the researcher observes the social situation under study.

**Focus groups:** Used for gathering feedback when qualitative researchers are interested in collecting data based on social interactions between participants and researchers. In art therapy research, focus groups are typically used to help evaluate art therapy approaches and provide feedback.

**Formal Elements Art Therapy Scale (FEATS):** A standardized rating procedure developed by Gantt and Tabone that enables art therapists to quantify formal elements in artwork by assigning a score to 14 variables of interest, such as *space* and *prominence of color*.

**Free association:** In arts-based research, a data collection procedure used that involves mining of the imagery and process for immediate symbols to delve beneath the surface of the artwork.

**Generalizability:** The usefulness of research findings for a larger group beyond the sample that participated in the study.

**Grounded theory:** A qualitative research method that is based on the idea of discovering a theory by scrutinizing concepts that are grounded in the data through identification of basic social processes in a particular situation. Theory is generated from participants' experiences and a step-by-step method using inductive and deductive reasoning is used in order for theory to develop based on a process, action, or interaction generated from the data (classic grounded theory). Modified grounded theory takes on a more emergent and inductive systematic approach to data analysis through coding; postmodern grounded theory and discursive grounded theory focus on analyzing discourse; and constructivist grounded theory allows for researchers and participants to be co-constructors of their interactive and iterative realities and subsequently the derived theory.

**Grounded theory analysis:** An iterative method of qualitative analysis that involves a *constant comparative* process to derive theory from the participants' experiences using the three main stages identified by Strauss and Corbin: (a) open coding (inspecting, comparing, abstracting, and ordering data), (b) axial coding (reconstructing data into categories based on relationships and patterns within and among the clusters identified in the data), and (c) selective coding (classifying and providing an explanation of the central or core category in the data). These stages are characterized by Charmaz as initial, focused, and theoretical, and involve saturation and the use of memos.

**Hermeneutic phenomenology:** Reflects the concept of the *hermeneutic circle* to describe the iterative and interactive relationship between the clients and the researcher's interpretation of their worldview. The researcher uses *spiraling* (questions prompted out of responses) as an open-ended form of dialogue to ensure a shared understanding created out of participants' experiences. Other types of phenomenology include *new phenomenology* and *empathetic phenomenology*.

**Heuristic phenomenology:** Emphasizes the personal experiences of the researcher, which inform the process of inquiry either through self-discovery or through a shared encounter with others using the following step-by-step process to derive findings: initial engagement, immersion, incubation, illumination, explication, and creative synthesis.

**Heuristic research:** An approach to qualitative research established by Clark Moustakas that involves discovery of the nature and meaning of experience through a process of internal search. In arts-based research, a self-inquiry method that involves immersion in artistic expression within an autobiographical framework that can lead to self-transformation.

**Homogeneous sampling:** A type of purposive sampling (nonprobability) that is used when the primary interest is in studying a group in depth, based on the desirability of seeking participants who are all similar in some way.

**Human Figure Drawing (HFD):** A constructive assessment of cognitive/neuropsychological and developmental level that involves drawing a person.

**Hybrid forms (of art):** A term used in arts-based research that describes the blending of art and social sciences with the goal of creating an artifact recognized as art that is used to spread research findings. Audiences are aware that the presented art is based on the artist's experience of the data, but the art is not expected to prescribe solutions.

**Hypothesis:** A testable prediction of a study outcome.

**Hypothesis, directional:** A hypothesis that predicts the specific way in which results will occur, such as "significantly more" or "significantly less."

**Hypothesis, nondirectional:** A hypothesis that an experiment will result in unspecified relationships between and among variables.

**Incremental validity:** Used to determine whether a new assessment will successfully identify a client's presenting problems and provide accurate diagnostic information better than an established test.

**Inductive lens:** An interpretive lens used in the process of qualitative data analysis that involves the researcher bracketing out his or her assumptions and approaching the data set with an open mind, to let the emerging findings be the driver.

**Inductive reasoning:** Thinking from the specific to the general, as in moving from understandings of individuals' unique experiences to theory development about a phenomenon.

**Informed consent:** The process by which a potential research participant is fully informed of all study procedures and risks, to assess whether or not to voluntarily participate.

**Inner consistency:** In arts-based research, ensuring the best match between the experience that a participant intends to communicate and the artistic product so that it conveys rootedness in the researcher's own voice and personal style.

**Integrative approach:** A method applied in the art therapy evaluation process that entails the combining of qualitative and mixed methods approaches to validating assessment that is considered to be a more humanistically oriented means of data collection.

***International Classification of Diseases*** **(ICD-10):** Published by the World Health Organization in 1992, this provides the foundation for the identification of health trends and statistics globally, and the international standard for reporting diseases and health conditions. It is the diagnostic classification standard for all clinical and research purposes.

**Inter-rater (inter-scorer) reliability:** The frequency with which two or more raters consistently assign the same scores to test results. To determine inter-rater reliability, it is recommended that three individuals who are trained in using the given rating procedure (such as the FEATS) score the samples (such as a set of PPAT drawings). The raters' sets of scores are then compared, and a determination is made as to how closely their scores match.

**Internal consistency (reliability):** The extent to which all of the items of a test measure the same latent variable, i.e., those not directly observed but statistically *inferred* based on other variables that are directly measured. It is determined through *split-half* reliability and coefficient *alpha*.

**Interval (Likert) scale:** A type of *continuous* scale used by researchers to measure variables of interest when the difference between a continuum of neighboring values is the same, and therefore meaningful, for purposes of statistical analysis. The FEATS scale #1, *Prominence of Color*, appears to be interval as it provides a range of values from 0 through 5, but because subjective interpretation plays a role, the numerical differences are imprecise (hence, equal-*appearing*).

**Intervention/Embedded design:** Mixed methods research in which either qualitative data are collected within a mainly quantitative study (typically a randomized controlled study) or quantitative data (such as scores on a standardized instrument) are embedded within a mainly qualitative study.

**Interview:** A qualitative data-gathering procedure that derives detailed and personalized accounts from study participants based on one-to-one engagement involving a line of questioning on topics such as background/demographics, knowledge, experience/behavior, opinion/values, feelings, and so on. A range of interview types exist on a continuum between highly structured and unstructured and are selected based on consideration of researcher style, study focus, and participant variables.

**Introduction (problem to be investigated):** A written section of the traditional research proposal and final report contained in Chapter I that typically includes background of the problem, statement of the problem, purpose of/rationale for the study, research questions and/or hypotheses, definition of terms, and brief overview of study.

**Instrumentation:** Instruments, tests, and procedures such as structured observation used for data collection.

**Justice:** This research principle embodies researchers' obligation to be fair regarding who participates in research versus who benefits from it.

**Literature review:** A written section of the traditional research proposal and final report contained in Chapter II providing an evaluative summary of selected published (and unpublished) sources. It reflects the researcher's familiarity with the previous work of others on their topic of interest based on what has already been accomplished, how it was accomplished, the quality of the published scholarship, and the extent to which each source is relevant to his or her research question.

**Maximal variation sampling:** A type of purposive sampling (nonprobability) that seeks to represent a wide variety among the participants, which is desirable when seeking to study a range of or vast differences within a sample of participants.

**Mean:** The average value in a set of numbers.

**Measurement error:** Refers to the approximation of the range within which a person's scores vary on an assessment instrument.

**Mechanisms of change:** Elements of psychotherapy treatment that are attributable to particular techniques and approaches resulting in the reduction of a patient's symptoms.

**Median:** The middle value in a set of numbers.

**Member checking:** A procedure used in qualitative research to ensure credibility of the findings by asking study participants to verify that different stages of the analysis process (i.e., individual or common themes) are an accurate reflection of their experiences.

**Methods (or Procedures):** A written section of the traditional research proposal and final report contained in Chapter III that details all the steps involved in carrying out an investigation.

**Methodology:** The processes involved in the research.

**Mixed methods research:** Research in which both quantitative and qualitative data are collected and integrated in specific ways to capitalize on the strengths of both types of data to answer research questions.

**Mixed methods research questions:** These questions address the effect of merging quantitative and qualitative results in mixed methods research.

**Mode:** The most frequently occurring value in a set of numbers.

**Multiphase program evaluation design:** Mixed methods research in which several phases of quantitative and qualitative data collection are implemented over time to evaluate the effectiveness of a program.

**Narrative analysis:** A method of qualitative analysis that requires *re-authoring* or *re-storying* dialogue to elicit how participants constructed meaning within a given incident. Various forms of narrative analysis exist, but a widely used approach in art therapy research emphasizes examination of how the self and identity are expressed through the participant's narrative.

**Narrative inquiry:** A qualitative research method that elicits life stories relating to social and cultural issues. It involves participants providing situated accounts in which they are the protagonists within a particular plot or storyline using their own metaphorical and symbolic language to convey the magnitude and multitude of the layered meanings within the account.

**National Institute of Clinical Excellence (NICE):** The UK entity that provides national guidance and advice to improve health and social care.

**National Institute of Mental Health (NIMH):** The lead federal agency for research on mental disorders. NIMH is one of the 27 institutes and centers that make up the National Institutes of Health (NIH), the largest biomedical research agency in the world. NIH is part of the US Department of Health and Human Services (HHS).

**Naturalistic data collection:** A method of gathering data that involves researchers immersing themselves in the field to understand how the participants construct their realities. Peripheral participation occurs when the researcher has no interaction with the participants; passive participation involves a bystander level of engagement, such as the researcher sitting in on an art therapy session; balanced (occasional) or active (full) levels of participation can involve functioning as both art therapist and researcher during an art therapy session; complete immersion occurs when the researcher is also the participant.

**Nominal scale:** A type of *discrete* (or *categorical*) scale used by researchers to measure variables of interest based upon categories in which order does not matter, for purposes of statistical analysis. The DDS scale *idiosyncratic color* is a type of nominal scale.

**Non-experimental research:** Research in which variables are not manipulated by the researcher, and therefore cause and effect cannot be determined, although relationships among variables can be discovered.

**Nonmaleficence:** This research principle means "do no harm" to research participants.

**Objectivity:** The positivist principle that researchers must remain distant from the mechanics of their own studies, to eliminate bias.

**Objectivity – projection:** One of five components or tensions from Eisner's model of determining credibility in arts-based research, underscoring the need for balance in honoring the subjectivity inherent in the methodology while building in sufficient checks for rigor.

**Ontology:** A branch of philosophy concerned with the nature of reality.

**Open-ended questionnaires:** Paper and pen or online questionnaires that involve using open-ended questions such as "please describe" or "tell us about" to elicit a lengthy response from a study participant.

**Operationalization:** In quantitative research, the way in which variables are defined so they can be measured.

**Ordinal scale:** A type of *continuous* scale used by researchers to measure variables of interest when the rank order of items in a scale matters, but not the difference between values, for purposes of statistical analysis. The DDS scale *color* is a type of ordinal scale.

***p*-value:** A percentage that expresses the statistical probability that a research result occurred due to chance or not. The smaller the *p*-value, the higher the likelihood that the result is not attributable to chance.

**Paradigm:** A world view or philosophy based on assumptions about the nature of reality, how knowledge is constructed, and procedures used to find answers to questions.

**Participatory Action Research:** A qualitative, action research method that emphasizes collective and social change among oppressed groups through exploring how power can be balanced, using a cyclical process that includes the following steps: *reflect*, *plan*, *decide*, and *implement*. Participants are regarded as co-researchers and the researcher-participant relationship is more egalitarian than in other methods. Change is derived through insights and decision making and strategies are implemented and identified through deliberate intention to develop new insights that improve practice.

**Particular – general:** One of five components or tensions from Eisner's model of determining credibility in arts-based research related to transferability of findings beyond a specific situation through reducing the bias imposed by egocentrism to advance knowledge while appreciating that researchers' insights into their study can inspire others in similar circumstances.

**Person Picking an Apple from a Tree (PPAT):** A constructive art therapy assessment of cognitive/neuropsychological and developmental level that involves the standardized use of Mr. Sketch markers and the directive (*Draw a person picking an apple from a tree*). PPAT drawings are scored with the Formal Elements of Art Therapy Scale.

**Phenomenology:** A type of inquiry that involves comprehending meanings, the *life world*, of particular phenomena by returning to the essence of pre-reflective understandings through bracketing or reductionism: bracketing out individual biases and outside distractions to suspend judgment and see a phenomenon clearly. Conversely, hermeneutic phenomenology focuses on how one experiences another's life world, based on the concept that, since one cannot be fully objective when observing the human experience, phenomena should be interpreted through the lens of one's own background and experience.

**Phenomenological analysis:** A method of qualitative analysis with different types that each prioritize unique ways of eliciting participants' lived experience. The *descriptive* approach focuses on the essential and rigorous nature of drawing out essences of the participants' lived experience, and the *interpretative* approach focuses on unpacking the participants' lived experience by making connections between cognitive, linguistic, affective, and physical states elicited within the data and, in turn, identifying the relationship between the participants' voices and their emotional and mental states.

**Philosophical worldview:** A fundamental set of beliefs espoused by an individual that forms the basis of all of his or her thoughts, perceptions, and actions.

**Poetry:** A data collection procedure used in arts-based research that allows for a creative interpretation that makes use of phrases that arise from the creative process and descriptive lines to describe elements of the artwork.

**Positivism:** A research paradigm that asserts that we can know only those universal truths which can be objectively observed and tested.

**Postpositivism:** A paradigm that emerged in response to positivism that values logic and deductive reasoning, and is based on the assumptions that complete objectivity is not possible in research, that universal truths cannot be entirely discovered, and that researcher bias is a given.

**Pragmatism:** The research paradigm most associated with mixed methods research, it implies applying the most logical combination of quantitative and qualitative data to answer research questions.

**Predictive validity:** An important sub-type of criterion validity that involves assessing clients on a particular construct (e.g., depression), and then comparing the results with those obtained from the same sample at a future point in time. It is most relevant when needing to determine course of treatment, assess potential for risk of a client engaging in self-harm, or advising a prospective employer about whether to hire a job candidate based on his or her likelihood of developing an emotional disorder.

**Process-based:** An approach to psychological assessment pioneered by Bornstein that contextualizes personality tests based on the psychological processes that occur as people respond to test stimuli. Associated terms include *constructive* and *performance-based* measures.

**Quasi-experimental research:** Research in which experimental research designs are used and variables are manipulated, but random sampling and random assignment are not, thus limiting generalizability of results.

**Random assignment:** The process of randomly assigning individuals in a sample to experimental and control conditions.

**Random sampling:** A procedure by which all members of a population (potential participants) are given an equal chance of being selected for the study sample.

**Ratio scale:** The most precise level of measurement available in the form of a *continuous* scale, for purposes of statistical analysis. A ratio variable has the same properties as an interval variable, but in addition, it uses a true, or absolute, zero. The FEATS scale #4, *space*, can be considered a type of ratio scale. The variable of *behavior* can exemplify a ratio scale when counting *frequency of observed behaviors*.

**Reliability:** The extent to which researchers can depend on the accuracy of a measurement based on estimating the degree of test variance caused by error. An assessment's reliability depends upon its ability to maintain consistency, accuracy, predictability, and stability. Four main methods are used to determine reliability: *test-retest*, *alternate-form*, *internal consistency*, and *inter-rater* (or *inter-scorer*) reliability.

**Reliability coefficient:** A reliability estimate used to explain the difference between people's scores on the same assessment at two different intervals or on two parts of the same assessment. If 0.80 or higher is attained, the difference between scores, whether time to time, form to form, or item to item, is more likely to result from a true difference than from chance fluctuation.

**Reliability (qualitative research):** As determined through critical appraisal standards and guidelines to ensure that the transcript is accurate, operational definitions are consistent, research team meetings are documented, cross-checking occurs regularly, and procedures are applied such as establishing consensus on coding.

**Replication:** Performing a study again, using the same design but with different participants or slight variations in specific aspects of the study.

**Research Domain Criteria (RDoC):** An initiative of the US National Institute of Mental Health, a project that promises to reshape the direction of psychiatric research with this new taxonomy that focuses on biology, genetics, and neuroscience. It enables scientists to define disorders by their *causes*, rather than by their symptoms. The RDoC integrates many levels of information (from genomics to social factors) for each patient to provide a precise characterization. The five RDoC construct domains consist of negative valence systems, positive valence systems, cognitive systems, social processes, and arousal and regulatory systems. The eight units of analysis by which these constructs are measured are: genes, molecules, cells, circuits, physiology, behaviors, self-reports, and paradigms.

**Research review board:** This entity, also called an institutional review board or research ethics committee, provides oversight of research that involves human participants to protect the public from unsound research practices. It is usually housed within universities or medical centers.

**Research question:** A question framed using process-oriented language and focused on understanding the *how* and *why* of a social interaction that the researcher is interested in studying. The researcher phrases the question in such a way that it is clear what type of knowledge she or he is hoping will be revealed by using a particular systematic method, while defining the study parameters within the question, to demonstrate that a satisfactory answer will be provided through the data collection and analysis process. In quantitative studies, research questions remain fixed from the beginning; in qualitative studies, the research question evolves through reflexivity and interaction with the participants, and in arts-based studies the research question aims to reveal the essence of a situation and retain an exploratory qualitative nature while maintaining a clear connection to art therapy theories, practices, and circumstances.

**Researcher stance:** The position taken by a researcher reflecting the theory of knowledge that informs and governs the research process to be undertaken. In arts-based research, embracing several positions is recommended, including that of the *artist*, the *scientist*, the *adventurer*, and the *witness*.

**Respect for persons:** Also called "autonomy," this ethical principle recognizes that individuals are capable of making their own decisions about participation in research studies, and, if incapable, they are entitled to protection in the form of a legally authorized representative.

**Results:** A written section of the traditional research proposal and final report contained in Chapter IV that reports the results of the collected data and analysis and displays these visually using figures (such as photographs of artwork) and tables. Such graphics are referred to and summarized descriptively in the text of the chapter.

**Risk/benefit ratio:** A determination made by research oversight committees regarding whether the potential benefits of proposed studies outweigh their inherent risks.

**Sampling:** Ways by which participants are recruited for a research study.

**Scientific method:** A way of knowing an objective truth through hypothesis testing, deductive reasoning, and rigorous systematic investigation.

**Self-inquiry:** In arts-based research, the exploration of personal experiences through the process of artistic expression to deepen understanding of more general experiences.

**Significance, statistical:** The degree to which results of a study are unlikely to have occurred by chance.

**Social justice/transformative design:** Mixed methods research in which a social justice or transformative lens informs all aspects of a study, which can utilize any appropriate mixed methods design (see also, "Transformative").

**Snowball sampling (recruitment):** A type of purposive sampling (nonprobability) that involves selection of participants based on participants' own recommendations for additional participants throughout the course of the study.

**Spill writing (free writing):** A data collection procedure used in arts-based research that involves continuous writing without attention to form.

**Split-half reliability:** A test that splits a single knowledge area into two parts and is then administered simultaneously to one group of test subjects, followed by computation of correlation to determine the relationship between the scores from both parts of the test.

**Standard deviation:** A value that represents how spread out numbers in a sample are from the mean.

**Standard error of measurement:** An index that helps describe, statistically, the extent to which test results change in different situations by providing an established range of possible scores that provide context for understanding how much variation, or error, is considered typical for a given test item.

**Statistics, descriptive:** Summarizing mathematical techniques that result in descriptions of data in numerical form or graphic displays.

**Statistics, inferential:** Statistical techniques that allow researchers to draw inferences from the results of their studies regarding relationships between variables and applicability of results to a larger population.

**Story or fairytale:** A data collection procedure used in arts-based research that involves the researcher engaging in fiction writing to encourage imagination.

**Test-retest reliability (time to time):** Is measured by comparing two (or more) of a set of a client's scores derived from an assessment taken at different time intervals that are carefully determined. If the scores are close, then the assessment is deemed to have test-retest reliability.

**Test selection:** Applies when a researcher's purpose is to design a study of a client population and requires use of a well-established pretest and posttest instrument.

**Textual-based:** Refers to a type of qualitative data collection that involves gathering knowledge on the research topic when the language used by the participants and how they interact within certain health, community, educational, and correctional cultures and systems is of interest, through use of written accounts and documents such as journal entries, client records, social media content, and the like.

**Thematic analysis:** A form of inductive qualitative analysis that involves extracting themes from data and demonstrating the relationships between the themes and how they address the research questions. These relationships can be displayed using visual maps. Unlike content analysis, in thematic analysis latent and manifest content are seen as co-dependent and inseparable.

**Therapeutic assessment:** A client-centered approach to psychological assessment developed by Stephen Finn, it incorporates traditional psychological assessment with various standardized instruments and techniques of *collaborative assessment* with an emphasis on individual narratives and anecdotal evidence to enhance the therapeutic relationship, inform clinical practice, and promote therapeutic change.

**Transformative:** A research paradigm that is also referred to as the *critical-ideological* paradigm, it acknowledges power imbalances, seeks social justice, and empowers the marginalized. Therefore, the researcher's proactive values are central to the study in order to collaborate and help change social conditions through working with the participants.

**Translation:** A data collection procedure used in arts-based research that involves the conversion of arts into narrative through three successive phases: (a) *formative* (documenting immediate reactions and responses), (b) *assemblage, construction, and interpretation* (amplifying fragments with narrative and structure), and (c) *final synthesis – interpretation, representation, and dissemination* (aesthetically reconfigured).

**Triangulation:** A technique used in research that serves to validate data through cross-verification from two or more sources.

**True experimental research:** Research in which random sampling and random assignment are used to assign participants to experimental and control conditions.

**Trustworthiness:** Applies to evaluation of quality in the interpretation of qualitative findings and the level of confidence that the study was conducted in a rigorous manner through provision of assurances that results are believable and provide an honest account, that the *transferability* of the findings beyond the participants in the study is clearly conveyed, and that the findings can be depended upon, can be confirmed, and have utility.

**Typical sampling:** A type of purposive sampling (nonprobability) that involves selection of participants based on how well they represent the phenomena that is being studied.

**Validity:** An attribute of the dependent variable used to determine the extent to which an instrument measures what it is supposed to measure. An assessment is valid only for a specific use, because validity is relative to the assessment's purpose and subject characteristics. Three main types of *evidential* (research-based) validity examine a test's ability to provide useful, accurate, and unbiased data: *content*, *criterion*, and *construct* validity.

**Validity coefficient:** Expresses a relationship between scores derived from the same people on two different tests.

**Validity, external:** The extent to which study results can be generalized.

**Validity, internal:** The extent to which results of an experiment are directly attributable to the experimental design and method.

**Variable:** A characteristic, attribute, or behavior that varies in at least two ways and can be measured.

**Variable, confounding:** A variable not manipulated by the researcher that affects its results and obscures the effects of the variables under study. (Example: amount of research participants' art education and art practice.)

**Variable, dependent:** A variable that is expected to be affected by the independent variable.

**Variable, extraneous:** An additional independent variable beyond those being tested in a study that unless controlled will prevent inferring cause and effect relationships.

**Variable, independent:** The variable that is assumed to affect the dependent variable under study.

**Variable, intervening:** A variable outside of an experiment that explains a link between study variables that exists separately from the study.

**Variability, measures of:** Statistical techniques that describe how widely values are dispersed across a sample.

**Work imaginatively – referential clarity:** One of five components or tensions from Eisner's model of determining credibility in arts-based research through determining *referential adequacy* – the extent to which the contents that the evaluator confirms is there can actually be identified.

# Index

*Note*: Page references to tables are in **bold**, while references to figures are in *italics*. References to notes are denoted by the letter "n" and the note number following the page number.

"68–95–99.7 rule" 73

AATA *see* American Art Therapy Association (AATA)
A-B single-subject design 63–64
A-B-A-B single-subject design 64
ABR *see* arts-based research (ABR)
Accreditation Council for Art Therapy Education (ACATE) 4
Acosta, I. 205
action research 94, 262
Adult Attachment Projective Picture System (AAP) 168
aesthetics – verisimilitude 135, 262
Agee, J. 84
Ainsworth, M. D. 223
Albert-Proos, D. 124
Allan, J. 159–160
Allen, P. B. 125, **126**
Alon, U. 202
Alter-Muri, S. B. 206
alternate-form reliability (form to form) 190, 194, 262, 276
American Art Therapy Association (AATA) 2, 3, 4, 8, 262; advocacy by 9; comparison of foundational and AATA ethical principles 26–27; Ethical Principles for Art Therapists 19, 24–25, 32–34, 167; Ethics and Research committees 32; membership surveys 66, 72; Values Statement 158
American Counseling Association, Center for Counseling Practice, Policy and Research 28

American Psychiatric Association (APA) 5, 266–267
American Psychological Association (APA) 19; Publication Manual 206, 219
Analysis of Variance (ANOVA) 76–77, 262
analytical integration 262
Andsell, G. 73–74
Ansara, Y. 20
Archibald, M. M. 122
Ardon, A. M. 184
Arnheim, R. 205
art: art for scholarship's sake 130, 262, 267; artistic inquiry 263; characteristics 234; creativity and artmaking 24; ethical use of in art therapy research 32–34; interpretation of artwork 205; power of, acknowledging by art therapists 21; process of artmaking 91; response art 133, 137, 139, 210, 237; storage or disposal of artworks 34; therapeutic implications of artmaking 23, 61, 66, 92; three-dimensional artmaking 43; using in art therapy research 31, 32–34; variability in artwork of children 205–206; versus arts 121; workshops, artmaking 94, 95, 133; *see also* Art Therapy-Projective Imagery Assessment (AT-PIA); arts-based research (ABR); arts-informed research
Art and Creative Materials Institute 33

art psychotherapy 61
art therapists/art therapy researchers 1–4, 8, 9; assessment research *see* assessments, art therapy research; ethical dilemmas 25, 28, 29, 30, 31, 36; experimenter bias 52; mixed methods research *see* mixed methods research (MMR); moral code 30, 32, 36; qualitative research *see* qualitative research; quantitative research *see* qualitative research; studies *see* studies, art therapy research; in United Kingdom 24, 25, 34, 67; validity concerns 53, 54; *see also* ethical considerations; research, art therapy
art therapy: as adjunct to Cognitive Processing Therapy (CPT) 2, 21–22, 155, 156; assumptions underlying the profession 42; dyad form 103; engagement in process 43; factors impacting growth of profession 3; meaning-making 205; origins 149; research *see* research, art therapy; theory 42; *see also* art therapists
Art Therapy Credentials Board 24
Art Therapy in the Community (ATIC) 159
Art Therapy-Projective Imagery Assessment (AT-PIA) 171, 183, 184, 262
a/r/tography 120, 121, 263; *see also* arts-based research (ABR)
arts, versus art 121
arts-based research (ABR) 10, 12, 119–146, 262–263; advantages 130–133; adventurer role 136–137; analysis 140; artist role 136; arts versus art 121; creative arts therapy experience 121; credibility in 133–136, 139, 265, 274; defining 120–122; documentation 139; encouraging creative inquiry 132; expanding audience reach 132–133; expanding knowledge 131–132; explication 122–124; free association 138, 269; and heuristics 125, **126**, 127, 135; honoring artistic knowledge 130–131; hybrid forms 130, 267, 270; increasing social awareness 133; making of art by researcher 121; poetry (data collection procedure) 93, 138, 275; presentation 140–141; procedures 138–139; research characteristics 127–130; research questions 137–138; scientist role 216; self-inquiry 124–127, 278; significance of actions within practice 121–122; as "soft-form" of qualitative inquiry 10–11; spill writing (free writing) 138, 278; steps for conducting 136–141; story/fairytale procedure 138, 275, 278; traditions 122–127; translation 138, 139, 279; *see also* evocative power; explication
arts-informed research 120, 121, 263; *see also* arts-based research (ABR)
assemblage, translation 139
assessments, art therapy research 167–200; assessment research 263; background 168–174; collaborative assessment 6, 170, 264, 279; collaborative assessment 170; Diagnostic Drawing Series (DDS) 171; drawings 171–174, **175**, 178, 179, 183–185, 187, 189, 191, 192, 194; Expressive Therapies Continuum (ETC) 42, 101, 172, 211, 268; Face Stimulus Assessment (FSA) 171, 172–173, 191, 192, 268; frequency of observed behaviors 179; integrative approach 169–174, 271; interval (Likert) scales 71, 178, 271; interviews 168–169; nominal scales 174, 176–177, 273; ordinal scales 71, 75, 77, 177–178, 274; process-based approach, psychological assessment 6, 167–168, 276; qualitative methods 170; quantitative measurement levels 174, **175**, 176–180; rating systems **175**; ratio scales 71–72, 75, 77, 178–180, 276; rigor in research, establishing 180–195; self-harm concerns 186, 187; therapeutic 279; *see also* Art Therapy-Projective Imagery Assessment (AT-PIA); Expressive Therapies Continuum (ETC) assessment; Face Stimulus Assessment (FSA); Person Picking an Apple from a Tree (PPAT) art therapy assessment
associational (correlational) research 67–68
Attachment Rating Scale (ARS) 75

attachment theory 223
Attachment to Mother scale (ATM) 75
Attard, A. 8
attrition (mortality) 52
audience reach, expanding 132–133
authenticity 105
Autism Spectrum Disorder (ASD) 98
autobiography 92–93, 270
autoethnography 93, 125, 127, 263, 267
autonomy (respect for persons) principle 19–20, 277
axial coding 269
axiology 10, 85, 263

Bach, J. S., *Magnificat* 65, 66
Badiee, M. 158
Barone, T. 121–122, 138
Bat Or, M. 195
Beck Depression Inventory (BDI) 168, 181
Belmont Report, 1979 19, 22, 263
beneficence principle 19, 21–22, 263
Bernier, M. 184
better questions – better answers 136, 263
Betts, D. J. 13, 107–108, 170, 172, 204, 208, 230
bias: experimenter 51–52, 55; selection 50, 54, 55
Bird's Nest Drawing (BND) 75, 76, 220–222, 224, 226, 263; assessments, art therapy research 171, 172, 189, 190
Boeije, H. 155
Boothby, D. 65–66
Borch, D. von der 95
Bornstein, R. F. 6, 167–168, 276
Bottorff, J. L. 103
Bowlby, J. 223
Boydell, K. M. 133
Braun, V. 100, 101
breast cancer treatment, art therapy for 103
Bresler, L. 106
bricolage 84, 88, 263
Brief Mood Introspection Scale (BMIS) 56
Bringing Research to Life! (research simulation experiential) 13–14, 77–78, 107–108, 140; art characteristics 234; art exhibit visit surveys 233; arts-based data analysis 142–143; baseline survey 232; developing proposal 208–212; informed consent 230–231, 271; materials packet 230–242; qualitative data analysis 100; quantitative research 56; relational aesthetics questionnaires 235; *see also* research simulation experiential materials packet
Brinkmann, S. 83
British Association of Art Therapists 24
Brittain, W. L. 173, 206
Brophy-Dixon, J. 139
Brown, R. J. 69
Burke, C. 35
burnout, professional 139
Buros Center for Testing 48
Burrell, S. S. 127
Bustamante, R. 153–154
Bute, J. J. 103

CAAHEP *see* Commission on Accreditation of Allied Health Education Programs (CAAHEP)
Caddy, L. 67–68
Cahnmann-Taylor, M. 130
Camic, P. M. 102
Campbell, D. 54
Campbell, M. 21–22, 155, 156
Canada: Art Therapy Association 24; First Nations adolescents in 20
Carolan, R. 129
case study method 89–90, 264; one-shot case study 55–56; practical guides 254; research report 215–216
categorical scale *see* nominal scales
causal comparative designs 68–69
central tendency measures 72, 264
characteristics of arts-based research 127–130, 128–129, 268; economy of means 129–130, 267; inner consistency 129, 271
Charmaz, K. 90, 91, 102
Chataway, C. J. 94
childbirth, fear of 96
Chilton, G. 119, 120, 122, 130–131, 136, 137, 138
chi-square 75, 194, 195
Choi, S. N. 103
Clandinin, D. J. 103

Clarke, V. 100, 101
Clausen, C. 186–187
client-centered approaches, psychological assessment 6–7
Clock Drawing Test (CDT) 173
cluster random sampling 46, 47
coding: axial 269; Declaration of Helsinki, 1964 19; ethical codes 25–27; Nuremburg Code, 1947 18; open 269; selective 269
coefficient alpha 192, 195, 271
Cognitive Processing Therapy (CPT) 2, 21–22, 155, 156
collaborative assessment 6, 264, 279
Collaborative Institutional Training Program 36
collage 55, 130–131, 137
Collie, K. 103
*color* (ordinal scale) 274
Commission on Accreditation of Allied Health Education Programs (CAAHEP) 201, 263–264; Standards and Guidelines for the Accreditation of Educational Programs in Art Therapy (S&Gs), 2016 3–4
Common Rule, US 35
communicative integration 264
compassion fatigue 139
complete immersion 99
conceptual integration 264
conceptual validity 190, 264
concurrent validity 185–186, 264, 266
Conduct Disorder 68
confounding variables 43, 280
Connelly, F. M. 103
consent *see* informed consent
consequential (impact-based) validity 264
conspiratorial conversations 129, 268
constant comparative process 102
construct validity 160, 187–190, 264, 280
constructive measures 276
constructivism 10, 12–13, 86–87, 147, 265; and postpositivism 149
content analysis 101–102, 265
content validity 181–184, 265, 268, 280
control groups, true experimental research designs: ethical considerations 21; nonrandomized pretest-posttest 61–62; posttest only 58–59; pretest-posttest 57–58; wait lists 22; *see also* true experimental research designs
convenience sampling 46, 47–48, 88, 265
convergent parallel design 151–152, 265
convergent validity 189, 264, 265
Coopersmith, S. 186
Coopersmith Self-Esteem Inventory (SEI) 186
Corbin, J. 90, 269
correlational research 67–68
Council for Higher Education Accreditation (CHEA) 263–264
Cox, S. 141
Crawford, F. 67–68
creativity principle: and artmaking 24; in arts-based research 133–136, 139, 265, 274; creative arts therapy experience 121; creative dialogue 138, 265; creative inquiry, encouraging 132; defining 265; in qualitative research 265–266; value of creativity 19, 21, 24–25
credibility: aesthetics – verisimilitude 135, 262; arts-based research (ABR) 133–136, 139, 265, 274; better questions – better answers 136, 263; mixed methods research (MMR) 160; objectivity-projection 136, 274; particular – general 135, 274; qualitative research 265–266; quality evaluation 104; working imaginatively – referential clarity 134–135, 280
Creswell, J. D. 105–106
Creswell, J. W. 105–106, 147, 151, 154–156, 158, 159
criterion validity 184–185, 266, 280
critical ethnography 93
critical research priorities 18
critical sampling *see* purposive (critical) sampling
critical social science 7
critical-ideological paradigm 87, 279
Cronbach's alpha 192, 195, 266
cross-sectional studies, surveys 66–67
Crotty, M. 92
cultural appropriateness 204–205
Curtis, E. K. 205

Daly, J. 106
D'Archer, J. 148
data: amount 178; distribution of 73–74; enhancement 123; hard 148; integration of 147; qualitative *see* qualitative research; quality of 161; quantitative *see* quantitative research; triangulation of 151–152, 265–266, 279
data analysis: arts-based 142–143; central tendency measures 72, 264; descriptive statistics 72–74; ex-post facto ("after the fact") studies 69; measures of variability 73, 280; numbers and measurement 70–72; qualitative 99–104; quantitative 69–77, 150; *see also* quantitative research
data collection: digital storytelling 93; field notes 99; interactive forms 95–97; interviews 95–97, 271–272; journal of reflections, use of 123; mixed methods research (MMR) 155–157, 159–160; naturalistic forms 98–99; participation 99; participatory action research (PAR) 94; poetry procedure 93, 138, 275; questionnaires 97–98; story/fairytale procedure 138, 275, 278; textual-based 97–98, 279; translation 138, 139, 279
data source integration 266
Davidson, L. 92
Davis, B. 91
Davis, T. 28–30
Day, J. 31
de Zárate, M. H. 93
Deaver, S. 8, 23, 72, 98, 148, 152, 169, 173, 183–185, 187–188, 205
deception, in research 24
decision-making: ethical 25–30, 36; models 27–30
Decker, K. 156
Declaration of Helsinki, 1964 19
deductive lens 266
deductive reasoning 266
DeGrace, B. W. 193
degree of error 191, 266
Dejkameh, M. 124
Delphi method 9, 148, 266; questionnaires 84, 98, 107
dementia, assessing 173

demographic questionnaires 53, 204
Denzin, N. K. 7
Department of Health and Human Services (HHS), US 273
dependent variables 43–44, 49, 64, 280
depression 7–8, 98; Beck Depression Inventory (BDI) 168, 181; mixed methods research (MMR) 150, 156
descriptive statistics 70, 72–74, 278
descriptive survey research 66–67
designs, mixed methods research 150, 151–160; advanced 151, 154–160; basic 151–154; convergent parallel 151–152, 265; explanatory sequential research design 152–153, 268; exploratory sequential research design 153–154; intervention/embedded design 154–156, 271; multiphase program evaluation design 158–160, 273; sequential designs 151, 152–154, 268; skills required 150; social justice 156–158, 278; triangulation 151
designs, qualitative research 84; case study method 89–90; ethnography 93; grounded theory 90–91; narrative inquiry 92–93; participatory action research (PAR) 94–95; phenomenological inquiry 91–92
designs, quantitative research 54–69; control groups 57–59, 61–62; factorial 64–66; non-experimental 66–69; nonrandomized control group pretest-posttest 61–62; one-group pretest-posttest 56–57; one-shot case study 55–56; pre-experimental 55–57, 77; pretest-posttest 57–59, 61–62; quasi-experimental 9, 48, 60–61, 276; single-subject 63–64, 72; Solomon 4-group 59–61; static group comparison 57; time-series 62; true experimental 57–64; *see also* quantitative research
*Diagnostic and Statistical Manual of Mental Disorders (DSM)* 5, 6, 266–267
Diagnostic Drawing Series (DDS) 171, 172, 174, 175, 266; Drawing

Analysis Form (DAF) 177; Drawing Inquiry Form (DIF) 184
dialectical pragmatism/dialecticism 149, 161
dialogue: creative 265; re-storying, in narrative analysis 273
dialogue groups 94
Dickson, R. 131–132
digital storytelling 93
directional hypotheses 44
discourse analysis 104, 267
discriminant validity 189, 264, 267
discursive grounded theory 90
discussion 267
distribution 267
distribution-free tests 75
distributive justice 22
"DO ART" model (Hauck and Ling) 31
Drabble, S. 155
drawing/drawings 7, 35, 133; assessment 171–174, **175**, 178, 179, 183–185, 187, 189, 191, 192, 194; Bird's Nest Drawing (BND) see Bird's Nest Drawing (BND); Clock Drawing Test (CDT) 173; content validity 183; diagnostic and screening tasks 172–173, 221, 223, 262; Diagnostic Drawing Series (DDS) 171, 172, 174, **175**, 177, 184; Drawing Analysis Form II 174; Face Stimulus Assessment (FSA) 172–173, 191, 192; Formal Elements Art Therapy Scale (FEATS) 179; House-Tree-Person (HTP) 186, 192, 225; Human Figure Drawing (HFD) 60, 171, 173, 179, 185–187, 192, 205, 225; Person Picking an Apple from a Tree (PPAT) 173, 174, 177, 178, 179, 185, 194; Person-in-the-Rain (PITR) projective drawings 185; quantitative research 48, 65, 66, 69, 70; self drawing 76; still life 213, **214**, 225
DSM see Diagnostic and Statistical Manual of Mental Disorders (DSM)

Eatough, V. 102
economy of means 129–130, 267
Edinger, E. F. 223
Edwards, D. 55
egocentrism 274
Einstein, T. 138
Eisner, E. 10–11, 121, 133–135, 263, 265, 274, 280
Elkins, D. 72
Ellingson L. 104
Elliott, R. 106
Elo, S. 101
embedded design 154–156
Emerson, P. 103
empathetic phenomenology 92, 270
epistemology 10, 85
Erard, R. E. 7–8
error: degree of 191, 266; measurement 191, 272; standard error of measurement 193, 278
ethical considerations 12, 18–40; art, ethical use of in art therapy research 32–34; beneficence principle 19, 21–22; codes 25–27; comparison of foundational and AATA ethical principles 26–27; creativity 19, 21, 24–25; decision-making 25–30, 36; ethical and moral responsibilities 106–107; ethical dilemmas 25, 28, 29, 30, 31, 36; ethical principles 26–27, 35, 36; Ethical Principles for Art Therapists (AATA) 19, 24–25, 32–34, 167; "ethics in practice" 30; fidelity principle 19, 21, 23–24, 268; foundational principles 18–19; institutional review boards (IRBs) 21, 23, 28; integrity principle 19, 23; justice principle 19, 22–23, 272; nonmaleficence principle 19, 21–22, 24; practical guides 258–259; presentation, in ABR 141; principle ethics 31, 267; research proposal 216–217; research review board oversight 34–36, 139; respect for persons see autonomy (respect for persons) principle; storage or disposal of artworks 34; virtue ethics 31, 267; vulnerable populations 21, 23; see also American Art Therapy Association (AATA)
ethnography 93, 267–268; autoethnography 93, 125, 127, 263, 267; critical 93
ethnorelativistic attitudes, of art therapists 20
Evans, K. 106
evidential validity 264, 280

Index   287

evocative power 128–129, 268
ex post facto ("after the fact") studies 268
experimental research designs: control 49–50; defining 268; practical guides 251–252; quantitative methods 48–50; quasi-experimental research 9, 48, 60–61, 77, 276; research proposal 215; true experimental research designs 48–49, 57–64, 77, 279; *see also* factorial designs; non-experimental research designs
experimenter bias 51–52, 55
expertise 268
explanatory sequential research design 152–153, 268
explication 122–124; analysis 124; data enhancement 123; defining 268; dissemination 124; field notes 123; memo-writing 123; research questions 122
exploratory sequential research design 153–154, 268
ex-post facto ("after the fact") studies 68–69
Expressive Therapies Continuum (ETC) assessment 42, 101, 172, 211, 268
external validity 53–54, 280; weak 63
extraneous variables 43, 204, 280
Eyde, L. 24

Face Stimulus Assessment (FSA) 171, 172–173, 191, 192, 268
face validity 182, 268
factorial designs 64, 66–69, 268
fairness 105
Farrant, C. 23
FEATs *see* Formal Elements Art Therapy Scale (FEATS)
Fenner, P. 139
fidelity principle 19, 21, 23–24, 268
field notes 99, 123, 269
finger paints 71
Finlay, L. 106
Finn, S. E. 6, 168, 170, 279
Fischer, C. T. 6, 106
Fish, B. J. 133, 137
Fleischman, P. 5
Flicker, S. 20
focus groups 127, 160, 269; qualitative research 90, 91, 94, 95, 97, 107

Forester-Miller, H. 28–30
Forinash, M. 138
Formal Elements Art Therapy Scale (FEATS): defining 269; developmental level scale 188–189; instrumentation 51; interval (Likert) scale 271; manual 177; mixed methods research (MMR) 154; modified 70; and Person Picking an Apple from a Tree (PPAT) assessment 173, 174, 177, 179, 274; and ratio scale 179, 276
Fowler, J. P. 184
Fox, K. 95
Fraenkel, J. R. 151, 206–208, 218–219
free association 138, 269
Frosh, S. 103
Fujiura, G. T. 106
funding agencies 7

Gantt, L. M. 154, 179, 186, 269; *see also* Formal Elements Art Therapy Scale (FEATS)
Gee, J. P. 104
generalizability 55, 148, 173, 269; quantitative research 42, 47, 49, 53, 77
Gerber, N. 122, 139, 149
Gibbs, G. R. 106
Gibson, D. 139
Gilfillan, P. 93
Gillam, L. 25, 30
Gioia, D. 151
Glaser, B. G. 90, 102
Gottfried, A. E. 66
Gottfried, A. W. 66
Gough, B. 7
graduate art therapy students 1, 3, 13, 167, 201, 206, 215
Graves-Alcorn, S. 172
Green, C. E. 192–193
Green, E. 172
Greene, J. 149
Groth-Marnat, G. 170, 186, 192, 225
grounded theory 90–91, 269; constant comparative process 102; constructivist 90, 102
Guardhouse Project (Klorer) 127, 132–133
Gubrium, A. 20
Guerin, D. 66

Guillemin, M. 25, 30, 141
Gussak, D. 195

Hacking, S. 194
Haeyen, S. 90, 101
Handler, L. 205
Hanson, W. 151
"hard science" 41
Harris, C. 98
Hartz, L. 61
Hartzell, E. 56–57
Hauck, J. 31
Haynes, S. N. *182*
Hegarty, P. 20
Heidegger, M. 91
hermeneutic circle/phenomenology 91, 269–270
Hess-Behrens, N. 205
heuristic phenomenology 92, 270
heuristic research 255, 270; arts-based research (ABR) 125, **126**, 127, 135; research proposal 216
HFD *see* Human Figure Drawing (HFD)
Hill, H. 20
Hinz, L. 31, 34, 101, 172, 195, 211
historic utilization 160
Hoffman, N. 141
Holmqvist, G. 72, 101
homogeneous sampling 88, 270
Hooren, S. van 90
House-Tree-Person (HTP) drawings 186, 192, 225
Howell Major, C. 89
Human Figure Drawing (HFD) 60, 61, 70, 205, 225, 270; assessment research 171, 173, 179, 185–187, 192
human subjects committees 21
Hunter, A. 124
Huss, E. 89
Husserl, E. 91
Hutschemaekers, G. 90
hybrid forms 130, 267, 270
hypotheses: conducting of study 222; defining 270; directional and nondirectional 44, 270; testing, in quantitative research 30, 44–45, 74
Hyun, H. 206–208, 218–219

ICD-10 *see* International Classification of Diseases (ICD-10)
*idiosyncratic color* (nominal scale) 174, 176, 177–178, 273

incremental validity 189, 270
independent variables 43, 49, 64, 280
inductive lens 270
inductive reasoning 270
inference transferability 161
inferential consistency 160
inferential statistics 70, 74–77, 278
information gathering 94
informed consent 19, 21, 230–231, 271
inner consistency 129, 271
Inner Working Models (IWMs) 220
inquiry form 243–246
Insel, T. 5
institutional review boards (IRBs) 139, 201; ethical considerations 21, 23, 28, 35
instrumentation 48, 51, 272; cultural appropriateness 204–205; design 94; development of 154; internal validity 51; research proposal and report 225
integrative approach 169–174, 271
integrity principle 19, 23
interaction effects, external validity 54
internal consistency reliability 190, 191–192, 276
internal review board (IRB) 106
internal validity 50–53, 280; attrition 52; experimenter bias 51–52; history 50–51; instrumentation 51; maturation 52; selection bias 50; single-subject research 64; statistical regression 52–53; unanticipated external events 50–51
International Classification of Diseases (ICD-10) 5, 271
interpretivism 265
inter-rater/inter-scorer reliability 177, 190, 194–195, 271, 276
interval (Likert) scales 71, 75, 77, 178, 179, 271
intervening variables 43–44, 280
intervention/embedded design 154–156, 271
interviews 95–97, 153, 271–272; assessments, art therapy 168–169; central tendency measures 72; ex-post facto ("after the fact") studies 69; face-to-face 96; mixed methods research (MMR) 153–155; semi-structured conversational style

96–97, 153–155; types 96–97; variability measures 73; *see also* qualitative research
intraclass correlations 195; *see also* coefficient alpha; percent agreement
IRBs *see* institutional review boards (IRBs)
Irwin, R. L. 121
Isaac, S. 206–208, 218–219
Ishai, R. 195
isomorphism 42

Jacobsen, M. H. 83
Jensen, R. E. 103
Johnson, B. 149
Johnson, K. M. 195
Johnson, R. B. 147, 162
journaling, visual 131–132, 139
Jung, C. 132; *Liber Novus (The Red Book)* 124–125
Junne, F. 8
justice principle 19, 22–23, 272; *see also* social justice

Kagin, S. L. 195, 211
Kaimal, G. 152
Kaiser, D. H. 75, 76, 98, 148, 168, 172, 220, 221, 223–226
Kalmanowitz, D. 137
Kapitan, L. 20, 23, 31, 94, 95, 121, 127, 135, 158
Kaplan, F. 148
Karkou, V. 98
Kay, S. R. 194–195
Keats, P. A. 103
Kellman, J. 92–93
Kim, G. 173, 191, 192
Kim, J. 173, 191, 192
Kimport, E. 56–57
Kleijberg, M. 101
Klorer, P. G. 127, 132–133
Knill, P. 130
knowledge: artistic, honoring 130–131; expanding 131–132; Standards and Guidelines for the Accreditation of Educational Programs in Art Therapy (S&Gs), 2016 3–4
Koppitz, E. M. 173
Kortesluoma, R. 183
Kramer, E. 128, 129–130
Kristiansen, S. 83
Kroger, R. O. 104

Kruskal–Wallis One-Way Analysis of Variance 76–77
Kuo, N. 64, 72
Kvist, L. J. 96–97
Kyngäs, H. 101

Laak, J. der 187
Lack, H. S. 185
Landgren, K. 96–97
language, and discourse analysis 104
Larkin, M. 8
Leavy, P. 105, 119, 120, 130, 133, 135–138, 265
Leech, N. 160
Lett, W. 95
Levi, N. 195
Levick, M. F. 206
life cycle, human 34
Likert scale *see* interval (Likert) scales
Lincoln, Y. S. 7
Linde, H. 127
Ling, T. 31
Litell, M. 94, 95, 158
literature reviews 138, 223, 272; practical guides 250; research proposal and report 202, 203, 206, 207, 213, 215, 223; *see also* research proposal and report
Long, B. C. 103
longitudinal surveys 66
Lowenfeld, V. 173, 206
Lusebrink, V. B. 195, 211
Lykes, M. B. 95
Lyons, A. 7

MacIntyre, D. J. 98
McLeod, J. 89
McNiff, S. 119, 120–122, 125, 127–130, 137, 138
McVittie, C. 34
Manders, E. 138
Manen, M. van 102
Matto, H. C. 186–187
maturation 52
maximal variation sampling 47, 88, 272
mean (average value in a set of numbers) 52–53, 72, 73, 272
meaning-reconstruction theory 125
Meara, N. 31
measurement error 191, 272
mechanisms of change 272

median (middle value in a set of numbers) 72, 73, 272
Medical Outcomes Study Short-Form Health Survey (SF-36) 58
member checking 272
membership surveys (AATA) 66, 72
memo-writing 123
mental illness: defining 5; dementia 173; depression 7–8, 98, 150, 156, 168, 181; Oppositional Defiant Disorder 68; personality disorders 90; philosophy of recovery 159; post-traumatic stress disorder (PTSD), veterans with 2, 18, 22, 155–157; psychosis/schizophrenia 67, 91, 98; *see also* Autism Spectrum Disorder (ASD); *Diagnostic and Statistical Manual of Mental Disorders (DSM)*; International Classification of Diseases (ICD-10)
mentalization-based therapy (MBT) 97
Mertens, D. 157
methodology 10, 85–86, 140, 272
methods/procedures 223–225; arts-based research (ABR) 138–139; defining 272; design, research 223–224; implications for clinical practice 6–9; instrumentation 225; quantitative research 48–54; research proposal and report 202, 203, 206, 207–208, 213, 214, 215–217, 223–225; selection of subjects 224; *see also* designs, mixed methods research; designs, qualitative research; designs, quantitative research; research proposal and report
Michael, W. 206–208, 218–219
Milgram, S. 24, 28
Miller, C. 62, 72
mindfulness-based art therapy (MBAT) program 58
Minnesota Multiphasic Personality Inventory (MMPI-2) 168, 169
mixed methods research (MMR) 10, 12, 147–166, 149; combining/integrating of quantitative and qualitative data 147–152; data collection 155–157, 159–160; defining 147, 272; designs 150, 151–160; dialectic paradigm for 149; evaluation of studies 160–161; exploratory sequential research design 268; interviews 153–155; mixed methods way of thinking 150; planning 161; pragmatism 148–149, 161, 162–163; questions 273; rationale for use 148; required skills 149–151; research questions 150–151, 273; skills required 150; stages of studies 161; statistics 152; strengths and weaknesses 161–162; thematic analysis 153, 155; as third research movement 147; transferability 160, 161; transformative 157–158; trauma research 155–157; underlying philosophy 148–149; *see also* qualitative research; quantitative research
MMR *see* mixed methods research (MMR)
mode 72, 73, 273
modified grounded theory 90
Monti, D. A. 2, 58, 61, 150
Moon, B. L. 34, 141
Mouradian, L. E. 193
Moustakas, C. 92, 125, **126**, 135, 270
Muldoon, K. 125
multiphase program evaluation design 158–160, 273
music therapy 59, 65
Myers-Coffman, K. 139

Naglieri, J. 173, 186–187
Nainis, N. 150
narrative analysis 103, 273
narrative inquiry 92–93, 273; identity issues, for personal storytelling 137
National Academies of Sciences, Engineering and Medicine 1
National Institute of Clinical Excellence (NICE), UK 6, 273
National Institutes of Health (NIH), US: National Institute of Mental Health (NIMH), US 5, 6, 169, 170, 273; Research Domain Criteria (RDoC) 5–6, 169, 211, 276
naturalistic forms of data collection 98–99
Naumann, E. 223

Nelson, J. 153–154
new phenomenology 92, 270
Nicaraguan communities, use of PAR with 94–95
Nikkonen, M. 183
Nishida, M. 55, 56
nominal scales 71, 75, 176–177; *idiosyncratic color* example 174, 176, 177–178, 273
nondirectional hypotheses 44
non-experimental research designs 66–69; causal comparative or ex post facto 68–69; correlational research 67–68; defining 273; descriptive survey research 66–67
nonmaleficence principle 19, 21–22, 24, 274
nonprobability (purposive) sampling 46, 265, 266, 270, 272, 278, 280
nonrandomized control group pretest-posttest design 61–62
normal curve 73–74
normal distribution 267
Nuremburg Code, 1947 18
NVivo (computer-based data analysis program) 100

obedience study (Milgram, 1963) 24
objectivity principle 42, 77, 148, 274
objectivity-projection 136, 274
O'Cathain, A. 155, 161
one-group pretest-posttest design 56–57
one-shot case study 55–56
online questionnaires 97, 98, 101
ontology 10, 85, 274
Onwuegbuzi, A. 147, 153–154, 162
open coding 269
open-ended questionnaires 84, 97–98, 107, 274
Open-Studio Process 125, **126**
operationalization 45, 274
Oppositional Defiant Disorder 68
order effects 53–54
ordinal scales 71, 75, 77, 177–178, 274
Orr, P. 101

Page, A. 67–68
painting: arts-based research (ABR) 127, 130, 133, 140; bottle paints 71; paint sticks 71; quantitative research 62, 71, 72; water color 71
paradigms, qualitative research 10, **11**, 84, 86–87, 148, 274
parametric tests 75
Park, S. W. 103
participatory action research (PAR) 94–95, 274
particular – general 135, 274
passive participation 99
Patterson, S. 67, 73, 90–91
Patton, M. 95–96
Pavlicevic, M. 73–74
Pearson product-moment correlation coefficient (Pearson's $r$) 75, 76, 184, 194
percent agreement 195
performance-based measures 276
peripheral participation 99
Person Picking an Apple from a Tree (PPAT) art therapy assessment 51, 171, 177–179, 185, 194, 271; and FEATS 173, 174, 177, 179, 274
personality disorders 90
personality tests 276
Person-in-the-Rain (PITR) projective drawings 185
Peterson, C. 58
Pfeifer, N. 60, 76
phenomenological analysis 102–103, 275
phenomenology: being in the world 91; bracketing 91; defining 275; descriptive method 102, 103; empathetic 92, 270; hermeneutic circle/phenomenology 91, 269–270; heuristic 92, 270; interpretive method 102–103; life world 91; lived experience 103; modified 91, 92; new 92, 270; reductionism 91; spiraling 91, 269–270; studies 87
philosophical assumptions, qualitative research 85–86
philosophical worldview 275
photography/photographs 139, 218, 231; digital 32, 33; ethical considerations 27, 32–35
Piaget, J. 205
Pierce, V. 156
Plano Clark, V. 151, 154, 156, 159
Plavnick, J. 64, 72
Pleasant-Metcalf, A. 63, 64

poetry (data collection procedure) 93, 138, 275
Polkinghorne, D. 103
positive psychology 170
positivism 41, 148, 275
postmodern grounded theory 90
postpositivism 10, 12–13, 42, 86, 275; and constructivism 149; mixed methods research (MMR) 147, 148, 149
post-traumatic stress disorder (PTSD), veterans with 2, 18, 22; mixed methods research (MMR) 155–157
Potash, J. 11, 12, 13, 107–108, 208, 230
power, evocative 128–129, 268
PPAT (Person Picking an Apple from a Tree) *see* Person Picking an Apple from a Tree (PPAT) art therapy assessment
practical guides: ethics 258–259; experimental design 251–252; literature reviews 250; program development and case study 254; qualitative research 253; quantitative research 251–252; research questions 248–249; rigor 260–261; sampling 256–257
practical wisdom 31
pragmatism 10, 12–13, 87, 152, 275; defining 149; dialectical 149, 161; mixed methods research (MMR) 148–149, 161, 162–163
predictive validity 186–187, 266, 275
pre-experimental designs 55–57, 77
presentation, in ABR 140–141
pretest-posttest research designs: control group 57–58; control group posttest only 58–59; nonrandomized control group 61–62; one group 56–57
Pretorius, G. 60, 76
principle ethics 31, 267
probability (inferential statistics) 70, 74–77, 278
probability sampling *see* random sampling
problem definition 94
process-based (PF) approach, psychological assessment 6, 167–168, 181, 276

program development: practical guides 254; research proposal 215–216
Prosser, J. 35
psychoeducation 59
psychological assessment: client-centered approaches to 6–7; process-based approach 6, 167–168, 276; *see also* assessments, art therapy research
psychological inquiry 124
psychosis 67, 91, 98
PTSD *see* post-traumatic stress disorder (PTSD), veterans with
Punamaki, R. 183
purposive sampling *see* nonprobability (purposive) sampling
*p*-value 74, 274

qualitative research 10–11, 12, 83–118; ABR as "soft-form" of qualitative inquiry 10–11; action steps (PAR) 94; art therapists' understanding of their role regarding artwork produced in clinical sessions 34; assessments 170; bricolage 84, 88, 263; case study method 89–90, 264; collective interpretation of results (PAR) 94; combined/integrated with quantitative research 147–152; compared to quantitative 29–30; content analysis 265; credibility in 265–266; data analysis *see* data analysis; data collection *see* data collection; designs 89–95; development of 84–88; dialogue groups 94; discourse analysis 267; ethical and moral responsibilities 106–107; ethnography 93, 267–268; focus groups 90, 91, 94, 95, 97, 107; grounded theory 90–91, 102, 269; interviews *see* interviews; narrative inquiry 92–93, 273; origins 7; paradigms 10, **11**, 84, 86–87, 148, 274; participatory action research (PAR) 94–95, 274; phenomenology *see* phenomenological analysis; phenomenology; philosophical assumptions 85–86; practical guides 253; quality, evaluation of 104–106;

questionnaires 84, 94, 97, 98, 101, 107, 108; relationship building 88–89; reliability 276; research proposal 215; research questions 84–85, 277; research report 215; sampling *see* sampling; skills required 149; strategies 105–106; textual-based data collection 279; *see also* arts-based research (ABR); mixed methods research (MMR); quantitative research
Qualitative Research Guidelines Report 30
quality, evaluation of 104–106; mixed methods research (MMR) 160–161
quality of life (QOL), health-related 58
quantitative research 10, 12, 41–82; combined/integrated with qualitative research 147–152; compared to qualitative 29–30; concepts and definitions 43–48; data analysis 69–77, 150; designs 54–69; drawing 48, 65, 66, 69, 70; generalizability 42, 47, 49, 53, 55, 77, 148, 269; hypothesis testing 30, 44–45, 74; inferential statistics 70, 74–77, 278; instrumentation 48, 272; internal validity 50–53, 280; linear approach 29–30; longevity and income link 44; measurement levels 174, **175**, 176–180; methods/procedures 48–54; and mixed methods research (MMR) 147, 149; objectivity principle 42, 274; operationalization 45, 274; practical guides 251–252; quantitative data analysis 69–77; questionnaires 45, 53, 61, 65; replication 42, 45, 276; research proposal 215; research report 215; scientific method 41–42, 278; skills required 149; variables 43–44; *see also* mixed methods research (MMR); qualitative research
quasi-experimental research designs 9, 48, 77, 276; Solomon 4-group design 60–61
questionnaires: Delphi method 84, 98, 107; demographic 53, 204; online 97, 98, 101; open-ended 84, 97–98, 107, 274; participatory action research (PAR) 94; qualitative research 84, 94, 97, 98, 101, 107, 108; quantitative research 45, 53, 61, 65; relational aesthetics 13, 14, 78, 108, 209, 235; self-esteem 61; stress 65

Ramanathan, D. 139
random assignment (randomization) 49, 51, 53, 59, 276
random sampling 46–48, 276
randomization *see* random assignment (randomization)
randomized controlled trials (RCTs) 2, 155; multi-site 9
range 73
ratio scales 71–72, 75, 77, 178–180, 276
RCTs *see* randomized controlled trials (RCTs)
reactivity, external validity 53
re-authoring/re-storying, in narrative analysis 103, 273
referential adequacy 280
reflexivity 20, 30, 104
regression, statistical 52–53
relational aesthetics questionnaires 13, 14, 78, 108, 209, 235
reliability 190–195; alternate-form 190, 194, 262, 276; concept/definition 190–191, 276; internal consistency 190, 191–192, 276; inter-rater/inter-scorer 177, 190, 194–195, 271, 276; qualitative research 276; split-half 271, 278; test-retest 190, 194, 276, 278; *see also* validity
reliability coefficient 276
reliable change index (RCI) 193
Rennie, D. L. 106
replication 42, 45, 276
research, art therapy 1–17; aim 2; art, ethical use of 32–34; assessment *see* assessments, art therapy research; completion of report 217–220; critical priorities 18; deception 24; designs *see* designs, mixed methods research; designs, qualitative research; designs, quantitative research; ethics *see* ethical considerations; experimental research *see* experimental research; factors impacting growth of art

therapy profession 3; guidelines for choice of approach 10–11; importance of 2–14; meandering 202; methodology 10, 85–86, 140, 272; obligations of art therapy researchers 36; prioritization of studies 18; proposal 206–217; research questions *see* research questions; research review board 34–36, 277; researcher stance 136–137, 277; researcher-participant dialogue 86; researcher-participant hierarchy 20; scales used in *see* scaling methods; schools 49; shaping of research by government agencies/other entities 3, 5–6; studies *see* studies, art therapy research; text organization 11–14; traditional model for report 202–203; training 36; trustworthiness of researchers 23, 104, 279–280; using art in 31, 32–34; *see also* qualitative research; quantitative research; research proposal and report

Research Domain Criteria (RDoC) 5–6, 169, 211, 276

research ethics committees (RECs), United Kingdom 35

research proposal and report 202, 206–217; completing the research report 203–204, 217–220; conducting of study 203, 220–226; curiosity and inquiry 210; developing 208–217; discussion 202, 218, 225–226; embarking on research 208–217; ethical considerations 216–217; Expressive Therapies Continuum (ETC) assessment 211, 268; guidelines for writing 202; heuristic and arts-based 216; introduction 202, 203, 206, 207, 210–212, 221–223; literature review 202, 203, 206, 207, 213, 215, 223; methods/procedures 202, 203, 206, 207–208, 213, *214*, 215–217, 223–225; overview 206–208; preparing for publication 219–220; program development 215–216; qualitative research 215; quantitative and experimental research 215; research question 212; research simulation experiential materials packet 208–212, 230–242; results 202, 218, 219, 225; rigor and integrity 217; sampling 216; *see also* studies, art therapy research

research questions: better questions – better answers 136, 263; conducting of study 222; defining 277; explication 122; formulating 150–151; mixed methods research (MMR) 150–151, 273; practical guides 248–249; qualitative 84–85, 277; quantitative 150; research proposal 212; sub-questions 84

research review board 277; oversight 34–36, 139

research review committees, US 35

researcher-participant relationship: dialogue 86; as hierarchy 20; participatory action research (PAR) 94

respect for persons *see* autonomy (respect for persons) principle

response art 133, 137, 139, 210, 237

results, research 225, 277

Richardson, L. 104

Riesmann, C. 103

Riethmiller, R. 205

rigor, research: practical guides 260–261; random assignment 49; reliability 190–195; research proposal 217; validity 180–190

risk/benefit ratio 21, 277

Robb, M. 32–33

Robbins, S. 65–66

Roberts, L. 186, 192, 225

Rorschach test 168, 185

Rosal, M. 64

Rose, D. 5

Rossetto, E. 91

Rübeling, H. 76

Rubin, J. A. 138

Rumbold, J. 139

sampling: convenience 46, 47–48, 88, 265; critical 88; defining 45, 278; homogeneous 88, 270; maximal variation 47, 88, 272; nonprobability (purposive) 46, 265, 266, 272, 278, 280; participants 88–89; practical guides 256–257; probability 46, 48; quantitative

research 45–48; random 46–48, 276; research proposal 216; research report 216; selling 88–89; snowball (recruitment) 88, 278; strata (subgroups), random sampling 46; typical 88, 280
Sandelowski, M. 106
Savin-Baden, M. 89
scaling methods 70–71; continuous types 177, 178; interval (Likert) scales 71, 75, 77, 178, 179, 271; nominal scales 71, 75, 174, 176–177, 273; ordinal scales 71, 75, 77, 177–178, 274; ratio scales 71–72, 75, 77, 178–180, 276; *see also* Attachment Rating Scale (ARS); Attachment to Mother scale (ATM); Brief Mood Introspection Scale (BMIS); self-concept scale, single-subject design; Sensory Processing Scale (SPS); Tennessee Self-Concept Scale (TSCS); Wechsler Intelligence Scale for Children-Revised (WISC-R)
schizophrenia 67, 91
Schmidt, L. 31
Schore, A. N. 168
Schreiber, E. 68–69
Schreiber, K. 68–69
scientific method 41–42, 278
Scotti, V. 130–131, 137
Scribner, C. 205
SD *see* standard deviation (SD)
selection bias 50, 54, 55
selective coding 269
self-concept scale, single-subject design 64
self-esteem questionnaires 61
self-harm 186, 187
self-inquiry 124–127, 278
self-narrative 267–268
semi-structured conversational style interviews 96–97, 153–155
Sensory Processing Scale (SPS) 188
Seo, S. 173, 191, 192
sequential research design: explanatory 268; exploratory 268
Shin, S. K. 103
significance, statistical 278
Silverman, M. 59
single-subject designs 63–64, 72

skills: artistic, controls for extraneous variables 204; mixed methods research (MMR) 149–151; Standards and Guidelines for the Accreditation of Educational Programs in Art Therapy (S&Gs), 2016 3–4
Slayton, S. 148
Smith, J. A. 102
Smith Stevens, S. 174
snowball sampling (recruitment) 88, 278
social awareness, raising 133
social justice 93, 156–158, 278
Solomon 4-group design 59–61; quasi-experimental designs 60–61
Spaniol, S. 94
Spearman's rho 76
spill writing (free writing) 138, 278
spiraling 91, 269–270
split-half reliability 271, 278
Springham, N. 5, 6, 102
St John, P. 64
St. Pierre, E. 104
Stake, R. E. 89
Stallings, J. 98
standard deviation (SD) 73, 278
standard error of measurement 193, 278
Stanley, J. 54
State-Trait Anxiety Inventory (STAI) 56, 193
static group comparison design 57
statistical regression (to the mean) 52–53
statistical significance 278
statistics 69–77; common tests 75–77; descriptive 70, 72–74, 278; inferential 70, 74–77, 278; mixed methods research (MMR) 152; purposes in research studies 70; *see also* quantitative research
still life 213, *214*, 225
story/fairytale (data collection procedure) 138, 275, 278
strata (subgroups), random sampling 46
stratified random sampling 46–47
Strauss, A. L. 90, 102, 269
stress questionnaires 65
Strobino, J. 55, 56
structured interviews 96

studies, art therapy research 12; artwork interpretation 205; background of problem 221; comparison 224; conducting 220–226; controls for extraneous variables of artistic skill and background 204; cultural appropriateness of art-based instruments/interventions 204–205; definition of terms 222; designing and executing 201–228; factors unique to, impacting study quality 204–206; flow chart 202, 203; methods/procedures 223–225; normative 224; prioritization of 18; purpose 221–222; research questions/hypotheses 222; results 225, 277; risks 21, 139; scientific justification 23; statement of problem 221; traditional model for report 202–204; variability in artwork of children 205–206; see also research, art therapy; research proposal and report

subjectivity, importance in psychological science 7

surveys: AATA membership 66, 72; art exhibit visit 233; baseline 232; descriptive 66–67; electronic software 153; longitudinal 66; Medical Outcomes Study Short-Form Health Survey (SF-36) 58; Survey of Public Participation in the Arts (SPPA) 152

Sweetman, D. 158

symptom reduction approach, moving away from 5

Symptoms Checklist Revised (SCL-90-R) 58

Tabone, C. 179, 186, 269
Temple, M. 34
Tennessee Self-Concept Scale (TSCS) 186
test selection 279
test-retest reliability (time to time) 190, 194, 276, 278
text organization 11–14
textual-based data collection 97–98, 279
thematic analysis 100–101, 279; mixed methods research (MMR) 153, 155

thematic maps/models 124
Therapeutic Assessment 6, 279
Thick, L. 61
Thompson, D. M. 193
time-series designs 62
Timm-Bottos, J. 158
Torres, A. 94, 95, 158
training, research 36
transferability 104, 279–280; mixed methods research (MMR) 160, 161
transformative design/research paradigm 87, 157–158, 278, 279
translation 138, 139, 160, 279
trauma research 155–157; see also post-traumatic stress disorder (PTSD), veterans with
triangulation of data 151–152, 265–266, 279
true experimental research designs 57–64, 77; control group posttest only 58–59; defining 48–49, 279; nonrandomized control group pretest-posttest 61–62; pretest-posttest control group 57–58; single-subject 63–64; Solomon 4-group 59–61; time-series 62; see also experimental research; quasi-experimental research designs
trustworthiness 23, 104, 160, 279–280
$t$-test for independent means 76
Tuskegee Syphilis Study, US 19
typical sampling 88, 280

United Kingdom: art therapists in 24, 25, 34, 67; British Association of Art Therapists 24; Delphi method questionnaires 98; group art therapy process, England 73; immigrants and asylum seekers in 158; National Health Service 67; National Institute of Mental Health (NIMH), US 6, 273; research ethics committees (RECs) 35
United States: American Art Therapy Association (AATA) see American Art Therapy Association (AATA); American Counseling Association 28; American Psychiatric Association (APA) 5, 266–267; American Psychological Association (APA) 19, 206, 219; Census Bureau 152; Code of Federal Regulations Title 45 Part

46 (45 CFR46) 23, 34–35; Common Rule 35; National Endowment for the Arts 152; National Institutes of Health (NIH) 5, 6, 273; Research Domain Criteria (RDoC) 5–6, 169, 211, 276; research review committees 35; Tuskegee Syphilis Study 19
Uttley, L. 2–3

validity 180–190; conceptual 190, 264; concurrent 185–186, 264, 266; consequential (impact-based) 264; construct 160, 187–190, 264, 280; content 181–184, 265, 268, 280; convergent 189, 264, 265; criterion 184–185, 266, 280; discriminant 189, 264, 267, evidential 264, 280; external 53–54, 63, 280; face validity 182, 268; incremental 189, 270; internal 50–53, 280; predictive 186–187, 266; *see also* reliability
validity coefficient 280
Van Lith, T. 92, 95, 96, 98, 103
variability: in artwork of children 205–206; measures of 73, 280
variables: confounding 43, 280; continuous 70–71; defining 280; dependent 43–44, 49, 64, 280; discrete 70–71; extraneous 43, 204, 280; independent 43, 49, 64, 280; interval (Likert) scale 71, 178, 271; intervening 43–44, 280; and measurement 70; media dimension 71; quantitative research 43–44; *see also* quantitative research
Vazzano, S. 206
virtue ethics 31, 267
visual journaling 131–132, 139
vulnerable populations 21, 23

Wahlbeck, H. 96–97
wait lists, control groups 22
Wallen, N. E. 206–208, 218–219
water color 71
Watkins, D. 151
Watts, P. 93
Wechsler Intelligence Scale for Children-Revised (WISC-R) 185
Weishaar, M. 140
Willis, P. 92
Wood, L. A. 104
Woodby, L. L. 140
words, situated meanings in 104
work imaginatively – referential clarity 134–135, 280
workshops 94, 95, 133, 141
Wykes, T. 5

Yin, R. K. 89

Zago, C. 99
Zappa, A. 20
Zhang, W. 155
Zipfel, S. 8
Zubala, A. 98
Zucker, D. 124

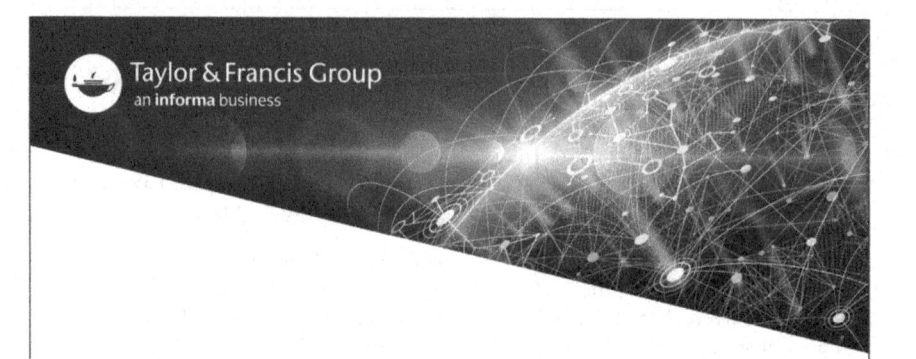